THE HISTORY
OF AMERICAN FUNERAL DIRECTING

Robert W. Habenstein & William M. Lamers

Ninth Edition

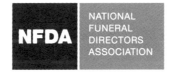

THE HISTORY OF AMERICAN FUNERAL DIRECTING

Ninth Edition

Published by the National Funeral Directors Association of the United States, Inc.

Copyright © 2018, 2014, 2010, 2007, 2001, 1996, 1995, 1981, 1962, 1955

All rights reserved. No part of this publication may be reproduced, stored in or introduced into a retrieval system or transmitted in any form or by any means, electronic, mechanical, photocopying, recording or otherwise, without the prior written permission of the copyright owner. The scanning, uploading or distribution of this book via Internet or via any other means without the permission of the publisher is illegal and punishable by law.

Address orders to:

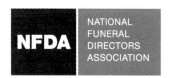

NFDA, 13625 Bishops Drive, Brookfield, WI 53005 USA
800-228-6332
www.nfda.org

ISBN 978-0-692-12056-9

Printed in the United States of America

Cover Design: Scott High
Editor: Chris Raymond

In memory of Howard C. Raether,
Executive Director of the National Funeral Directors Association, 1948-1983.
Howard was a friend and mentor to many in funeral service.

Table of Contents

List of Plates 9

List of Figures 14

Acknowledgments 16

Preface to the Ninth Edition 19

Part One: Early Mortuary Behavior

1. Pagan Roots of Modern Funeral Practice 23
FUNERAL CUSTOMS OF THE ANCIENT EGYPTIANS: Death Beliefs; The Threat of Plague as a Burial Motive; Embalming; Coffins; Undertaking Specialists and the Ritual of Embalming; Influence of Egyptian Death Customs. FUNERAL CUSTOMS OF THE ANCIENT GREEKS: Death Beliefs; Burial Practices; Coffins and Tombs. FUNERAL CUSTOMS OF THE ANCIENT ROMANS: Roman View of Death and the Importance of Burial; Roman Burial Customs; Early Funeral Directing; Influence of Roman Burial Practices.

2. Early Hebrew, Christian and Scandinavian Burial 53
FUNERAL PRACTICES IN EARLY HEBREW CULTURE: Death Beliefs; Burial Customs; Mourning Customs; Place of Burial; Interment the General Practice. FUNERAL BELIEFS AND CUSTOMS OF THE EARLY CHRISTIANS: Death Beliefs; The Resurrection of the Body and Cremation; Christian Equality in Death; Death as "Sleep"; Burial Customs; The Role of the Family in Early Christian Funerals; Other Christian Funeral Customs; Washing the Corpse; The Wake in Early Christian Funeral Practices; The Funeral Procession; Early Christian Cemeteries; Early Christian Burial Practices Grow More Complex; Early Christian Funeral Functionaries. FUNERAL BELIEFS AND CUSTOMS OF THE ANCIENT GERMANS AND SCANDINAVIANS: Cremation as a Protection from the Dead; Cremation to Free the Spirit of the Dead; Some Common Elements in the Mortuary Beliefs of Early Peoples.

3. Death and Burial Through the Middle Ages & Renaissance 77
CHRISTIAN INFLUENCE UPON FUNERAL BEHAVIOR DURING THE EARLY MIDDLE AGES: Funerals; Church and Cemetery Burial in the Middle Ages; Disposal and Contagion; The Purgatorial Doctrine and the Formation of Leagues of Prayer and Other Pious Practice; The Wake During the Middle Ages; Funeral Feasts; Funerals of State During the Middles Ages and the Use of

the Effigy; Sepulchral Monuments; The Plagues; The Plagues Overload the Cemeteries; Coffined Burial Becomes the Custom. SOCIAL DEVELOPMENTS AND FUNERAL PRACTICE: Funeral Ostentation Grows Among the English Middle Classes; The Development of Burial Clubs; The Shroud in England Changes from Linen to Wool; The Free Distribution of Mourning Clothes; English Burial Fees During the Waning Middle Ages; Mourning Colors; The Widow During the Middle Ages — Her Lot and Her Raiment; Local Customs Add Color; Medieval Preoccupation With the Physical Side of Death; The Sexton Emerges; Independent Heart Burial; Independent Bone Burial; Embalming in the Middle Ages; The Surgeon and the Anatomist Take Over; The Reformation and Christian Funeral Beliefs and Practices.

4. *Medical Embalmers and the Rise of English Undertakers* 117
Embalming and the Growth of Medical Science; The Role of the Barber-Surgeons in Embalming; The Emergence of the Funeral Undertaker; Feudal Funerals; Coffins, Funeral Goods and the Early Undertaker; Tradesman Undertaker and Medical Embalmer; Clergy and the Undertaker; Burial and Sanitary Reform.

Part Two: The Rise of American Funeral Undertaking

5. *American Colonial Funeral Behavior* 141
Ideological Framework for Colonial Funeral Practices; Burial Practices; Social Change in Late Colonial America.

6. *Early American Funeral Undertaking* 161
Tradesmen Undertakers; Performers of Personal Service; Religious Functionaries; Municipal Officers.

7. *Coffins, Burial Cases and Caskets* 179
17th- & 18th-century Coffined Burial in America; Early Coffin Shops and Coffin Warehouses; Variation in Early Function and Type; Stone and Metal Coffins; The Fisk Metallic Coffin; The Large-scale Manufacture of Metallic Burial Cases; From Pragmatic to Aesthetic; The Metallic Burial Casket; Cloth Burial Cases; "Also-rans" in 19th-century Burial Receptacles; Life Signals; Burial Vaults and Outside Boxes; Balance Sheet on Wood, Cloth and Metal.

8. *Preservation: The Ice Age Into Embalming* 219
Customary Aspects of Preserving the Dead; Corpse Coolers and Cooling Boards; The "Airtight" Receptacle; Chemical Embalming by Injection and Its Innovators; Thomas Holmes and the Eruption of Civil War Embalming; Embalming Devices, Fluids and Techniques; "Schools," Fluid Houses and the Spread of Embalming.

9. *Transportation: Carriage to Gas Buggy* **255**
Funeral Processions and the Hearse; Colonial Hearses; Hearses with Horses, 1850-1910; Chassis; Hearse Sizes and Colors.

10. *The Pattern of Late-19th-Century Funerals* **279**
First Responses to Death; At the House; Funeral Arrangements; The Funeral; The Funeral Cortège; At the Cemetery; Rural Variations; Late-19th-century Mourning Symbols; Aesthetically Pleasing Mourning Symbols; Sepulture and Memorialization; The Changing Functions of the Undertaker.

11. *The Associational Impulse* **315**
BACKGROUND FACTORS: Occupational Organization; Socio-Cultural Movements — The General Public-Health Movement; Socio-Cultural Movements — The Specific Movement for the Cremation of the Dead. 19TH-CENTURY ASSOCIATIONAL DEVELOPMENT AMONG FUNERAL DIRECTORS: Origins and Early Developments; Pressures, Interests and Motives; Characteristics of Early Leadership; Code of Ethics; Communication Within the Trade; Growth, Problems and Change; 20th-century Traces of Professionalism.

Part Three: Organization of Modern Funeral Service

12. *Institutional Growth and Modern Associational Developments* **353**
Mortuary (Funeral Service) Education: (1. Schools; 2. Agencies, Conferences and Councils; 3. Interest Group Committees; 4. Licensing Laws); Developments in Mortuary Law; Multiplication of Associations; Economic Growth and Developments; Integration and Stabilization.

13. *The Panorama of Modern Funeral Practice* **383**
THE FUNERAL PATTERN IN MODERN AMERICA: Responses to Death; The Funeral Director — Death Call to Disposition of the Body. OPERATING THE MODERN FUNERAL HOME: The Contemporary Funeral Establishment; THE FUNERAL: OPTIONS & ALTERNATIVE SELECTIONS: The Changing Scene; RECENT DEVELOPMENTS: FUNERAL OPTIONS OR ALTERNATIVES: In the 21st Century; RECENT DEVELOPMENTS: REGULATIONS AND ENTITLEMENTS; RECENT DEVELOPMENTS: MANDATORY AND VOLUNTARY CONTINUING EDUCATION; THE FUTURE: AN OVERVIEW.

Index **403**

List of Plates

Plate		Page
1A	Aerial View of Pyramids at Gizeh. From *Antiquity*, IX (1935), facing page 5	29
1B	Canopic Jars — Containers of Vital Organs. Courtesy of the Chicago Natural History Museum	29
2A	Canopic Chest, Tut-ankh-Amon. Courtesy of the Cairo Museum	32
2B	Egyptian Outer Coffin Inscribed with Magical Texts. Courtesy of the Chicago Natural History Museum	32
3A	Modeled Outer-Coffin and Coffin, Showing Use of Cartonnage. Courtesy of The Chicago Natural History Museum	33
3B	Gold Mask, Tut-ankh-Amon. Courtesy of the Cairo Museum	33
3C	Coffin Portrait. Courtesy of the Fitzwilliam Museum	33
4A	Preparation of Egyptian Mummy, a Painting. Courtesy of the Bettmann Archives	37
4B	Examples of Mortuary Mummy Bandaging. Courtesy of the Chicago Natural History Museum	37
4C	The Dawn of Conscience: Weighing of the Heart by Anubis. Courtesy of The British Museum	37
5A	Attic Black-Figured Plaque. Courtesy of the Walters Art Gallery	41
5B	Lekythos of Amasis, Used in Greek Funerals. From *Athenische Mitteilungen 59*, 1939, Plate 4	41
5C	Mourning Scene, Greek Lekythos. From originals in The British Museum	41
6A	Funeral Procession, Painted on Grecian Pottery. From Puckle, *Funeral Customs*, facing page 112	43
6B	Farewell Scenes, Greek Lekythoi. From the Oberlander Museum, Reading, Pennsylvania, and the Kerameikos Museum, Athens	43
6C	Stele of Aristion. From Stobart, *The Glory That Was Greece*. Original in National Museum, Athens	43
6D	Restored Grecian Funeral Lot. From Brueckner, *Friedhof am Eridonos*, page 71, Figure 43	43
7A	Funeral Procession; Relief from Amiternum. From Quasten, *Musik und Gesang in den Kulturen der Heidnischen Antike und Christlichen Frühzeit*, Plate 31	47
7B	Roman Burial Urn. Courtesy of the National Foundation of Funeral Service, Evanston, Illinois	47
7C	Tomb of Cecillia Metella, Appian Way	47
7D	Columbarium, Vigna Codini. From Lanciani, *Pagan and Christian Rome*, facing page 260	47
7E	Funeral Urn Depicting the Conclamatio. Thermaen Museum, Rome, from Rush, *Death and Burial in Christian Antiquity*	47
8A	Divine Service, Catacombs of St. Calixtus, A.D. 50. From Davey, *A History of Mourning*, page 19	65
8B	Vault in Catacombs of Rome. From Puckle, *Funeral Customs*, facing page 138	65

9A	Early Christian Sarcophagus. From Wilson, *The Clothing of the Ancient Romans*, facing page, 81, photograph, Alinari, Florence.	67
9B	Tomb of Innocent VIII. From Lanciani, *Pagan and Christian Rome*, facing page 242.	67
10A	Mourning Scene, Gallo-Roman Bas-relief. From Davey, *A History of Mourning*, page 15.	71
10B	German Funeral Sacrifice, a Painting. From the Fairchild Collection, National Foundation of Funeral Service.	71
11A	Funeral of Archduke of Brussels, 1622. From Davey, *A History of Mourning*, Page 57.	81
11B	Funeral Procession of St. Edward the Confessor, from an 11th-century Tapestry. From Davey, *A History of Mourning*, page 23.	81
12A	Anglo-Saxon Widow, 9th Century. From Davey, *A History of Mourning*, page 21.	87
12B	Death Criers, French Costumes, 17th Century. From Davey, *A History of Mourning*, page 30.	87
12C	Funeral of an Abbess, 10th Century. From Davey, *A History of Mourning*, page 27.	87
13A	"Corpse Bearer," 18th Century, England. From Smith, *The Cries of London*, facing page 20.	93
13B	Coffin Pall, Church of Folleville, France, Late Renaissance. From Davey, *A History of Mourning*, page 31.	93
13C	Funeral Scene in Hogarth's "The Harlot's Progress" Showing Rosemary Sprigs. Early steel engraving.	93
14	Funeral Procession of Queen Elizabeth, 1603. From Davey, *A History of Mourning*, page 45.	97
15A	Death Devouring Man and Beast, Tapestry Design of the Middle Ages. From Davey, *A History of Mourning*, page 64.	103
15B	Bones of All Men, an Early Woodcut by Holbein. From his *Danse Macabre*.	103
15C	Angels Praying Over a Skull, 16th-century Bas-relief. From Davey, *A History of Mourning*, page 29.	103
15D	"Danse of Death," Nohl. From his *The Black Death*.	103
16	Portion of a Treatise on Embalming, d'Argellata, 15th Century. From his *Chirurgia*.	111
17A	Early 18th-century English Funeral Invitation. From Ashton, *Social Life in the Reign of Queen Anne*, page 37.	125
17B	Corpse Lying in State, 18th-century Drawing. From Ashton, *Social Life in the Reign of Queen Anne*, page 36.	125
17C	Part-time Undertaker, 18th-century English Tradesman's Card. From the Fairchild Collection, National Foundation of Funeral Service.	125
18A	Trade Sign, Four Coffins and Heart, c. 1720. From Heal, *The Signboards of Old London Shops*, page 45.	129
18B	Whight Hart and Coffin. From Heal, *The Signboards of Old London Shops*, page 174.	129
18C	Precursor to Furnishing Undertaker, Tradesman's Card of 1740. From Heal, *London Tradesmen's Cards of the XVIII Century*, page xcvi.	129
19	Title Page of Early Work on Embalming, Published 1705.	131
20	Portion of Colonial Broadside. From U.S. Library of Congress.	147

21	Broadside of Funeral Hymn Showing Burial Dress and Coffin. From U.S. Library of Congress	149
22	Facsimile Portion of Broadside Elegy, Written by a Slave Girl. From U.S. Library of Congress	151
23	"Monkey Spoons" Used by Early Dutch Colonists. By special permission from Mrs. J.C. Mitchell, Boca Raton, Florida	153
24A	Knorr Undertaking Establishment, Germantown, Pennsylvania, Mid-19th Century. From photographs provided by Kirk & Nice, Germantown, Pennsylvania	165
24B	Late-18th- and Mid-19th-century Bills for Coffins and "Attendance." From photographs provided by Kirk & Nice, Germantown, Pennsylvania	165
25	Advertisements of Mid-19th-century Tradesmen & Undertakers and Their Combination Establishments. From *The American Funeral Director*, November 1952, pages 65 ff	167
26	Early Combination Business.	169
27	Furnishing-Undertakers Advertisements, 1860 and 1870. From *The American Funeral Director*, November 1952, pages 65 ff.	171
28A	Undertaker, Manufacturer and Sexton, 1849. From U.S. Library of Congress	173
28B	Undertaking as Part-time Work. Advertisement in Charlestown, Massachusetts, directory, 1838. From U.S. Library of Congress	173
28C	Early Advertisement Indicating Use of English-style Trade Sign by American Undertaker. Baltimore city directory, 1845. From U.S. Library of Congress	173
28D	Livery Stable Keeper and Undertaker, Baltimore, 1847. Baltimore city directory, 1847. From U.S. Library of Congress	173
28E	Advertisement Showing Use of Term "Funeral Undertakers," Boston, 1873. Boston city directory, 1873. From U.S. Library of Congress	173
29	Boston Funeral Bill, Itemized on Form Supplied by City Registrar. Courtesy of Edwin A. Christ, Columbia, Missouri.	177
30A	Early Metallic Burial Case, "Ogee" Design to Reduce Excess Space. Patent Sketch	191
30B	End Seal Airtight Burial Casket, Patent Sketch, 1877	191
31	Examples of the Casket-maker's Art, Late-19th Century. Courtesy of *Casket and Sunnyside* and Crane & Breed Mfg. Co.	195
32	"The Grant State Casket," Used in Funeral of President U.S. Grant. Courtesy of the National Casket Co.	199
33A	Eisenbrandt "Life Signal," 1843, Patent Sketch	203
33B	Life Signal to be Used with Electrical Alarm, Patent Sketch	203
34	Life Detector, Mechanical Principle, 1871, Patent Sketch	205
35	Grave-Signal by Albert Fearnaught, 1882, Patent Sketch	206
36	"All Weather" Device for Indicating Life in Buried Persons, 1882, Patent Sketch	207
37A	Boyd Metal Grave Vault, 1879, Patent Sketch	209
37B	Burial Safe, to be Lowered Into the Grave, 1878, Patent Sketch	209

38A	Handmade Glass Caskets, Built About 1900, Found in Bozeman, Montana. Courtesy of Howard Nelson, Bozeman, Montana	211
38B	Casket After 65 Years Underground, Showing Protection of Metal Vault	211
39	Catalogs of Coffin and Casket Manufacturers, Late-19th Century	213
40	Ornamental Casket Trim and Hardware, From a Manufacturers Catalog, Late-19th Century. Courtesy of Harry C. Hill, Flint, Michigan	215
41	Corpse Cooler of Frederick and Trump, 1846, Patent Sketch	223
42A	Advertisement of Co-inventor of Corpse Cooler, 1847. Boston city directory, 1847. From U.S. Library of Congress	225
42B	Refrigerator-type Corpse Cooler, 1870, Patent Sketch	225
42C	Body-lifting Device, 1880, Patent Sketch	225
43A	Cement-filled Corpse-preserving Coffin, 1867, Patent Sketch	227
43B	Apparatus for Filling Blood Vessels of Dead Bodies, 1861, Patent Sketch	227
43C	Portable Elastic Receptacle for Shipping Body, 1863, Patent Sketch	227
44	Facsimile of First Patent for Embalming Process, 1856	237
45	Page from Ledger of Hudson Samson, 1870, Showing Charge "Embalming & Services."	243
46	Cooling Boards and Improved Ice Caskets, Late-19th Century	244
47	Advertisement for Embalming Supplies, 1880, *The Casket*	245
48	Early Advertisement for Non-Poisonous Embalming Fluid, 1909, *Western Undertaker*	247
49A	Embalming-supply Salesman's Business Card, About 1900. New York Historical Society, Bella C. Landauer Collection	249
49B	Advertisement of Pioneer in Embalming, Auguste Renouard	249
50A	Wrought Iron Hearse of Renaissance Era. From Puckle, *Funeral Customs*, facing page 227	257
50B	Drawing of an Early English Bier on Wheels	257
50C	Hand-built Early American Hearse, 1787. Courtesy of William Sirlin Mortuaries, Pittsburgh, Pennsylvania	257
51A	A Pioneer Hearse	261
51B	American Hearse of the 1850s. From *The Sunnyside*, March 15, 1913, page 14	261
51C	Hearse Used During and After Civil War. From *The Sunnyside*, March 15, 1913, page 14	261
51D	The Return to a Rectangular Design, About 1884. From *The Sunnyside*, March 15, 1913, page 15	261
52A	Hand-carved Wooden Drape Hearse, About 1898.	264
52B	Model of Ornate Child's Hearse, Late-19th Century.	264
53	Processional Hearse, Exhibited at Chicago World's Fair, 1893. From *The Sunnyside*, March 15, 1913, page 14	265
54A	"Ready for the Funeral," a Well-appointed Hearse of the Late-19th Century	267
54B	Mosque Deck-style Popular Through the 1900s. From *The Sunnyside*, March 15, 1913, page 15	267
54C	Chicago Funeral Trolley Car, World War I Period	267
55	Patent Sketch of an Early Auto-Hearse Passenger Vehicle	269

56A	One of the First Auto-Hearses Marketed, 1909. From *The Western Undertaker*, June 1909, page 1	271
56B	Improved, More-ornate Version of 56A. From *The Western Undertaker*, August 1909, page 1	271
56C	Undertaker's Auto Built in 1905	271
56D	An Early Motor Ambulance, 1900. From *The Western Undertaker*, December 1909, inside back cover	271
57A	Rear-loading Funeral Car of the Early 1920s. From a Sayers & Scovill Co. catalog, 1922	273
57B	Two-tone-finish Funeral Car, 1922, as Lighter Colors Gain Favor in Succeeding Decades. From a Sayers & Scovill Co. catalog, 1922	273
57C	Hearse Body on Auto Chassis, 1908	273
57D	Post-World War I Hearse Showing Persistence of Black in Funeral Vehicles	273
58A	Funeral Limousine, c. 1922. From a Sayers & Scovill Co. catalog, 1922	275
58B	Funeral Hearse Used by Chinese in America. Acme Photo	275
58C	Matched Funeral Vehicle Procession, Early 1920s	275
59A	Side-service Funeral Car Used in 1946	277
59B	An Ambulance Used in 1934. Courtesy of The Superior Coach Corporation	277
59C	A Side-servicing Car of the 1920s	277
59D	Style-setting Funeral Car, 1932. Courtesy of The Superior Coach Corporation	277
60	Funeral Notice, Late-19th Century	288
61	Mourning Card, Memento of the Deceased	289
62	Harbinger of Death — the Letter Edged in Black	291
63	Funeral Badges — Indispensable to the Late-19th-century Funeral	299
64	Burial Robes Sold by Undertakers, 1880. From a Crane & Breed Mfg. Co. catalog	311
65	"Black Book" Notice of Early Philadelphia Undertakers Association. From *The Keystone State Echo*, June 1931, page 99	323
66	Front Cover of First Issue of *The Casket*, May 1876. Courtesy of *Casket and Sunnyside*	337
67	Front Cover of First Issue of *Embalmers' Monthly*, April 1892. Courtesy of *Embalmers' Monthly*	339
68	Portions of Front Covers of Early Undertaking Trade Journals. Courtesy *American Funeral Director* and *Casket and Sunnyside*	341
69	Additional Front Cover Titles of Early Undertaking Trade Journals. Courtesy *American Funeral Director* and *Casket and Sunnyside*	343

List of Figures

Figure		Page
1	Buried in Woolen Affidavit, 18th Century, England.	
	Courtesy of the New York Historical Society, Bella C. Landauer Collection	98
2	Early Colonial Letter to Editor Protesting Extravagances, Especially at Funerals.	
	Courtesy of Massachusetts Historical Society	146
3	Trade Card of Furnishing-Undertaker, Post-Civil War Period	164
4	"Professional" Card, Mid-19th Century.	
	Courtesy of the New York Historical Society, Bella C. Landauer, Collection	168
5	Females Who Performed Undertaking Tasks, Philadelphia city directory, 1810.	
	From U.S. Library of Congress	170
6	Late-18th-century Funeral Bill, Showing Participation by Female in Arranging for Services	170
7	Charlestown, Massachusetts, Town Undertaker, 1838, Advertisement in City Directory.	
	From U.S. Library of Congress	175
8	Early 19th-century Funeral Bill.	
	Courtesy of the New York Historical Society, Bella C. Landauer Collection	183
9	Patent Sketch of Fisk Metallic Burial Case, 1848	186
10	Mid-1860s Illustration of Crane, Breed & Co. Factory:	
	"Stoves, Hollow-ware, Fisk's, Crane's & Barstow's Patent Metallic Burial Cases and Caskets"	187
11	Fisk Mummy Case, Style of 1853. Courtesy of the Crane & Breed Mfg. Co.	188
12	Cloth Covered, "Bronzed Case," 1854. Courtesy of the Crane & Breed Mfg. Co.	189
13	"Plain or Octagon" Metallic Burial Case. Courtesy of the Crane & Breed Mfg. Co.	189
14	Zinc "Shoulder Casket" Burial Case, 1857. Courtesy of the Crane & Breed Mfg. Co.	192
15	Casket, Modern Rectangular Form, About 1860. Courtesy of the Crane & Breed Mfg. Co.	192
16	Workmen of the Stein Manufacturing Co. in 1873. Courtesy of the National Casket Co.	196
17	Stein "Style F State Casket," Similar to President U.S. Grant's Casket.	
	From an early Stein Mfg. Co. catalog	197
18	Terra Cotta Coffin, 1855, Patent Sketch	198
19	Wood and Cement Coffin, 1839, Patent Sketch	198
20	Coffin of Glass Plates and Iron Bands, 1859, Patent Sketch	200
21	Glass Coffin, Airtight, with Rib-Flange Construction, 1880, Patent Sketch	201
22	Glass Casket, Late-19th Century. From *The Keystone State Echo*, June 1931, page 28	201
23	Cross-shaped Casket, 1877.	
	From an 1877 issue of *The Casket*, in *The Keystone State Echo*, June 1931, page 30	202
24	Cement Mold Type of Burial Case, 1872, Patent Sketch	208
25	Metal-clad Wood Mold for Concrete Vaults.	
	Courtesy of the National Concrete Burial Vault Association	210
26	Finished Outside Boxes, Used in Late-19th Century. From an early Stein Mfg. Co. catalog	216

27	Corpse Cooler Consisting of Several Ice Cases, 1870, Patent Sketch	224
28	Early 19th-century Ad of the Liveryman-Undertaker	259
29	Itemized Bill for Luxury Funeral, 1886. Courtesy of the New York Historical Society, Bella C. Landauer Collection	283
30	Door Badges, Late-19th Century. From Hohenschuh, *The Modern Funeral: Its Management*	284
31	Professional Dress. Left, Coachman; Center, Undertaker; Right, Undertaker's Liveried Assistant. *The Casket*, April 1877	293
32	Couch-style Casket. From Hohenschuh, *The Modern Funeral: Its Management*	300
33	The Many Businesses of Dutch Charley. *The Casket*, 1879	330

Acknowledgments

The publishers and agents noted below have kindly granted permission to use quoted material:

Blades, East & Blades, London, *Annals of the Barber-Surgeons of London*, c. 1890, by Sidney Young.

B.T. Batsford, London, *London Tradesmen's Cards of the XVIII Century*, c. 1925, by Ambrose Heal; and *The Signboards of Old London Shops*, c. 1947, by Ambrose Heal.

Cambridge University Press, Cambridge, England, *A History of Epidemics in Great Britain*, c. 1891, by Charles Creighton; *The Road to Hel: A Study of the Conception of the Dead in Old Norse Literature*, c. 1943, by Hilda Ellis.

Catholic University of America Press, Washington, D.C., *Death and Burial in Christian Antiquity*, c. 1941, by Alfred C. Rush; *Ecclesiastical Sepulture in the New Code of Canon Law*, c. 1923, by John A. O'Reilly.

Columbia University Press, New York, *Medieval Handbooks of Penance*, c. 1938, by John T. McNeil and Helena M. Gamer.

Crane and Breed Casket Company, *The Evolution of the Modern Casket*.

Curtis Publishing Co., Philadelphia, *Saturday Evening Post*, "Their Last Words Had a Punch," by Charles L. Wallis, April 17, 1954.

Frederick A. Stokes Co., New York, *Funeral Customs, Their Origin and Development*, c. 1926, by Bertram S. Puckle.

George Allen & Unwin, London, *Heart Burial*, c. 1933, by Charles A. Bradford.

H.S. Eckels and Company, Philadelphia, "The Funeral Director in Grandpa's Time," *Clinical Topics*, May 1938, by Frederick A. Frantz.

Harvard University Press, Cambridge, Massachusetts, "Cremation and Burial in the Roman Empire," in *Harvard Theological Review*, XXV, October 1932, by Arthur D. Nock.

Houghton Mifflin Company, Boston and New York, *Economic and Social History of New England 1620-1789*, 2 vols., c. 1890, by William B. Weeden.

Indiana University Press, Bloomington, Indiana, *Main Street on the Middle Border*, c. 1954, by Lewis Atherton.

Alfred A. Knopf, Inc., New York, *A History of Medicine*, c. 1947, by Arturo Castiglioni.

The Macmillan Company, London, *Life and Labor of the People of London*, 9 vols., c. 1895, Charles Booth, editor.

The Macmillan Company, New York, *Spiritism and the Cult of the Dead in Antiquity*, c. 1921, by Lewis B. Paton; by special permission of Katharine H. Paton.

Macy-Masius, New York, *Samuel Sewall's Diary*, c. 1927, Mark Van Doren, editor.

Massachusetts Historical Society, Boston, Massachusetts, *Proceedings*, Vol. 17.

Methuen & Co., Ltd., *The Life and Times of Sir Edwin Chadwick*, c. 1952, by Samuel E. Finer.

New York Historical Society, New York, *The Arts and Crafts in New York*, c. 1938.

New York University Press, New York, *The Colonial Craftsman*, c. 1950, by Carl Bridenbaugh.

Oxford University Press, New York and Oxford, *Stories on Stone*, c. 1954, by Charles L. Wallis; *Burial Reform and Funeral Costs*, c. 1938, by Arnold Wilson and H. Levy.

Random House, New York, *The Persian Wars*, c. 1942, by Herodotus, George Rawlinson, translator.

F.C. Riddle & Bro. Casket Company, St. Louis, *Funeral Customs Through the Ages*, published in 1929.

The Ronald Press Company, now Alfred A. Knopf, Inc., New York, *Cities in the Wilderness*, c. 1938 by Carl Bridenbaugh.

Charles Scribner's Sons, *Social Life in the Reign of Queen Anne*, c. 1925, by John Ashton; *Dawn of Conscience*, c. 1946, by James H. Breasted; *Customs and Fashions in Old New England*, c. 1894, by Alice M. Earle; "Death and Disposal of the Dead," in *Encyclopedia Religion and Ethics*, c. 1912, John Hastings, editor.

University of Chicago Press, Chicago, *The Merchant Class of Medieval London*, c. 1948, by Sylvia Thrupp.

Yale University Press, New Haven, *Colonial Folkways*, Vol. VIII of The Chronicle of America Series, c. 1918, by Charles M. Andrews; *After Life in Roman Paganism*, 1923, by Franz Cumont.

William Wood & Co., New York, now Williams & Wilkins Co., Baltimore, *Outlines of Greek and Roman Medicine*, c. 1914, by James S. Elliott.

Preface to the Ninth Edition

Since its initial publication more than 60 years ago, *The History of American Funeral Directing* by Robert Habenstein and William Lamers has proven indispensable to funeral service professionals, mortuary science students and scholars alike.

Plumbing the depths of the historical record, the authors examine numerous cultures across time and place that contributed the many rich and varied threads forming the fascinating history of how we, as a species, have faced both the concept and the reality of mortality. Drawing from a wealth of sources, the authors further tailor this epic narrative to reflect the variety of influences — from individuals and institutions, to wars and whims — that woven together form the uniquely *American* fabric of funeral service on this continent.

This ninth edition — fully edited, updated and newly organized to enhance readability and comprehension — continues the mission established long ago by the National Funeral Directors Association of chronicling and sharing the crucial role played by the select group of men and women who care for both the living and the dead — then, now and always.

Chris Raymond, Editor
May 2018

PART ONE:
Early Mortuary Behavior

Chapter 1

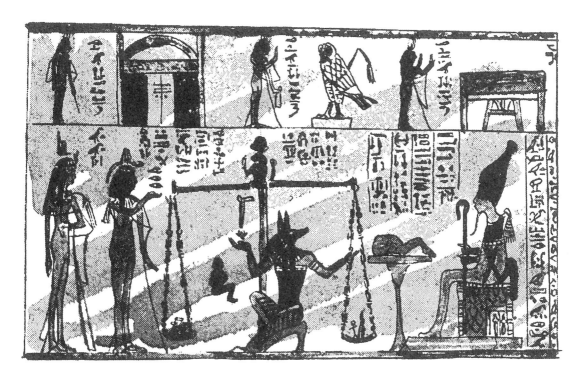

Pagan Roots of Modern Funeral Practice

Americans today are of a common mind with regard to many matters. They take it for granted that every man has a right to "life, liberty, and the pursuit of happiness." They believe without questioning that equality before the law is a part of their natural birthright, and that people should be permitted to select their places of residence, their mates, their occupations, and freely make the most of their own critical life decisions. They hold that every child has the right to a common school education, to be provided, if the parents so desire, at public expense. Although less often popularly expressed, but nonetheless firmly taken for granted, is the assumption that every person, no matter what the circumstance, has the right to a decent burial.

    This bundle of common beliefs — what people take for granted, the opinions that become the firm premises upon which they base their final group thinking and their individual judgments without questioning the broad underlying assumptions — these constitute the core of any social institution. An example might serve to clarify the point. Assume that we are confronted with the dead body of a man. What disposition shall we make of it? Shall we lay it in a boat and set it adrift? Shall we take the heart from it and bury it in one place and the rest of the body in another? Shall we expose it to wild animals? Burn it on a pyre? Push it into a pit, naked, to rot with other bodies? Boil it until the flesh falls off the bones, and then throw the flesh away and treasure the bones?

Such questions provoke others that we might not consciously articulate, such as: "What do people generally think this body is?" and, "What do they think is a proper way of dealing with it?"

Complicated individual and group processes gradually build-up laws, customs, traditions and fashions. And once people begin to think and act in a certain way, it is hard to make them change their minds. As a result of a long, slow development, with its roots deep in the history of Western civilization, it is the common American mindset today that the dead merit personal funeral services from a lay occupational group. These services include embalming; the preparation of the body for final viewing; a waiting period between death and disposition; the use of a casket that is attractive and protects the remains; a dignified and ceremonious service with consideration for the feelings of the bereaved; and an expression of the individual and group beliefs. Finally, convention demands burial in the ground or other disposition in a dignified place and manner that reaffirms those beliefs, insofar as not contrary to public health, expresses the esteem of the bereaved, and satisfies them that they are acting in accord with their means and that esteem.

All this is to be in the nature of personal services rendered by an occupational group set apart to serve these functions, and supplementary to the service that might be offered by the clergy as an independent occupational group. In a word, a "decent funeral" is a universally accepted part of American thought and life, and it is generally taken for granted that the funeral director's services are to be used in the burial of the dead.

What lies behind these contemporary American beliefs and practices? In dealing with their dead, why do Americans today strive to provide a certain type and standard of burial and call upon an occupational group to take the leading role in the laying away of the dead?

Obviously, some part of the so-called "reverential roots" of American mortuary belief descends from humanitarianism — the doctrine that our obligations are limited to and dependent alone on the individual and human relations — which developed as an outgrowth of the later Pagan Renaissance (as distinguished from the earlier Renaissance, which was Christian).

But to stop here would clearly commit the error of over simplification of historical origins. Humanitarianism alone neither explains nor accounts for the basic social interpretations of life and death in which the funeral customs of our day are anchored. To discover these, and to find out why people act as they do toward their dead, we must look to early Christian behavior and, beyond this, to the funeral behaviors of certain earlier civilizations. The long backward glance will show not merely customs that are related in the direct line, but also interesting resemblances, unrelated but born out of a common need. Thus, if two peoples, separated by thousands of years and half the globe, both use a litter to carry a body to the grave, it is likely that the same necessity in each case was the independent mother of invention, and that the practice of the latter group, in spite of its similarity, might be entirely unrelated to the practice of the earlier.

With these and other common-sense reservations before us, we propose to examine the most pertinent and common of ancient and medieval funeral practices in an effort to develop backgrounds for an improved understanding of present-day American methods of caring for the dead.

In spite of some variants in the formula, repeated so frequently that it has become a historical truism, the larger part of Western culture today is a composite of Greek aesthetics and philosophy, Roman law and administrative genius, and ancient Teutonic vigor, superimposed upon the dominant Judeo-Christian tradition. Nevertheless, the largest determinant in modern American funerary practice stems from the Christian tradition.[1] In turn, the rudiments of the Christian funeral outlook are in the main derived from Hebrew religious and ethical concepts. These, again, were undoubtedly influenced by the death beliefs and mortuary practices of the early Egyptians and other ancient civilizations. Before these, in the uncounted ages of prehistory, were practices whose nature we can only guess, guided in part by the practices of later primitive peoples of whom we have some knowledge.

To the new doctrines of Christ, the early Christian Church added interpretations having significance for funeral beliefs and practices still with us today. To a much lesser extent, contributions were made by the mystical and philosophical beliefs of the Greeks and Romans. Some pagan customs prevalent during the period of the early Christian Church undoubtedly were absorbed in the Christian burial complex. To understand better this original Christian complex and the contemporary American funeral beliefs and practices that stem from it, we will look backward along a few of the roads that lead to it.

FUNERAL CUSTOMS OF THE ANCIENT EGYPTIANS

Of all the great civilizations of ancient times springing up in the general area surrounding the Mediterranean basin — that is, Southern Europe, Western Asia, Northern Africa and, among others, the Babylonian, Assyrian, Chaldean and Persian — that of ancient Egypt has had perhaps more influence than any other upon civilizations intermediate to our own and, through these, upon the modern Western world. For that reason, and without denying that other ancient civilizations might have contributed indirectly to modern funeral practices, Egyptian civilization is singled out for consideration.

For five thousand years in the Nile Delta and southward along its flood plain, there flourished a culture in which the fine and practical arts, and the abstract and applied sciences, reached an early advanced development. Here, too, in the ordering of human affairs there appeared, perhaps for the first recorded time, a morality of group life based on internal conscience rather than on external authority supported by force.[2]

Although it is hazardous to attempt to settle such matters with finality at a distance of as much as six or seven thousand years, we are fortunate in that of all ancient civilizations, the material culture of the Egyptians is best preserved. Its magnificent cities, now in ruins, its monuments, tombs, pyramids and the wealth of objects made by human hands — all these testify to the splendor of a remarkable era. Archaeologists, who dig into the sands and reconstruct from the remains the life of those who made a civilization, have not exhausted the cultural treasures of the Nile country. Newer discoveries, plus an intensified interest in the social life of the ancient

Egyptians,[3] have led to a sharper appreciation of the high social, political, economic and religious achievements attained during five thousand years of Egypt's historical development.

Death Beliefs: One of the most persistent themes to pattern the thought and culture of the ancient Egyptians was that of death and the life beyond. The theologies of both Sun worship and the cult of Osiris — god of the underworld and judge of the dead — were profoundly affected by the idea of death. In a dry, warm climate, where the elements dealt benignly with the bodies of the dead and natural mummification was often the result, the earliest settlers of the Nile Valley were stimulated to ponder the prospects of continued life in and beyond the grave. One of the universal responses to death has been to attribute some life to the body lying in the grave, while believing at the same time that an element or aspect of the dead person resides elsewhere, apart from the grave.

The Egyptians attributed a divine origin to the soul; they held that, throughout life, it was engaged in a struggle with good and evil; and that, after life, its final state was determined by judgment, according to its behavior on earth. Those who were justified before Osiris passed into perpetual happiness; those who were condemned, into perpetual misery. The justified took the name of Osiris, the judge, under which name they indeed already had appeared for judgment.

Evidence found in tombs indicates that everyone who could afford a sculptured record was described as justified; every mummy was already an Osiris. It is probable that the performance of ceremonies and the whole process of embalming, together with charms attached to the mummy and prayers said by those who visited the tomb, were held necessary to secure future happiness. The practice of embalming attained major importance from the belief that the deceased would resume his normal, everyday activities in the afterlife. Thus, in the earlier periods, it was not unusual to sacrifice servants and make presentations of food and money to aid the soul on its journey to the Sun.

The Egyptians believed that the Sun was the center, the focus, of the universe, from which all things emerged and to which they returned. The death beliefs of the Egyptians pivoted around the idea that the complex elements that joined to make a person could be reassembled in the body of the dead. These elements included The Ba (Soul), The Yakhu (Shining One), The Name, The Shadow, The Heart (as the seat of the intellect and emotions), and the Ka.[4] The last is most significant, as it remained by the dead and demanded attention from the living. In earlier times, this attention took the form of food offerings, but later it was reduced to the saying of prayers.

Central to the Egyptian concept of life after death was the belief in bodily resuscitation. Although at death the various elements of the dead person were thought to depart, it was believed that they could be reconstituted or brought together again (as was the case in the miracle of Osiris) through a series of ritualistic actions. The body itself was therefore to be preserved in natural form so that the restoration of *the person* in its complex parts — the bringing together of the elements which at death had been separated — might take place.

Thomas Greenhill, a surgeon who worked in London and authored *The Art of Embalming*, published in 1705, ascribed human fastidiousness to the soul, saying that it left the body only when the body was "corrupt and putrified, as abhorring so loathsome an habitation; whereas on the contrary, it never forsook it when it was incorrupt and entire... By its being dressed in fine linen (the body) might court and incline its best companion, the soul, to cohabit with it."[5]

To this end, the art of embalming was employed and, as is commonly known, reached an amazing state of perfection. James H. Breasted, who has made extensive studies in the history of Egypt, notes, however, that "it is... not correct to attribute to the Egyptians a belief in the *immortality* of the soul... or to speak of his ideas of immortality."[6] It would be more accurate instead to say that the soul, in a sense, had to be "mortalized" by being brought back to the body. When soul and name and shadow and heart and body were joined, the "person" was restored.

Among the oldest of Egyptian funeral ceremonies are those associated with offering the dead such fare as various kinds of cakes, oils, beer and wine. To provide for this offering, a regular portion of a man's estate was set aside. While the food generally was permitted to decay, or was consumed by attendants on the theory that it nourished "the shade" (the deceased's spirit) spiritually even though eaten by the living, a tube down which food could be passed was sometimes extended from the exterior of the grave to the mouth of the corpse.[7]

Yet, despite the elaborate ritual and the practical provisions taken toward the dead to secure reconstitution of the person, continued attention to the grave and spirits of the dead by surviving relatives was thought necessary. The need for protecting the body, the coffin and funeral treasures gave impetus to the building of tombs. In consequence, tomb chaplains or priests, to whom the necessary ritualistic actions on behalf of the dead were delegated, entered Egyptian funerary customs. The most enduring monuments in the world, the great pyramids, were both memorials and tombs for the rulers of Egypt. (***See Plate 1***.)

Thus for nearly four thousand years, Egyptian society at every level, from the Pharaohs down to the least slave, was given over in great part to the task of preparing and caring for the dead. Appreciation of this fact led Breasted to remark:

> In no other land, ancient or modern, has there ever been such attention to the equipment of the dead for their eternal sojourn in the hereafter. The beliefs which finally led the Egyptian to the devotion of so much of his wealth and time, his skill and energy to the erection of the "eternal house" are the oldest conceptions of a real life hereafter of which we know.[8]

After the burial, offerings were made at stated times throughout the year by the family, and the chief inscription on the tomb begged the passerby to say a prayer for the good of the inhabitant thereof. The making of prescribed offerings at the tomb must have been most inconvenient.

Possibly because of this, burial grounds became peopled by a tribe of mercenary professional embalmers and lesser priests, who made their living not only by their profession, but also by fraud and even theft. Yet all in all, we must admire the generosity with which the Egyptians lavished their riches upon this mode of affection, to be repaid not only by a natural satisfaction, but also by the wholesome recognition that there are unselfish and unproductive uses of wealth.

The Threat of Plague as a Burial Motive: Combined with the religious motive, the concern of the ancient Egyptians for the proper disposal of the dead had some kind of sanitary purpose. Like the ancient Chinese, they sometimes used dry burials to keep the products of putrefaction from seeping into the soil and thus generating plague. In dry burial, bodies were shrouded in coarse cloth and laid upon beds of charcoal under six or eight feet of sand on the edge of the great plain at Memphis, and above the reach of the flooding Nile. The dry air and nitrous soil provided for their slow and inoffensive decomposition, and they were as well preserved from putrid decay as if they had been embalmed.

For the great masses of Egypt, this disposal practice (and not cavity embalming) was also an economic necessity, and tends to reinforce the theory that the national practice of elaborately ritualized embalming and entombment originated in the utilitarian purpose of sanitation as much or more than in primarily religious and ceremonial ends. Dry burial was in effect a cheaper form of embalming available to the Egyptian masses. Herodotus observed that the people of Egypt felt themselves continually menaced by some great epidemic scourge and took precautions accordingly.[9]

Against this backdrop of beliefs concerning death and the afterlife, specific Egyptian death customs come to have meaning and logic, even though over the course of nearly five thousand years, and through successive historical epochs, they grew and changed, responding to fashion and, possibly, even to outside influence. Some, such as the dismemberment of the body, passed out of existence completely. Yet, in spite of superficial changes, the basic beliefs remained unchanged. There was life after death, no matter what form it might take. This demanded not only the preservation of the body in its natural appearance, but also ritualistic actions to restore the elements that, along with the body, formed the person in the hereafter.

Embalming: As practiced during the peak of artistic performance in the New Kingdom period (1738-1102 B.C.), embalming presents one of the most universally interesting aspects of Egyptian care for the dead.[10] Later classical writers, Herodotus and Diodorus in particular, have described the process fairly accurately, noting that three grades of embalming were in vogue, these varying by the amount of time, attention and the quality of materials used in the operation.

For the well-to-do and those of high rank, the most elaborate and expensive process was used: the brain and the viscera were removed, embalmed or preserved separately, and placed in a series of four canopic jars, or burial vases. (***See Plate 1.***) In the New Kingdom period, these jars had four heads, representing the four Children of Horus, the hawk-headed god of day. Mestha, the manheaded, protected the stomach and large intestines; Hapi, the dog-headed, guarded the small intestines; Tuamutef, the jackal-headed, watched over the lungs and heart; and Qebhsennuf, the hawk-headed, protected the liver and gall bladder.[11] The cavities in the head and body were washed clean and filled with spices and resins. The body was then immersed in a soda solution for forty days, after which it was wrapped in fine linen.

PLATE 1

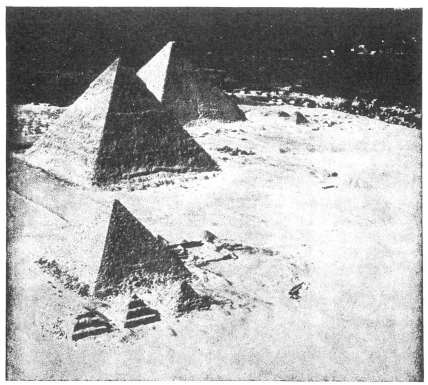

1A. Aerial View of Pyramids at Gizeh.

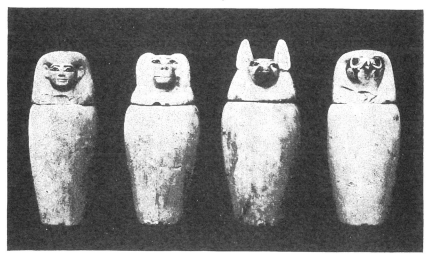

1B. Canopic Jars — Containers of Vital Organs.

A less costly method called for injecting cedar oil without evisceration. The body was laid in natrum or natron (a fixed alkali) for the prescribed period, after which the cedar oil, now dissolved in the soft organs, was released and the body, its flesh dissolved by the natron, was reduced to preserved skin and bones.

The third mode, practiced for the poorer classes, comprised purging the intestines and soaking the body in a soda solution for seventy days. The use of bitumen, or pitch, was a later development and resulted in the hard, black mummy that tended to last almost indefinitely. It is the type that constitutes the popular image of an Egyptian mummy in the Western mind. Bodies embalmed with expensive unguents, spices, oils and resins quickly lost their preserved condition when unwrapped and were not likely to remain long on public display.

The most celebrated description of Egyptian embalming was written by Herodotus (484 to 424 B.C.), a Greek and the "Father of History." He writes in *The Persian Wars* that, in Egypt:

> ...There are certain persons appointed by law to the exercise of the profession of embalming. When a dead body is brought to them, they exhibit to the friends of the deceased different models highly finished in wood. The most perfect of these they say resembles one whom I do not think it religious to name in such a matter; the second is of less price, and inferior in point of execution; another is still more mean; they then require after which model the deceased shall be represented; when the price is determined, the relations retire and the embalmers thus proceed. In the most perfect specimens of their art, they draw the brain through the nostrils, partly with a piece of crooked iron, and partly by the infusion of drugs; they then with an Ethiopian stone make an incision in the side, through which they extract the intestines; these they cleanse thoroughly, washing them with palm wine and afterwards covering them with pounded aromatics; they then fill the body with powder of pure myrrh, cassia, and all other perfumes except frankincense. Having sewn up the body, it is covered with nitre for the space of seventy days, which time they may not exceed; as at the end of this period it is washed, closely wrapped in bandages of cotton, dipped in a gum which the Egyptians use as a glue; it is then returned to the relations, who enclose the body in a case of wood, made to resemble a human figure, and place it against the wall in the repository of their dead. The above is the most costly mode of embalming. They who wish to be less expensive adopt the following method: they neither draw out the intestines nor make any incision in the dead body, but inject an unguent made from the cedar; after taking proper means to secure the injected oil within the body, it is covered with nitre for the time specified above; on the last day they withdraw the liquor before introduced; which brings with it all the bowels and intestines; the nitre eats away flesh, and the skin and bones only remain: the body is returned in this state, and no further care taken concerning it. There is a third mode of embalming appropriate to the poor. A particular kind of ablution is made to pass through the body, which is afterwards left in nitre for the above seventy days, and then returned. The wives of men of rank, and such females as have been distinguished by their beauty or importance, are not immediately on their decease delivered to the embalmers:

they are usually kept for three or four days, which is done to prevent any indignity being offered to their persons. An instance of this once occurred.[12]

Coffins: The desire to keep bodies from touching the earth was characteristic not only of the Egyptians but of most early African peoples. Mats and skins, and reed, wooden and earthenware baskets, had been employed to this end during the earlier periods of Egyptian history. As concern with perfection in preservation developed, so did the art of producing more elaborate coffins. From the XIth Dynasty (about 2500 B.C.) down to the days of the Empires, coffins play an important role in Egyptian burial. In the earlier historical periods they were rectangular and tended to be massive, along the lines of a sarcophagus. Hieroglyphic inscriptions covered the exterior and were devoted to prayers, genealogies, and religious and magical texts intended not only to help the restoration of the body, and thereby the reconstitution of the person, but also to aid and give power to the dead in the afterlife. (***See Plate 2***.)

Between the XIIth and XVIIIth dynasties, the shape of the coffin was changed, probably as a result of the growth of the cult Osiris, and the anthropoid (man-resembling) coffin came into use.[13] Here, the face of the dead was reproduced, first by wood carving and later by "cartonnage" — a mixture of linen and stucco painted in lifelike resemblance. (***See Plate 3***.) Usually this outer casing was given the appearance of a laborer bearing the implements of husbandry, with only the face and hands exposed, while the rest of the body was painted with subjects relating to the future state and bore the principal inscription, giving the name and titles of "the Osiris justified."

The final development of this form is seen in the portrait coffin, developed under the Romans about the second century A.D., in which, instead of a modeled head, the face was painted on a wooden panel held in place by bandaging.[14] (***See Plate 3***.) The realism and representational quality of the portraiture far surpasses the earlier Egyptian art with its unresolved problem of perspective and proportion. Budge describes these painted coffins in some detail:

> The finest and most beautiful painted coffins found in Egypt date from the XVIII dynasty, and the nobles and priests of Amen-Ra were provided with most luxurious funerary equipment. It was no uncommon thing for a great noble to be buried in three coffins, the outermost serving as a sarcophagus. The coffins are well shaped and well made, and both inside and outside are covered with Vignettes and long texts from the Theban Book of the Dead, and from the Book of Gates, the Book "Ammi Tuat" and scenes from the work describing the passage of the dead Sun-god Afu-Ra through the hours of the night. Numerous small scenes, in which the deceased is seen adoring Osiris and his company of gods of the dead, and various forms of the Sun-god, are painted on every available space. Vignettes and texts were painted in bright colours upon the layer of plaster with which the coffin was overlaid, and the whole coffin, both inside and out was given a thick coat of yellowish varnish. The passage of thirty-four centuries has diminished the brightness of the colours... but when such a coffin left the hands of the scribe and artist the effect of this medley of hard uncompromising colours and disconnected subjects must have been somewhat crude and startling.[15]

PLATE 2

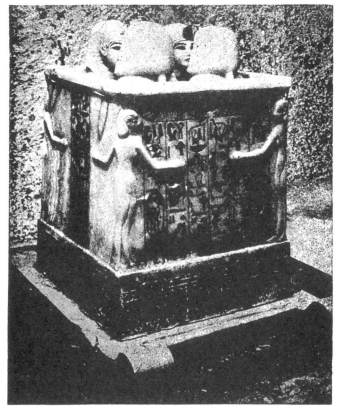

2A. Canopic Chest, Tut-ankh-Amon.

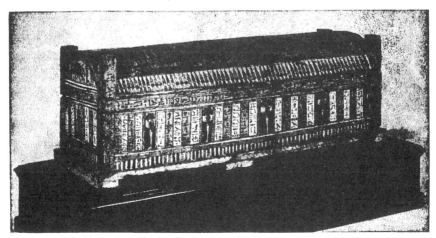

2B. Egyptian Outer Coffin Inscribed with Magical Texts.

PLATE 3

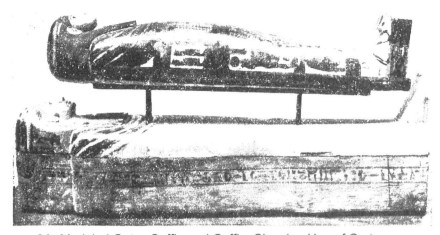

3A. Modeled Outer-Coffin and Coffin, Showing Use of Cartonnage.

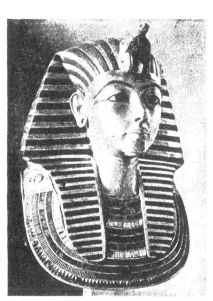 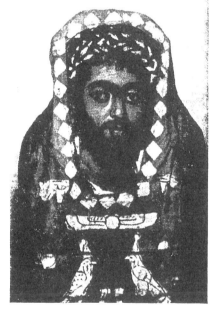

3B. (Left) Gold Mask, Tut-ankh-Amon.
3C. Coffin Portrait.

Some of the most opulent of these coffins had rich inlays of lapis lazuli, variously colored opaque glass, mother of pearl, and semi-precious stones. That of Tut-ankh-Amon was made of gold and jewels. (***See Plate 3***.) Although the nobility occasionally used stone and granite coffins, such materials were generally reserved for the massive sarcophagi, which in turn were also engraved with appropriate scenes and texts.

Undertaking Specialists and the Ritual of Embalming: In a society where so much time, energy and materials were expended on the disposal and care of the dead, it was necessary to develop an elaborate division of labor with the usual accompanying specialization of tasks and offices. While it was primarily the duty of the family and relatives to take the necessary measures to ensure the appropriate immediate and continued care of the dead, wealth and rank permitted these duties could be delegated to specialists. As the Egyptians succeeded in meeting the economic and social problems of life on this earth, they increasingly tended to let these specialists handle the complexities of securing an agreeable afterlife for the dead. It followed, then, that as a family's wealth and prestige grew, so did the luxury and costs of its funerals, as well as the number of specialists who were engaged in them.

For an Egyptian of rank, most arrangements and operations necessary to appropriate burial were *undertaken* by various classes of occupational specialists. The setting of death and burial was overwhelmingly sacred, combining magical and religious elements, and the actions toward the dead took place at all stages within a thoroughgoing ritualistic context. Upon the death of the head of the house, women of the household "rush frantically through the streets, beating their breasts, and from time to time clutching at their hair, which is sprinkled with the thick dust of the streets, and uttering wailing cries of grief."[16] The *Kher-heb*, or priest, who superintended embalming and funeral arrangements was called, and, with his assistants, arrived as quickly as possible. The body was then removed to the embalming chambers while the priest discussed the method of preserving it. Arrangements also got underway for final entombment, to take place some two or three months later. Meanwhile, the tomb was properly inscribed or plastered with texts and scenes of the departed's life; tomb furniture was built; and, among other things, a group of professional mourners was immediately organized to sing funeral dirges throughout the city.

In the embalming chamber, the *Kher-heb* was in complete charge, and, under him, the surgeon and his assistants proceeded with the embalming operations. Since embalming basically had a ritualistic and symbolic aspect representing the dismemberment and restoration of Osiris, each step in the operation was taken in conjunction with prayers and protective formulas. One assistant, the scribe, indicated the path of the incision. Another, using a sacred stone knife, made the incision and might be subject to ritualistic stoning for any violation of the sacred body. Other assistants completed the evisceration, the washing, and the application of spices, unguents and gums. Next, the viscera were preserved and placed in canopic jars, while the body was soaked in a tank of natron solution.

Following this, the intricate task of bandaging began once the body had been properly filled with spices and preservatives. Bandaging was invariably accompanied by a vast number of ritual actions, and the mummy cloth was inscribed with passages from various texts and formulas to give power to the dead in the afterlife. In the process, hundreds of yards of bandages were used by the specialists, and weeks were consumed in completing the task. Meanwhile, scarabs, amulets and useful artifacts and ornaments were put inside the body, within the bandages, or in the coffin or tomb. (***See Plate 4***.)

In the entire history of the preparation of the human body for burial, it is unlikely that so many specific functions have ever been assigned to so many separate functionaries as among the ancient Egyptians. Thomas Greenhill,[17] a surgeon writing at the very end of the 17th century, with the works of Herodotus, Diodorus and other ancient authors before him, finds that Egyptian embalming required five distinct specialists, each performing a separate office: "A *Designer* or *Painter*, a *Dissector* or *Anatomist*, a *Pollinctor* or *Apothecary*, an *Embalmer* or *Surgeon*, and a *Physician* or *Priest*." The last functionary was a "great philosopher" and "instructed others in these ceremonies."[18]

Describing the specific functions, Greenhill points out:

> The *Surgeon*, Who was the chief *Embalmer*, generally directed and took care to see the several Operations perform'd in due order, and sometimes did them himself; for tho' the *Curatores Corporis*, that were his Assistants and Servants, commonly Dissected, Embowell'd, Wash'd, Anointed and *Embalm'd* the Bodies of the meaner sort of People, yet when any Prince or Nobleman was to be *Embalm'd*, after the richest and most curious manner, he perform'd the chief part of the Work himself, and this he was the more capable of as being both an exquisite *Anatomist*, and well vers'd in the Nature of all *Balsamic* Medicines, whether *Galenical or Chymical*, and tho' he might be something inferior to the *Physician*, yet in conjunction with him, was he both the better able to consider the Nature of the deceas'd Person's Distemper, or Cause of his Death, and accordingly to proceed in his *Embalming*; and lastly he was very dextrous and knowing in the *Art of Bandage*, whereby it appears his chief Business was to *Embalm* and Roul up the Body... so was there (also) a greater occasion for skillful Apothecary, to take care of and see to the compounding the *Aromatic Powders, Oils, Balsams, Ointments, Cerecloths, Tinctures, Spirits*, and the like analogous Things, and their Application, according to the Directions of the *Doctor*; and as the *Surgeon* had under him a *Dissector*, &c. who embowell'd and wash'd the Body, and did the like inferior Business, so had the *Apothecary* Servants under him to make up the Medicines, administer Clysters and Injections, and to Anoint the Body, thence call'd *Pollinctors*. Thus was the chief Concern of the *Embalming* a Body manag'd by the Advice and Assistance of the *Physician, Surgeon* and *Apothecary*, as indeed it ought also to be perform'd at this Day, and not to have ignorant *Undertakers* direct and act all things at their pleasure.[19]

The funeral procession was also under the organizing genius of the *Kher-Heb* who, with his assistants, arranged for the transportation of the mummified corpse in its inscribed and ornamented coffin, as well as for all the funeral paraphernalia. The mummy was placed on a sledge drawn by oxen or men, and the procession with its burdened, wailing servants, professional mourners simulating anguished grief, religious functionaries, and relatives set out for the place of entombment. When it reached the river or came to a sacred lake that had to be crossed, the mummy was removed to a sacred boat, which bore the principal mourners and was towed by another boat, which was, in turn, followed by still others bearing lesser mourners, offerings and all other goods and equipment necessary for the burial.

When the family tomb was reached, in the case of the wealthier, the tomb priests and their assistants directed interment. Under their directions, the sarcophagus was placed in a sepulcher, usually at the bottom of a pit, but decorated as lavishly as the family could afford. Offerings were then made for the welfare of the deceased in a chapel in the upper part of the tomb. One tomb sufficed for each family, and sometimes for several generations of the same family. In the case of the less wealthy, many were buried in the sepulchral chambers of a single pit, above which was reared no structure or grotto. When the mummy had been laid away, masons closed the grave for eternity.

According to Diodorus, a legal tribunal judged everyone before the right of burial was permitted, and of this there might be a survival in the practice of the modern Egyptians, which prescribes that a witness must answer for the character of the deceased before his burial.

Influence of Egyptian Death Customs: It is not proper to conceive of the Egyptians as devoting all their talents and energies to the disposal and care of their dead. Having brought their civilization to a relatively high peak of economic and social development, luxurious treatment of the dead became a potentiality that, it must be admitted, was most fully realized. After the rise of the cult of Osiris, belief in a prosperous afterlife, under special conditions, spread over most of Egyptian society. As noted, the basic reason underlying the practice of mummification was the belief that it was necessary to preserve the body in the most perfect form in order that it might be rejoined by the complex entities that make up the total personality or person. Although this belief did not make its way into Christian theology, such was the depth and scope of Egyptian culture that Christians in Egypt were embalmed and mummified as a matter of custom.

The Egyptians of the Osiris cult believed that while entry into the world beyond depended in lesser part upon magical and mystical procedures, basically it was contingent upon the candidates having lived a life free from evil. The selective process was symbolically represented by the Egyptians in the popular scene of the "Balance," where the heart of the dead man was weighed by the god of death, Anubis, against a feather. (*See Plate 4*.) Should the balance be unfavorable, the heart was devoured by the monster Ament, and the dead man's desire for the glorious otherworld of Osiris remained unattained. The implications of this belief were felt in the Hebrew and early Christian religions and represented one of the earliest introductions of a sense of inner values, or conscience, which served to control ancient man in his relations to his fellow man.

PLATE 4

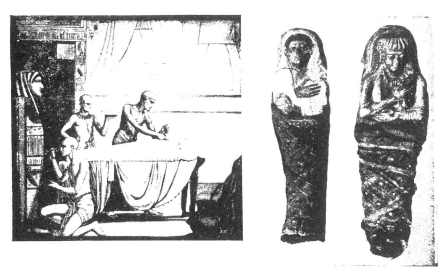

4A. (Left) Preparation of Egyptian Mummy, a Painting.
4B. Examples of Mortuary Mummy Bandaging.

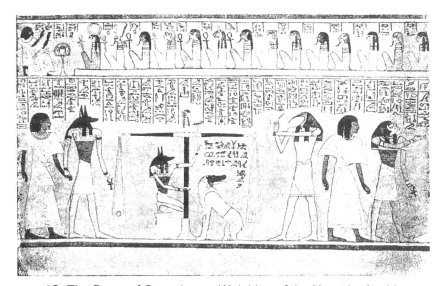

4C. The Dawn of Conscience: Weighing of the Heart by Anubis.

The Egyptian custom of embalming the dead was rooted in a system of religious beliefs whose content, by and large, has not been incorporated into modern Western civilization. Nevertheless, from earliest times until now, Egyptian embalming has continued to rouse lively interest and admiration, and from ancient Egypt to the present, neither the idea nor the practice of embalming has ever been lost; nor, for that matter, was there ever an eclipse of knowledge as to the general procedure that the Egyptians used.[20]

In considering Egyptian embalming practices, we should remember again that the embalmers belonged to the priestly class, and that embalming was a religious ritual, as well as a physical operation. This double function of embalming was not carried along into later Western funeral practices, even though certain other aspects of burial continued to have both a physical and religious significance.

FUNERAL CUSTOMS OF THE ANCIENT GREEKS

During the two thousand years between the Golden Age of Mycenae (1600 B.C.) and the closing of the University of Athens (A.D. 529, which marked the final extinction of Grecian culture on the homeland), on an almost uninhabitable Mediterranean peninsula there arose a magnificent Greek civilization — much of whose cultural heritage has long since been incorporated into the basis of Western thought and action. Though not as rich in historical depth as Egypt, perhaps, the pinnacle of Greek cultural achievement reached in the 5th century B.C. stands above the comparable development of any other ancient civilization. Art, philosophy and political activity found ample room for the highest development in this classical or "golden" age. Our review of the death beliefs and mortuary customs of the ancient Greeks will focus on this period.

Death Beliefs: To the Greeks, death was always conceived as one of the harsher lots of mankind. The writings of the classical period used stern and severe epithets for death, although ancient Greek literature is not without consolations for it.[21] Although the belief in a future existence persists in vague form throughout Greek literature, earlier beliefs conceived of the dead as living a bodily existence under the earth. Later, in Homeric times (circa 700 B.C.), this belief gave way to the concept of a shadowy afterlife peopled by disembodied souls — a belief not uncommon to ancient Mediterranean peoples generally.

To A. Rohde, a close student of Greek mortuary customs, this belief in a disembodied existence accounts for the introduction of cremation.[22] But this theory does not explain the fact that cremation first appeared on the Greek peninsula itself three centuries earlier during the Bronze Age, when the Greek states were loosely organized into the Achaean empire under the leadership of Mycenae. The practice of burning the dead had been brought down into the peninsula from the north by less-civilized Greeks, who had contact with neighboring barbarians, and who, with their iron weapons, conquered their weaker cousins. Although infrequently practiced at first, its acceptance increased in the Protogeometric period, and it took the place of earth burial shortly before the beginning of the historical period, around 700 B.C.[23]

At its highest point of development, the Greek conception of the afterlife involved the separation of the soul from the body and its ascent, or journey, into an eternal and immortal afterlife. Rush writes:

> The worship of Dionysius, [the god of wine] originating in Thrace, must have sown the first seed of the belief in an immortal life of the soul. The rites of this cult were intended to produce a wild excitement in which the limitations of ordinary life seem to be abolished. In such an ecstasy or *alienatio mentis* the soul was supposed to have left the body and winged its way to union with the god.[24]

Despite the popularity of this cult, with its Oriental overtones, it is fair to say that the general response of the Greeks to the thought of death was one of resignation rather than anticipation of the glorious afterlife. The translation of the individual to the Elysian Fields, or the union of the soul with the cult god, were beyond the expectations of the many and, only under special circumstances, the lot of the few.

At the pessimistic end of the spectrum of Greek death beliefs, hopelessness and despair prevailed, as revealed in the revulsion for death expressed by the classic writers. The revolting character of death in this concept is seen from the fact that Euripides refers to it as "the sable-vestured King of Corpses, Death."[25]

But, whatever the belief as to the mode of afterlife (and *some* form of such was always conceived), the general and overriding concept was materialistic in the sense that the soul was not forever freed of a bodily counterpart. Death was real; it was bad, evil and possibly terrifying. Consequently, the funeral ritual and the attention given to the grave and the memory of the departed played an important role in the mode by which the living related themselves to the dead.

Burial Practices: Reverence for the dead permeates Greek burial customs through all the ages.[26] Not only was it customary to give the dead a fitting burial, but, in classical times, the law of Athens required burial, or at least the covering with earth, of the corpses of strangers. Neglect of the dead was condemned and even urged as a disqualification for office.

Greek literature offers many examples to show how important burial was to the Greeks. In the play *Antigone* by Sophocles, for instance, when the tyrannical King Creon forbids the burial of the rebel Polynices, Antigone, the sister of the dead man, demands the privilege of giving at least symbolic burial to the corpse so that its shade (spirit) might cease to wander disconsolate upon the earth and enter into the Elysian Fields. When permission is refused, the girl scatters dust upon her brother's body and so brings death upon herself by violating the royal decree. In the *Iliad* by Homer, when Hector, the hero of the Trojans, is vanquished by Achilles, the champion of the Greeks, he drops to his knees — not to ask that his life shall be spared, but to beg that his enemy will take the gold he knows his father, Priam, king of Troy, will offer for his body so that it may be given burial.

Lest the dead remain unburied, the Athenians cremated them on immense pyres erected on the battlefields where they had fallen and, gathering the bones, returned them to Athens to be entombed splendidly and with due honor and ceremony. There is a legend of the mourning parents who stood before the Council of Athens and successfully demanded the execution of the victorious general who had returned in such hot haste to the city to claim his triumphal honors that he had left his dead, the son of the petitioners among them, unburied on the field of glory.[27]

Although the earlier Greeks might have included human sacrifice in their burial rites, this practice was later reduced to a symbolic offering, and, as Graves has pointed out, "almost everything connected with the interment of the dead seems essentially modern."[28] As soon as death occurred, the eyes and mouth of the deceased were closed by relatives or friends. Greek funerary urns often depict the scene; usually it is the female performing the act or possibly the children. (*See Plate 5*.) Since passage into the netherworld required crossing the river Styx, a coin (obol) was placed in the dead man's mouth for Charon, the ferryman. Without such fare, the unlucky shade was doomed to wander a hundred years along the shores.

Family members generally prepared the body for burial. Female next-of-kin performed the washing of the body with warm water because it was thought that those only "apparently dead" might be revived in the process.

Laying out and dressing the corpse was a sacred duty, entrusted in like manner to female relatives. While the body was anointed with oils, perfumes and spices, in keeping with the belief of the shadowy afterlife of the disembodied soul, no serious attempt at embalming was made.

From the earliest times in Greek history, it was customary not to bury the dead naked, but with clothing.[29] Plutarch refers to the fact that the tendency to be extravagant in clothing the dead caused Solon to decree that only three burial robes could be used. These were the covering for the funeral bed, the garment in which the corpse was enveloped, and the outer covering.[30] This early instance of sumptuary law is not, historically, an isolated case. Later periods in Western civilization, including the early American Colonial period, reveal sumptuary decrees and legislation dealing with excessive funerary display.

Flowers, woven into wreaths, were furnished for the dead by relatives and friends of the deceased. Included with the corpse was a honey cake for the dog Cerberus, the three-headed guardian of the entrance to Hades. While mourning was indicated by dark, subdued colors, the dead were robed in white.

Within a day after death, the body — washed, anointed, dressed and ready for burial — was laid out in state. Friends and relatives then viewed the corpse, a practice that partly served to guarantee death had actually occurred (*see Plate 5*) and that the corpse might not have suffered violence. Meanwhile, ritualistic wailing by female mourners began.

After one day of lying in state, unless the social prestige of the dead was such as to require extension of up to seven days, a funeral procession was formed to accompany the body to the tomb. The procession usually set out one hour before dawn and consisted of the corpse on a bier carried by the relatives or friends, or possibly hired "corpse bearers,"[31] as well as female mourners, fraternity members (either immediately preceding or just behind the corpse), and hired

PLATE 5

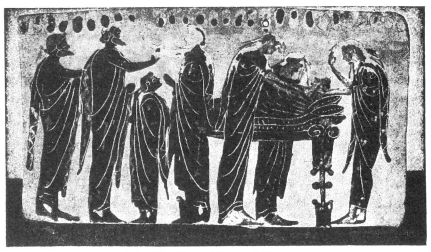

5A. Attic Black-Figured Plaque.

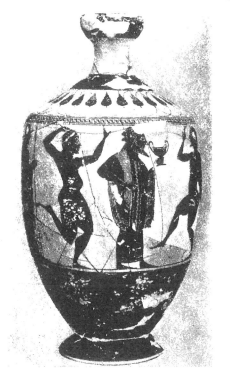
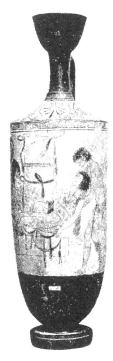

5B. (Left) Lekythos of Amasis, Used in Greek Funerals.
5C. Mourning Scene, Greek Lekythos.

dirge singers. (***See Plate 6***.) Curiously enough, any *man* might join in the dismal march to the grave, but every *woman* was denied the melancholy privilege unless she had passed her sixtieth year, or was connected to the deceased by blood and was over sixteen years of age.[32]

As noted earlier, cremation of the dead began in Greece about 1000 B.C. as a burial form adopted from the immigrant Greek-speaking people from the North. At first rarely used, its acceptance increased through subsequent historic periods until, during Homeric and classical times, it was the predominate mode of disposition. While at no time was earth burial entirely superseded, the belief in the power of the flame to set the soul free acted as a strong impetus to the practice of cremation. It should be noted, however, that the ashes of the dead were still conceived to have personal or spirit characteristics.[33]

Although a choice of inhumation (burial) or cremation was available during all late-Greek periods, the obsequies at the burial universally indicated a conception of a disembodied soul, or shade, in sharp contradistinction to the Egyptian belief in the reanimation of the dead by restoration to the body of the complex elements that, together, formed the person.

Coffins and Tombs: Wood, stone and baked-clay coffins were in use at various periods of early Greek history. Those of baked clay, representing the earlier eras, tended to be rudely fashioned, although some were decorated with painted floral designs. Chests of cypress wood were used in the later periods, yet stone was perhaps the most popular material, although its weight precluded its being carried in the funeral procession. The body was borne on the bier and, if not cremated, was deposited enclosed in the coffin, in the tomb.

Frank P. Graves has classified these tombs into four major groups: (a) *stelae*, or shafts, (b) *kiones*, or columns, (c) *trapezae*, or square-cut tombs, and (d) *naidia*, or temple-like structures.[34] The *stelae*, which were actually upright slabs of stone, and other tombs were often covered with figures carved in bas-relief and finished off with painting. (***See Plate 6***.) Scenes were apt to be lifelike, showing the deceased on the deathbed or at work in his home. In a relief found at Athens, some kind of a repast or feast is shown in which a bearded man reclines upon a couch and holds a plate or saucer in his hand; his wife is seated at his feet; a naked cup-bearer is near at hand; a friend stands at the head of the couch; and the dog lies under it.[35]

Inside the tomb, and sometimes inside the coffin, there were placed practical and artistic ornaments, jewels, vessels, wreaths, painted vases, and articles of toilet, war and play. As in the case of the Egyptians, preparations were often made by the individual before his demise for the continued care of the tomb. Family tombs were also used.

The final steps were the funeral feast, which broke the fast that the bereaved had been keeping, and the offering of sacrifices at the sepulcher on specified days. Although in early times these sacrifices took the form of blood propitiations to the appropriate gods, the Greeks later substituted offerings of food, wine and various libational mixtures. Thus, the Greeks of antiquity kept alive their relationship to the dead and to the dreary afterlife that they believed was the common lot of man.

PLATE 6

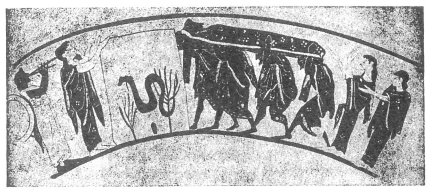

6A. Funeral Procession, Painted on Grecian Pottery.

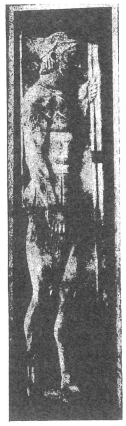

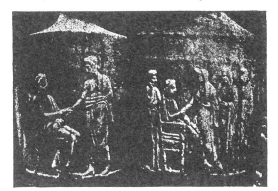

6B. Farewell Scenes,
Greek Lekythoi.

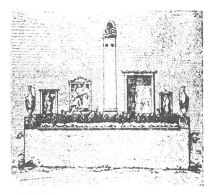

6C. (Left) Stele of Aristion.
6D. Restored Grecian Funeral Lot.

Herodotus tells us that the primitive Greeks sometimes slaughtered slaves and horses to provide servants and beasts for the dead in the material hereafter. This practice of so equipping the dead with all the goods and services needed in a happy life beyond is found in the funerary cultures of many peoples. Suttee — self-inflicted or group-inflicted cremation of a Hindu widow — though now illegal, is still practiced in India on very rare occasions. When facts grow difficult, symbols tend to replace them. Thus, when the Egyptians discontinued the custom of sacrificing slaves to be buried in the tomb with their masters, they substituted small clay figures.[36]

In considering objects buried with the dead, we should always bear in mind the fact that while some of these are designed to serve the dead, others are placed there primarily as symbols. The many clay scarab beetles found in Egyptian tombs, for example, had no utilitarian purpose in the afterlife but symbolized resurrection. To the Egyptian who watched the scarab beetle lay its eggs in dung, which it rolled into balls, and who saw the next generation of scarab beetles emerge from corruption, the meaning was clear: new life springs from decay. The Egyptians likewise saw in wheat a respected funerary symbol: life lies dormant, ready to grow from the germ. Wheat on Christian tombs added a sacramental meaning to this resurrection symbolism. Grapes and wheat represent wine and bread, the appearances under which Christ offers Himself and is received by the faithful on Christian altars.[37]

FUNERAL CUSTOMS OF THE ANCIENT ROMANS

In the 1,200 years from 753 B.C., when Romulus became the first king of Rome, to A.D. 476, when the barbarian Odoacer deposed Romulus Augustus, the last of the Roman emperors of the West, Roman civilization emerged, flourished, underwent major political, social, economic and religious changes before finally disintegrating rapidly under the onslaught of the barbarians from without and moral decay from within. Left behind was a residue of political, economic and social institutions to serve as models for the Western world in the administration of human affairs.

Although the Romans borrowed and adapted much of their culture in the areas of the practical and expressive arts from the Greeks, their contributions to the science and art of administration are substantially their own. Many details of Roman funeral and undertaking operations foreshadowed corresponding operations today. Of particular importance were the emerging role of the secular undertaker, as distinguished from the religious, and the assignment to him of specific tasks. Roman burial practices thus mark a major step in defining the status, character and occupational role of the modern funeral director.

Roman View of Death and the Importance of Burial: Belief in the afterlife among the Romans varied in the course of changing times. In earlier centuries, an animistic view (the doctrine that the soul is the vital principle) held that the soul of man, although separated at death from the body, hovered around the place of burial for its continued peace and happiness, and required constant attention from the descendants in the form of offerings of food and drink. Should the offerings be discontinued, the Romans thought that the soul would cease to be happy

Pagan Roots of Modern Funeral Practice

and might even become a spirit of evil to bring harm upon those who had neglected the proper rites.[38]

Starting about 300 B.C., contact with the Greek civilization bought to the Romans new religious and philosophical beliefs concerning death and the afterlife. The mystery cults of Greece and the Oriental East emphasized the spiritual aspects of the afterlife, and included the hope of joining with the cult god in a pleasant, wondrous or ecstatic existence in eternity. Opposed to this joyful lot was another world of torment, gloom and continued unhappiness.

A more philosophical conception, proposed by the Epicureans, was that the body and the soul, composed of atoms, simply disintegrated at death. Thus, the afterlife of man was no different than the before-life. However, what was originally a philosophy of moderation became vulgarized into a scheme of life that was characterized by St. Paul as meaning, "Let us eat and drink for tomorrow we shall die."[39]

Maecenas, writing during the Augustan age (43 B.C. to A.D. 14) revealed in poetry not only some of the dreaded maladies of the period but also the grimness with which the Romans held onto the life of the here-and-now:

> Though racked with gout in hand and foot,
> Though cancer deep should strike its root,
> Though palsy shake my feeble thighs,
> Though hideous lump on shoulder rise,
> From flaccid gum teeth drop away,
> Yet all is well if life but stay.[40]

The emergence of Christianity as the dominant religion of the Roman Empire, a phenomenon well underway by the year A.D. 300, made widespread for the first time a theological or religious orientation to death. Death had a meaning given it in terms of an organized set of beliefs about man and his maker, and Christians patterned their death customs, for the most part, after the mode of the sepulture (interment) of Christ.

In light of these different orientations to death and the disposal of the dead, it is difficult to make generalizations, but the Romans essentially envisioned some sort of afterlife at all times. Even Epicurus left instructions in his will that offerings should be made in perpetuity to his dead relatives and for celebrations of his birthday. Moreover, no matter what form of afterlife was conceived, the relation of the living to the dead was held to be continuous and of vital importance, to the quick and the dead alike.

Roman Burial Customs: At various times, the Romans practiced both cremation and earth burial. Cremation was the normal practice during the period of the Republic and the first century after Christ, but, under the Roman empire, fire burial was replaced by inhumation (burial). The causes for this change have been attributed to the spread of Oriental mystery cults and their abhorrence of fire; to the rise of Christianity, with its emphasis upon the hallowed nature of the body; and to the operation of fashion.[41]

For reasons of sanitation, burial within the walls of the city of Rome was prohibited, and so it followed that the great roads outside were lined with elaborate and costly tombs erected by the well-to-do. (***See Plate 7***.) Although most of these were for families, monuments or public memorials that, strictly speaking, were not tombs honored individuals occasionally. For the poor of Rome, of course, there was no such magnificence. Corpses of slaves and aliens were laid in the *commune sepulchrum*, the common burial pit, outside the walls.[42]

Great tombs, or *columbaria* filled with niches for the urns holding ashes of the cremated dead, were often erected by speculators who rented urn space to those unable to afford appropriate resting places of their own. In imitation of these structures, others were erected on the same plan by burial societies formed by members of the artisan class, and others still, as baths and libraries, were erected and maintained by benevolent men for the public good.[43] (***See Plate 7***.)

Although burial of the *misera plebs* (the wretched poor) eventually became a function of the state, burial societies were possibly the first agencies to assure appropriate burial for the poorer classes of workers. At Lanuvium between A.D. 100-200, the regulations of one such association indicate that social and festive affairs were likewise included in its official functions.[44]

There was little alienation of the dead — that is, avoiding the facts of death or hurriedly putting the dead out of sight — in Roman funeral behavior. A person died in the presence of the immediate family. Under ordinary circumstances, the body was washed with warm water, anointed, laid out in a white toga, and decorated with whatever insignia of rank the dead had achieved in life. The body was then put upon a funeral couch, feet to the door, to lie in state for a period of three days to a week, depending upon the prestige of the person in life. Flowers were strewn about the funeral couch, incense was burned, and, outside the door, cypress or pine boughs were set as a warning of the possible pollution by death.

In the case of the well-to-do, the care and laying out of the body was delegated to professional undertakers, who also took charge of the arrangements for the funeral procession and burial. Among the Romans, the corpse needed preservation not for eternity, as with the Egyptians, but only long enough to lie in state without putrefaction. Added attention signified that the dead had been a person of importance and therefore required a long period of lying-in-state.

In the scattered references to Roman burial, the role of the physician is not altogether clear. For example, while Pliny remarks that it was customary among the Egyptians to preserve bodies by the physician's art, it does not appear among Greeks and Romans that the physician served as embalmer. Although Roman embalming seems to have consisted for the most part of a superficial anointing of the corpse with spices and perfumes, cavity embalming was sometimes practiced, particularly for rich or important people.

Such as it was, embalming was delegated to the *pollinctores*, who were either slaves or employees of the *libitinarius*, the Roman equivalent of the head undertaker. The latter was so called because he exercised his business at the temple or grove of *Libitina*, the goddess of corpses and funerals. Deaths were also registered at this temple.[45]

PLATE 7

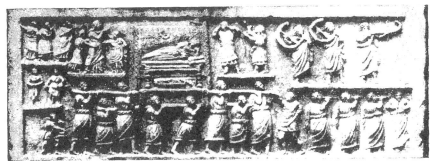
7A. Funeral Procession; Relief from Amiternum.

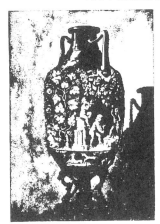
7B. Roman Burial Urn.

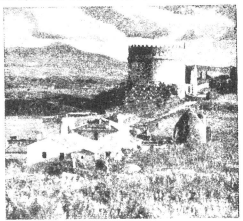
7C. Tomb of Cecillia Metella, Appian Way

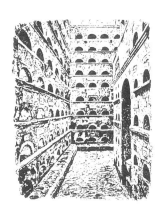

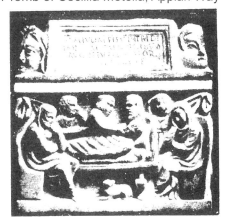

7D. (Left) Columbarium, Vigna Codini.
7E. Funeral Urn Depicting the Conclamatio.

In addition to the *pollinctores*, another sub-category of undertaker was the designator, who acted as master of ceremonies and director of the funeral procession.[46] The *praeco* or crier was a special functionary who summoned the participants to a public funeral. Interestingly enough, the social status of these tradesmen and functionaries was not high, as indicated by the fact that they were excluded from participation in political life. Should they resign their office, however, they could be elected to the highest magistracies.[47]

Early Funeral Directing: The *libitinarius*, apparently, is the direct ancestor not only of the undertaker but also of the modern funeral director. In addition to providing anointing or embalming, he supplied hired mourners, mourning costumes and other accessories for funeral pomp, and arranged services designed to ease the grief of the bereaved.

One of his more important functions was to arrange with his assistant designator the details of the funeral procession, which, among the Romans, had far more importance than it has now. Today, one funeral procession is much like another and attracts little attention. The Roman procession, on the other hand, gave persons of wealth and importance an opportunity to display their social and economic position by costly public parade. Johnston describes such a procession:

> The funeral procession of the ordinary citizen was simple enough. Notice was given to neighbors and friends. Surrounded by them and by the family, carried on the shoulders of the sons or other near relatives, with perhaps a band of musicians in the lead, the body was borne to the tomb. The procession of one of the mighty, on the other hand, was marshaled with all possible display and ostentation. It occurred as soon after death as the necessary preparations could be made, as there was no fixed intervening time. Notice was given by a public crier in the ancient words of style: "This citizen has been surrendered to death. For those who find it convenient, it is now time to attend the funeral. He is being brought from his house." (*Author's translation*.) Questions of order and precedence were settled by an undertaker (*designator*). At the head of the procession went a band of musicians, followed, at least occasionally, by persons singing dirges in praise of the dead, and by bands of buffoons and jesters, who made merry with the bystanders and imitated even the dead man himself. Then came the imposing part of the display. The wax masks of the dead man's ancestors had been taken from their place in the *alae* and assumed by actors in the dress appropriate to the time and station of the worthies they represented. It must have seemed as if the ancient dead had returned to earth to guide their descendant to his place among them. Servius tells us that six hundred *imagines* were displayed at the funeral of the young Marcellus, the nephew of Augustus. Then followed the memorials of the great deeds of the deceased, if he had been a general, as in a triumphal procession, and then the dead man himself, carried with face uncovered on a lofty couch. Then came the family, including freedmen (especially those made free by the testament of their master) and slaves, and next the friends, all in mourning garb, and all freely giving expression to the emotion that we try to suppress on such occasions. Torchbearers attended the train, even by day, as a remembrance of the older custom of burial by night.[48]

In selecting the buffoon to portray the dead man, an effort was made to obtain the services of an actor who resembled him. This travesty was intended to show that the departed members of the family had come back to escort the newest recruit to the ranks into the underworld. The waxen masks were carefully preserved as heirlooms, to be used only at funerals.[49]

While ordinary funerals were nighttime affairs, persons of higher status were buried by day. Torchbearers attended the day processions, however, as a remembrance of the custom of nocturnal burial. A funeral oration in the Forum was included in the funeral of those with sufficient prestige to be honored publicly. The body was then moved outside the city to the tomb where cremation or earth burial took place. At this point, the ceremony included the consecration of the burial site, the purification of those assembled, and the casting of earth upon the remains.

Subsequently, a mourning period was observed, offerings were made to the gods, and the memory of the dead was kept alive through later memorial festivals.

Fear that the dead might be jealous of apparent neglect by the living, who bore grief stoically, led both Greeks and Romans to introduce professional mourners into their funeral processions. Hired women shrieked and beat their breasts with abandon. As the ceremony drew to a close, the frenzy of their simulated sorrow mounted and climaxed with a triple ceremonial farewell, the *conclamatio mortis*, or calling out of the dead, as — tearing their hair, rending their garments and scratching their faces until they drew blood — they thrice encircled the coffin, shrieking out the name of the deceased.[50] (**See Plate 7**.)

By the time of Constantine, the first Christian emperor (A.D. 314-379) municipal authority had been extended to include the public disposal of any Roman who needed a proper burial but could not afford one. Companies of functionaries were established to prepare the religious procession, to carry the bier and to dig the grave. Sumptuary laws prohibiting excessive spending were enacted at the time, and overcharging for funeral paraphernalia was declared illegal. "Every person who needed it," writes Puckle, "was to have a coffin without payment, whilst even the poorest were to be followed to the grave by a cross bearer, eight monks, and three acolytes."[51]

From this period through the Middle Ages, the management of funerary behavior becomes increasingly the province of the Church, and for the next 1,500 years, the secular undertaker remains an occupational casualty to the revolution of Western culture.

Influence of Roman Burial Practices: Roman influence upon contemporary funeral beliefs has been slight, on the whole. The *conclamatio mortis*, for example, was not taken up by the Christian Church as a formal rite and must not be confused with occasional spontaneous outbursts of grief during Christian burials.

Some direct impact is to be found, however, in how the splendor, pomp and ceremony with which the Romans expressed their social hierarchy during their funerals influenced the uniform simplicity of early Christian funerals. Nock points out the operation of *fashion* in Roman funeral behavior, and he ascribes the decline of cremation to the desire of Romans to indicate their social position and wealth more advantageously through earth burial:

By fashion we mean the habits of the rich, which gradually permeated the classes below them. Burial seems to have made its appeal to them because it presented itself in the form of the use of the sarcophagus. This was expensive and gratified the instinct for ostentation. The richest could build mausolea. Many whose resources would not suffice for that, could afford sarcophagi, which might well appear a more solid and adequate way of paying the last honors to the dead... the sarcophagus re-established the popularity of burial, and then burial then came in its own right to be the dominant custom of the poor.[52]

Roman influence upon modern funeral practices is to be regarded in the last instance not so much for the *content* of those death beliefs, which might have been transmitted to the Western world, but for the *occupational models* useful to mass societies exhibiting an urban way of life. Most important from the point of view of this study is the secular functionary — the Roman "undertaker" — who, as arranger, manager and director of funeral affairs, as well as supplier of mortuary paraphernalia, established a pattern of occupational behavior meaningful to modern funeral directors.

Additionally, Roman administrative measures have suggested to today's societies that a body of mortuary law might be necessary to ensure adequate public protection in the disposal of the dead.

CITATIONS AND REFERENCES FOR CHAPTER 1

1. For detailed treatment of this subject, see Alfred C. Rush, *Death and Burial in Christian Antiquity* (Washington, D.C.: The Catholic University of America Press, 1941); Bertram S. Puckle, *Funeral Customs, Their Origin and Development* (New York: Frederick A. Stokes Co., 1926); Lewis B. Paton, *Spiritism and the Cult of the Dead in Antiquity* (New York: The Macmillan Co., 1921); and Edwin Mitchell, "Death and Disposal of the Dead," John Hastings (ed.), *Encyclopedia of Religion and Ethics* (New York: Charles Scribner's Sons, 1912).

2. The emergence of a morality of conscience in early Egypt was described by the eminent Egyptologists James H. Breasted, *The Dawn of Conscience* (New York: Charles Scribner's Sons, 1946), and W.M.F. Petrie, *Religion and Conscience in Ancient Egypt* (London: Methuen and Co., Ltd., 1898).

3. See, for example, Margaret A. Murray, *The Splendour That Was Egypt: A General Survey of Egyptian Culture and Civilization* (New York: Philosophical Library, 1949).

4. After Murray, *Ibid.*, p. 189.

5. Thomas Greenhill, *The Art of Embalming* (London: Printed for the Author, 1705), p. 106.

6. Breasted, *op. cit.*, p. 49.

7. Puckle, *op. cit.*, p. 101.

8. Breasted, *A History of the Ancient Egyptians* (New York: Charles Scribner's Sons, 1903), p. 65.

9. Charles Creighton, *A History of Epidemics in Britain* (Cambridge: At the University Press, 1891), Vol. I, p. 160.

10. Sir E.A. Wallis Budge, *The Mummy: a Handbook of Egyptian Funerary Archaeology* (2nd ed.; Cambridge: At the University Press, 1925). For the chemicals used, see Simon Mendelsohn's "The Mortuary Craft of Ancient Egypt," *Ciba Symposia*, Vol. 6, No. 2, May 1944, pp. 1795-1804.

11. For the hieroglyphic representation of these gods, see *A Guide to the Egyptian Collections in the British Museum* (London: Harrison and Sons, 1909).

12. Herodotus, *The Persian Wars*, translated by George Rawlinson (The Modern Library ed.; New York: Random House, 1942), Book 2, Ch. 85-90, pp. 155-158.

13. Budge, *op. cit.*, p. 428.

14. Murray, *op. cit.*, p. 189.

15. Budge, *op. cit.*, p. 428-429.

16. *Ibid.*, p. 340. The description of these burial proceedings follows Budge, pp. 336-351.

17. Greenhill, *op. cit.*, pp. 177-179.

18. *Ibid.*, p. 177. Italics in the original.

19. *Ibid.*, pp. 283-285. Italics in the original.

20. For a description of Egyptian embalming techniques and extensive bibliography, see Edward Johnson's *A History of the Art and Science of Embalming* (New York: Casket and Sunnyside, 1944).

21. Sister Mary Evaristus, *The Consolations of Death in Ancient Greek Literature* (Washington: National Capital Press, n.d.).

22. A. Rohde, *Psyche, The Cult of Souls and Belief in Immortality Among the Greeks*, pp. 19-24, quoted in Rush. *op. cit.*, p. 3.

23. See Martin P. Nilsson, *The Minoan-Mycenaean Religion and Its Survival in Greek Religion*, second revised edition (Lund Norway: C.W.F. Gleerup, 1950), p. 617, *passim*, for indications that the primitive belief of continued life in the grave (basic to the cult of the dead) does not immediately give way as the practice of cremation increases. See also Martin P. Nilsson, *A History of Greek Religion* (Oxford: At the Clarendon Press, 1925), p. 99 ff. Although the early Semitic and Mediterranean peoples generally held the belief in an underground community of departed spirits, unlike the Greeks, many resisted cremation. Thus, it is not safe to conclude that cremation of the dead is a logical and necessary product in ceremony and ritual of a certain set of death beliefs when these same beliefs are seen to lead to other funeral practices. The persistence of earlier beliefs and customs into newer practices is seen in the bottomless vases found by archaeologists in tombs of the Homeric period containing cremated remains. Offerings poured into such containers ran into the tomb, an indication that side by side with the Greek belief of the shadowy afterlife, the belief in the bodily afterlife still lingered. See also, Nilsson, *Greek Popular Religion* (New York, Columbia University Press, 1940), p. 22 ff.

24. Rush, *op. cit.*, pp. 3-4.

25. *Ibid.*, p. 5. The use of the term "sable" (black) crops up in the late-Reformation period with reference to the earliest undertakers. Steele, in the comedy "Grief a la Mode," uses the expression to indicate an occupational classification.

26. For a scholarly study devoted solely to Greek death customs, see Frank P. Graves, *The Burial Customs of the Ancient Greeks* (Brooklyn: Roche and Hawkins, 1891). More-recent data from the findings of classical archaeologists should be added, however, to bring the picture up to date. Recommended particularly are the works of Martin P. Nilsson: *op. cit.*

27. Puckle, *op. cit.*, pp. 237-238.

28. Graves, *op. cit.*, p. 20.

29. Rush, *op. cit.*, p. 125.

30. *Ibid.*, p. 126.

31. Graves, relying upon a passage in Pollux, accepts the fact of professional "buriers," whose sole business was pallbearing. *Op. cit.*, p. 40.

32. *Ibid.*, p. 42.

33. Nilsson, *Greek Popular Religion, op. cit.*

34. Graves, *op. cit.*, p. 53.

35. *Ibid.*, p. 57.

36. Puckle, *op. cit.*, p. 58.

37. *Ibid.*, p. 53 *seq.*

38. Harold W. Johnston, *The Private Life of the Romans*, Revised ed. (Chicago: Scott, Foresmen & Co., 1932), p. 41. The authors are indebted to this work, especially Chap. XIV, pp. 375-394.

39. Isaiah 22:13; I Cor. 15:22.

40. Quoted by James S. Elliott, *Outlines of Greek and Roman Medicine* (New York: Wm. Wood & Co., 1914), p. 66.

41. Arthur D. Nock, "Cremation and Burial in the Roman Empire," *The Harvard Theological Review*, XXV (October 1932), pp. 321-360.

42. See *Burial Reform and Funeral Costs* by Arnold Wilson and H. Levy (London: Oxford University Press, 1938), p. 6.

43. Johnston, *op. cit.*, p. 378.

44. See Ludwig Friedlander, *Roman Life and Manners Under the Early Empire*, translated by J.H. Freese (3 vols., 7th ed.; London: George Routledge & Sons, 1913), Vol. I, pp. 151-154.

45. William Smith, *et al.*, *A Dictionary of Greek and Roman Antiquities* (2 vols., 3rd ed.; London: John Murray, 1890), pp. 890-893, *passim*.

46. Ethel H. Brewster, *Roman Craftsmen and Tradesmen of the Early Empire*, Menasha, Wisconsin: George Banta, 1917), pp. 44-52.

47. *Ibid.*, pp. 49-50.

48. Johnston, *op. cit.*, pp. 390-391. For a more extended discussion of the role of crier (*praeco*), see Ethel H. Brewster, *op. cit.*, pp. 44-52. The most comprehensive treatise in English bearing on the social life of the Romans is Ludwig Friedlander's *Roman Life and Manners Under the Early Empire, op. cit.* See especially "Luxury in Funerals," II, pp. 210-218, for evidence that Roman extravagance in funerals far outstripped the display of modern times.

49. Puckle, *op. cit.*, p. 66.

50. *Ibid.*, p. 68.

51. *Ibid.*, p. 33.

52. Nock, *op. cit.*, pp. 321, *passim*.

Chapter 2

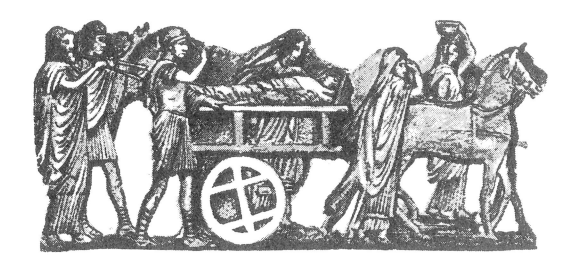

Early Hebrew, Christian and Scandinavian Burial

The resemblance of many pagan funeral customs to our own is so striking that it suggests that the funeral practices of Western civilization today are largely drawn from earlier, non-Christian sources. While some connection certainly exists between them, it is worth remembering that some of these resemblances are accidental, and that the basic system of concepts underlying present Western funeral practice is centrally rooted in Judeo-Christian mortuary beliefs. Although specific rituals and practices within this Judeo-Christian framework resulted from the rise of sects and denominations — and even within these, some modifications took place due to local and national customs, fashions and even whims — the basic ideological underpinning of Christian orientation to the dead and the provisions for their disposition remain essentially and substantially unchanged today.

FUNERAL PRACTICES IN EARLY HEBREW CULTURE

Death Beliefs: Like other Semitic peoples, the early Hebrews regarded human beings as composed of two elements: *basar*, or flesh (the same word used for the flesh of slaughtered animals), and *nefesh*, or breath.[1] The breath was a spirit-like substance that dwelt in life within the flesh, or, more particularly, within the blood. At death, the flesh returned to dust, while the breath or spirit persisted.

The Hebrews believed that the dead not only retained in large measure their former powers of thought and feeling, but also added to these certain supernatural powers, such as the ability to take possession of stones or images, or even the bodies of men. In addition, the ghosts of the dead looked, acted and dressed like the bodies they had left, although they were as shadows, or weakened images, so that Isaiah could say of them that they "grope as those who have no eyes and stumble at noon as in the twilight."[2]

Like other Semites, the Hebrews believed that the soul kept a close connection with the dead body so that, when the corpse was hurt, the soul suffered. In like fashion, the early Hebrews generally held that the soul led a shadowy afterlife in a netherworld called *Sheol*. This belief seems to have been arrived at later, for earlier specific cults of the dead tended to emphasize the return of the spirits of the dead to the grave, or to the place of residence in life.

By the end of the Babylonian captivity (597 to 547 B.C.), however, monotheism (a belief in one god) as distinguished from polytheism (a belief in many gods) had developed as a set of organized beliefs and centered on the figure of Yahweh, excluding other primitive forms of worship. In early Hebrew death beliefs, the soul was not seen as a completely discarnate element, since the close blood-flesh-spirit relation of human beings to Yahweh made a clear-cut separation of the body and soul difficult for the Hebrews to conceive.

Also, earlier conceptions of resurrection proposed that, in a manner similar to Egyptian belief, the breath or spirit was to be put back into the body. By about 150 B.C., in consequence of two hundred years of Persian domination, and well over a century of Greek domination, Hebrew death beliefs were basically these: upon death, the souls of the righteous, bereft of fleshy adornment, passed directly into a blessed existence; the souls of the wicked were sent into a state of punishment; and both would be raised from the netherworld at the day of the last judgment to receive their final rewards and punishments.

Burial Customs: Immediately after death, the eyes and mouth of the dead were closed, and the body was washed, anointed with sweet-smelling spices and dressed in its best attire. In the very early days at least, it was bound up in the position of an unborn child.[3] Although, at the time of Christ, the body was wrapped in linen after it was washed and anointed with spices, such shrouding seems to have been a later development because it is not mentioned in the Old Testament. The Jewish belief that the dead could be recognized by their garments in the underworld suggests that they had been buried in their customary daily apparel. In keeping with a practice that the Jewish historian Flavius Josephus (A.D. 37-100) describes as ancient, Jewish officials and kings were buried with spices, ornaments, and gold and silver.

Burial commonly took place on the evening of the day of death. This seeming haste was founded on hygienic necessity; in the warm climate of Palestine, putrefaction began quickly and spread rapidly.

The early Hebrews buried their dead without coffins, which first came into limited use after the Babylonian Captivity (597-547 B.C.). The body was borne to the place of interment on a bier. When the grave was reached, the poor were laid on the ground or in a shallow trench, and over them a mound of earth was shoveled. The rich were interred in natural caves or in artificial sepulchers hewn out of rock.

Mourning Customs: When death occurred, the nearest of kin "rent their garments." While originally it seems to have been the practice of the mourner to remain naked until the burial rites were completed, as civilization advanced and social awareness increased, the ceremonial rending became a stripping down to a loincloth of goat or camel hair, and, later, a removal only of the upper garment. Sandals were discarded, and, for a long time, bare feet remained a symbol of death.

Although the Hebrews removed their clothes, they did not uncover their heads but instead kept them draped or, in lieu of a drape, covered them with their hands. Although later forbidden, cuttings in the flesh once were practiced as a sign of grief. Earlier Hebrews cut off a generous tuft of hair between the eyes or shaved off a beard to parade their sorrow. Their descendants reduced the practice to a symbolic plucking of a few tufts.

Similarly, the custom of throwing oneself in the dust was later symbolically represented by sitting in the dust or placing dust upon the head. Fasting for the dead, which began at the moment of death, ordinarily terminated at evening on the day of death.

Lamentation for the dead was a regular and important rite among the Hebrews. Hired mourners swelled the wailing of the family. Although the professionals had a considerable repertory of lamentations, all addressed to the dead, they prepared special dirges for special persons. Practices that seemed to contain vestiges of earlier ancestor worship, or appeared closely allied to it, were stamped out by the later Hebrews over time.[4]

Place of Burial: The Jewish belief that family ties were not necessarily severed by death was important in determining their place of burial, inasmuch as family members who were buried together remained together in Sheol.[5] For this reason, the earliest tombs were placed upon the family's lands or near its dwellings, and burial therein was restricted to family members.[6] To be buried apart from one's kin was a catastrophe and regarded as a manifestation of the judgment of Jehovah. The early Hebrews sought to lie with their fathers and placed offerings in and before family tombs, which were generally easy to access. For example, Abraham's stood at the edge of his field; that of Joseph of Arimathea was in his garden; those of the kings of Judah were in Jerusalem in the royal gardens; and Samuel and Joab were given burial in their own houses. Not all sepulture, however, was so convenient; Aaron, Eleazar and Joshua were buried in mountains, and Rachel on the highway from Jerusalem to Bethlehem.[7]

While the kings of Judah erected tombs for their families in Jerusalem, these tombs were generally placed beyond the walls of the city for reasons of sanitation even in early times. Gradually, the belief crystallized that they were filled with uncleanness and therefore would defile. By the time of Christ, they were whitened with lime so that their ceremonial impurity might be recognized at a distance and shunned. Speaking to the Pharisees, Christ says, "Woe unto you, because you are as sepulchres that appear not, and men that walk over and are not aware."[8]

Unlike their neighbors, the Egyptians and the Phoenicians, who erected tombs of lavish and monumental splendor, the Hebrews preferred simple tombs — natural or artificial chambers, unadorned, and even without inscription, making it difficult to date them. At the root of this severity lies not only the general lack of interest of the ancient Jews in the "plastic arts" (three-dimensional art or visual representations) but also their stern opposition to ancestor worship. An adorned tomb of this period is generally an indication of Greek or some other foreign influence.

Hebrew graves divide themselves into four varieties: the grave as described below; the sunken grave with a stone cover; the bench grave; and the trench grave. The oldest and commonest form is the single chamber containing recess graves — oblong excavations, one-and-a-half-feet square and six feet long, hewn lengthwise into the chamber wall. Tombs might be a single chamber with a single grave; a single chamber with several or more graves; or several connected mortuary chambers. The above-ground tomb in Palestine is of later construction and of foreign origin and use.[9]

Among early Hebrews, ancestral burial places were sacred and used for worship, making vows and for sanctuary. Sacrifice to the dead was a practice that continued for a long time. Among offerings made were treasures, incense, spices and food. A double portion of inheritance was given to the firstborn male because the duty of bringing sacrifice and of making libation to the dead was his by law and custom. The anxiety of the ancient Hebrew lest he should not have a son originated, in part, in the fear that without a male heir, no one after his death might provide the gifts necessary so his soul could rest.

Interment the General Practice: During all historical periods, the ancient Hebrews interred their dead. While embalming was rarely practiced, both Jacob and Joseph were embalmed,[10] according to a custom that was foreign rather than strictly forbidden.

No such tolerance was accorded cremation, however. When cremation took place, it was frowned upon as an indignity to the corpse. In addition, by both venerable custom and the priest-code, it was regarded as a means of intensifying the disgrace of the death penalty.[11] At the root of this dislike was the age-old belief that, even after death, there was a bond between the soul and the body, and that the spirits of the unburied on earth, the cremated among them, wandered disconsolate, and in Sheol — the underworld, the abode of the dead — found no rest, but in pitiable conditions were driven into nooks and corners. Thus, the grave localized the soul in the body so that it there rested secure from harm. To remain unburied was therefore not only a disgrace but also a misfortune.[12] For these reasons, it was a sacred duty for all to bury an unburied body. Criminals who had been stoned to death were considered buried beneath the mound of stones that had slain them.[13]

Men dreaded the thought that they might remain unburied, and worse was the possibility that wild animals might devour one's corpse. Interment was denied as a punitive act only to foreign enemies. To violate a grave and to destroy its contents were considered great outrages. For strangers, criminals and the extremely poor, a public place of burial was provided. When Urias was brought out of Egypt and slain by King Joachim, "he cast his dead body into the graves of the common people."[14] The chief priests took the pieces of silver used to bribe Judas, "and after they had consulted together, they bought with them the potter's field, to be a burying place of strangers."[15]

FUNERAL BELIEFS AND CUSTOMS OF THE EARLY CHRISTIANS

Early Christian beliefs regarding death and the disposal of the dead were built upon the general mortuary ideology of the Hebrews, as vivified and expanded by the teachings of Christ.

Death Beliefs: To Hebrew conceptions of the "flesh and blood" relationship of human beings to God, of an afterworld from which the body is to be resurrected, and of the eventual divine judgment in which each individual must give an accounting for his or her life on earth and be punished or rewarded in the life hereafter, Christ and the Church He founded made significant additions. To the Hebrew doctrine of the fatherhood of God, Christ added the great commandment of love, and the concept of the "sonship of man" and, therefore, the brotherhood of man. To external conformity to the law, He added internal conformity to its spirit.

More significantly, He preached *the infinite and equal value of every human soul*. The soul was both spiritual and immortal, and not destined in the afterlife to be a discarnate spirit. There could be no annihilation of the soul in death; no soul could be totally destroyed. The teaching of Christ went beyond that of the Hellenistic Jews of Alexander and the *Book of Wisdom*. In Paton's words:

> Wisdom and all the Hellenists maintain that the future life is purely incorporeal, that there is no resurrection of any sort but that the body is evil and a clog to the soul from which it is delivered by death. This is not the conception of Jesus... He says "I am the resurrection and the life." This must indicate... that the soul is provided at death with a new body adapted to the new environment upon which it is entering.[16]

The Resurrection of the Body and Cremation: In the resurrection, the glorified body is patently to be, "a superior body, like unto those worn by the angels of God."[17] The resurrection concept of the Christians, therefore, certainly offered more than the promise of pagan immortality, which signified only the continued life of some aspect of the person. Because Christians held that it was the power of God that transformed the body on the day of judgment, many felt that the dead must necessarily be buried in the earth. Cumont remarks:

> If the Christians of the first centuries no longer feared that they would go to join the shades who wandered on the bank of the Styx, they were still pursued by the superstitious dread that they would have no part in the resurrection of the flesh if their bodies did not rest in the grave.[18]

Yet, in St. Paul's memorable passage — "...For this corruptible must put on incorruption and this mortal must put on immortality... then it shall come to pass the saying that is written, death is swallowed up in victory. O grave where is thy victory. O death where is thy sting."[19] — there is more than the suggestion that the disposition of the body after death by any one mode of sepulture was a matter of indifference. The resurrection was the *miracle* of God: bodies burned, buried or lost at sea shared equally in the miraculous transformation, although the Church held it revolting that the human body, "once the temple of the Holy Spirit, once sanctified and refreshed spiritually by the Sacraments" should be burned, except in "well-defined, isolated instances when because of disease or epidemic, cremation is absolutely necessary to prevent the disease."[20]

The principle involved here is that of the common good. Cremation, too, has been frowned upon because of its pagan associations, and because, in later suspicion of foul play, it rendered an official examination of the body difficult.[21]

Customarily, then, Christians buried their dead, although the practice of cremation was currently prevalent in Greek and Roman culture. There does not seem to have been a rigidly compelling doctrine prohibiting cremation, and Christians *were* occasionally cremated. But there was the example of the master: "Those who imitated Christ during their lives," Rush observes, "also wished to imitate Him in death and be buried after the manner of His burial."[22]

Although cremation was prohibited finally in Christendom during the reign of Constantine the Great, (A.D. 306-337), Christianity as a whole has never taken a final single stand in the matter. Today, some of the more "secularized" religious groups, such as the Unitarians, actually favor the practice.[23]

Christian Equality in Death: The doctrine that, in death, all men are equal, and that the eternal rewards they gain are not to be assigned according to earthly rank, is a central Christian death belief. While the Egyptian cult of Osiris and the Grecian belief in the Elysian Fields might have contributed to the Christian concept of the afterlife, these theories were basically aristocratic. Not all members of society could hope to share equally in the next-world comforts they offered. Rush comments that the Egyptians, "Seeing the differences among people in this life argued that there must be differences in the afterlife. They imagined there must be a special afterlife of happiness for chosen souls and especially the king."[24]

For the Greeks, the shadow-life afterworld, with the separation of soul from body, was a belief more likely born of resignation than of hope; it was the inevitable end to life's journey. The miracle that elevated one's afterlife to the Elysian Plain was beyond the expectation of all but a chosen few. "As an heroic myth it was more likely to capture the fancy of the poet than the allegiance of the average Greek."[25]

These aristocratic concepts of the afterlife are in strong contrast with Christian belief. Christ Himself held out to all men an equal hope of the kingdom of heaven, with the joy therein to be in no way allotted according to earthly title or position, but only as each — king or beggar alike — became as a little child.[26]

Death as "Sleep": The tone and direction of Christian funeral practices were set by the Christian belief in the resurrection of Christ. To non-Christians and the very early Hebrews, death was an uninviting reality in which the promise of an agreeable or intolerable afterlife was, at best, given only to a select few. The changed outlook produced by Christianity is to be clearly seen in the new metaphor in which death is represented as sleep. The "cemetery" by its etymology designates a sleeping place, where the dead rest for a while in Christ until they rise with Him in the general resurrection.

The concept and terminology of death as sleep have carried through almost 2,000 years into modern funerary usage. Death is not only sleep, but it is also a summons by Christ, or by His angels, who bear the souls of the elect to heaven. Under another metaphor, death to the early Christian became a kind of birth into eternity and a triumphal transition, and therefore not an event calling for hopeless and unconfined grief.[27]

Burial Customs: Primitive Christian burial customs, like those of the early Hebrews, were simple, unpretentious and organized within the context of community living by a group of people to whom the commandment "Little children love one another" represented a way of life in which the supreme law was, "Thou shalt love the Lord thy God with thy whole heart, thy whole soul, and thy whole mind" and "Thou shalt love thy neighbor as thyself." To bury the dead was one of the seven great enumerated corporal works of mercy enjoined upon all Christians.

Early canon law laid down simple requirements for the burial of the dead, asking only that the body should be decently laid out, with lights beside it; that it should be asperged with holy water and incensed at stated times; that a cross should be placed upon the breast, or, in lieu of a cross, the hands should be folded; and that it should be buried in consecrated ground. No regulation required that the dead must be buried in a coffin. A decree of the Council of Auxerre forbade the priest to bestow the ceremonial kiss upon the dead, and prohibited the practice of clothing the corpse in rich raiment.[28]

The Christian doctrine of the equal and inestimable worth of every soul found funerary outlet in the provision that even the poor should receive a befitting burial. According to Aristides, "when one of the poorer members of Christianity passes out of this world each one of the Christians, according to his ability, gives heed to him, and carefully sees to his burial."[29] The early Christian community provided its own burial services as a corporal work of mercy without hired pallbearers or other assistants — even in times of plague, when deaths were heavy and the funerary duties onerous.

Rush comments on this fact:

> During the time of plague and public calamity the bearing of the dead to burial was the work of private friends and charitable Christians. This is exemplified in the conduct of Christians during the plague which swept over the Roman Empire in the third century. Eusebius, describing the conduct of the Christians during this trying time, says: "Thus they would take up the bodies of the saints in their open hands to their bosoms, and close their eyes and mouth, and carry them on their shoulders and lay them out."[30]

The Role of the Family in Early Christian Funerals: Early pagan peoples generally closed the eyes and mouth of the dead as one of the first acts after death. Significantly, this intimate duty was not delegated to outsiders but performed by the husband or wife, children or other close relatives of the deceased. Wives and mothers are mentioned in Greek and Roman writings as carrying out the task and, among early Christians, the family administered to the dying and took charge of the care of the dead.[31]

Summing up early Christian funeral practice, Mitchell notes:

> When death ensued, the eyes were closed, the body washed, the limbs swathed, the whole body wrapped in a linen sheet with myrrh and aloes, and laid upon a couch in an upper room. (Acts 9:37 F.; Mark 15:46; John 11:44) These acts were performed by the elder women — kindred and friends of the family. Relatives and intimates were admitted to view the face of the deceased, and an interval of eight or more hours was required before burial.[32]

Among the Hebrews, certain women of the community were assigned the task of assisting in the laying out of the body. This task was considered a contaminating influence, a legal defilement, and, consequently, not to be undertaken by priests or members of the priestly class.[33]

This taboo did not extend into Christian funeral practice, however. Rather, the Christian "Kiss of Peace" marked a major break with Jewish tradition. Christians touched the dead, and since the body was considered sacred and holy, it was possible for the laity and even the clergy to handle it without fear of legal defilement or need for ritualistic purification. Even beyond such permissive touching of the corpse, Christians "developed a formal liturgical rite in their burial service which involved contact with the dead, namely imparting the Kiss of Peace."[34] The practice survives among the laity to this day in the final kiss sometimes given to the corpse immediately after death, or sometimes before the closing of the casket. Among the clergy it has been long since discontinued.

Rush notes other funeral rites in the primitive Church:

> Certain rites were performed before death which were intimately linked with each other, namely, the stretching out of the feet of the dying, the administration of the *Viaticum*, the catching of the last breath and the imparting of the final kiss. The first two were helps intended to aid the dying person. The stretching out of the feet was a help in the natural order; while the *Viaticum* was a help mainly in the supernatural order.[35]

The naive, disregarding the spiritual nature of the soul, somehow fancied that it would leave the body from the feet, progressing to the mouth. They therefore stretched out the feet to facilitate its egress and, incidentally, the laying out of the body upon death. The *Viaticum* was the Communion or Eucharist administered to the dying as a means of giving them strength on the journey into eternity. The word originally signified an allowance of money for transportation and supplies made to Romans sent on duty into the provinces.

Other Christian Funeral Customs: Although on the whole the early Christians anointed the corpse, especially in Rome and in the Holy Land, they showed a tendency to take over the burial practices in vogue in the countries in which Christianity was becoming established. Thus, in Egypt, without in any way accepting basic Egyptian religious beliefs, they embalmed their dead. In other localities, they sometimes practiced cremation.

Interestingly enough, the conventional pagan mourning colors of red, black and purple were rejected by early Christians. Basing their reasoning on the belief that the soul went forth into immortality clothed in white, they favored the use of white mourning garments (although the practice of mourning was originally discouraged). The return to the conventional dark colors represents one instance where customary usage was not successfully displaced in light of a new death belief.

With regard to the clothing of the dead by the early Christians, Rush writes:

> The manner in which the Christians clothed their dead can be traced back to similar practices in Jewish and other ancient burial rites. At times, linen garments were employed; at other times the corpse was clothed with the best kind of garments worn during life.[36]

Washing the Corpse: The mortuary customs of the early Greeks and Romans stressed the importance of having the family lay out the body. In both cultures, female relatives washed the corpse. While the ablution of the dead was a purification rite among the Jews, among the Greeks and Romans, the washing of the body with warm water was a test measure to guarantee that life was extinct.

The Christians borrowed from the Jews certain funerary customs associated with Christ, among them the washing of the corpse. Puckle believes that this custom originated in the "dim ages" and was part of the preparation to make the dead appear to best advantage in the afterlife. Among the Jews, this task was assigned to the eldest son and signified that the dead, being cleansed of sin, might enter into heaven. The Christians took over the rite with the interpretation unchanged. The body of Christ had been washed immediately after the descent from the cross. The practice, as St. John Chrysostom observed (died A.D. 407), was "hallowed in the person of our Lord."[37] Even during the visitation of the plague during the third century, Christians continued to wash the corpse, although they risked contamination by doing so.[38]

The Hebrews, unlike the Egyptians, did not embalm the corpse but instead anointed it with oils and spices. The purpose behind anointing in a preservative manner, or perfuming, or, on occasion, burying the body in lime, was to prevent speedy contamination and to counteract the odor of decay. Again, in reverential imitation of Christ's burial, the practice was followed among early Christians of perfuming the dead body in commemoration of the spices with which Jesus was wrapped. The pagans did not approve of this custom, thinking it foolish for the living to waste expensive ointments on the dead, which they thought they might better employ in anointing themselves.[39]

The Wake in Early Christian Funeral Practices: Among early Christians, as noted earlier, relatives and intimates were admitted to view the face of the deceased, and an interval of eight or more hours was required before burial.[40] Ancient peoples, including some Asiatic and pre-literate groups, had long observed the custom of keeping the corpse laid out after death and of keeping a "watch" or "wake" over it.[41]

Puckle gives a functional interpretation to this practice, holding that this delay between death and burial, varying in length according to custom and climatic conditions, served both a psychological need in gradually conditioning friends and relatives to the changed conditions brought about by death; and a physical need in providing an opportunity for continued close observation of the corpse, in the hope that it might return to consciousness.[42]

The old Jewish custom of "watching" or "waking" the dead was rooted in a genuine concern by relatives and friends that no person should be buried alive. To ensure against such a terrible contingency, the sepulcher was left unsealed for three days so that the corpse might frequently be scrutinized for signs of life. This practice was taken over by the early Christians, who used the occasion to gather and say prayers for the repose of the deceased, under the scriptural injunction that it is a "holy and wholesome thought to pray for the dead that they may be loosed from their sins."

Those Christians who believe in the purgatorial doctrine still observe the custom of praying for the dead.[43]

Gebhart adds a second purpose to the wake: to give comfort to the bereaved family.[44] During the night, psalms were occasionally sung, as they were sung on the vigils preceding the feasts of the martyrs.

The Christian wake manifests contributions and adaptations from several burial cultures. Instead of the wailings of the mourners, who might have been hired for the purpose by the Hebrews, or the shouts of the Roman *conclamatio*, outbursts of grief among the Christians were held in check. The grimness of death, for the latter, had lost its edge; the dead were "asleep in Jesus." While the Hebrew wake took the form of a vigil at the grave or in the sepulcher, the Greek custom was to wait three days before burying the dead. The Romans borrowed this practice from the Greeks, and the Christians from the Romans, so that the Christian wake became transferred from the grave to the home or the church. The element of time, however, remained flexible, varying with the prestige of the dead and the amount of money available for the preservation of the corpse.

If early Christian burial took place in the forenoon, the Requiem Mass was said and Holy Communion distributed; if it took place in the afternoon, the ceremony was limited to the singing of psalms and the saying of prayers, accompanied by the special service of the dead. This service consisted of hymns of thanksgiving for the deceased, and prayers by the living that they too might enter upon eternal life. The bishop pronounced thanks that the dead brother had persevered in his faith and in his Christian warfare, even to death, while the deacon read portions of scripture giving promise of resurrection. A hymn was sung on the same theme.[45]

The Funeral Procession: The early Christian funeral procession reflected in some degree the customs of the localities in which Christians lived. The funeral procession and the wake had been important parts of the burial complex of most peoples. While for the Egyptians, Greeks and Romans, these occasions varied with the social status of the deceased, the display lavished upon them is legendary and has intrigued ancient and modern writers, painters and sculptors alike.[46]

It should be noted that the impulse to display emotion at funerals, whether originating in uncontrolled feelings or in sentiment collectively evoked by the social demand of the situation, was subjected to social controls that sometimes crystallized into law. Greeks, Romans, Hebrews and Christians, Rush notes, at some time or other developed formal restraints to funeral behavior.[47]

In the earlier periods, the emphasis in Christian funeral processions was upon the maintenance of a subdued and reverent attitude, tinctured by a latent sense of triumph and exhilaration, since death was a victory, marking the beginning of a better life. Instrumental music, actors, buffoons, *praecos* and the like were excluded from the Christian funeral procession. Noisy exhibitions of grief were shunned. Young men, not for pay but as a corporal work of mercy, carried the bier to the place of interment outside the city or village — "A natural cave, or a tomb hewn in a rock hillside or in a subterranean chamber, or in a simple grave," as local conditions determined.[48] We read in *The Acts of the Apostles* that when Anais died, "the young men rising up, removed him and carried him out and buried him."[49]

The early Christian funeral procession was limited to the corpse, its bearers, and the family and friends of the dead. As it passed solemnly and quietly to the grave, psalms and hymns were sung. If possible, the funeral took place in the daytime to emphasize the belief that the dead person was entering into eternal light and life and not into gloom. Torches were carried at the head of the procession — not to light the way, since such function was not needed, but as befits the progress of a victorious combatant. Lights carried before the dead symbolized both the glory into which it was hoped he had come and the triumph of his new state. Many instances are recorded of the use of daytime torches in early Christian funeral processions. Lamps were employed as substitutes. When the body of St. John Chrysostom was removed from Comana to Constantinople, so many persons bearing lamps came out in ships to meet the corpse that the "sea was covered with lamps." When the abbeys of York were demolished, lamps were found whose light could not be extinguished by wind and water.[50]

Although the funeral sermon, as we know it today, does not seem to have been part of the funerary practice of the early Christians, the funeral oration honoring those of merit was taken over from non-Christian practice and, after the persecution era, was customarily included in the burial services for leaders or saints. Alms, in the form of food and money, were distributed to the poor at the grave and public prayers were offered for the dead, in keeping with purgatorial doctrine.

It should be noted that even in the primitive Church, the third, seventh or ninth, thirtieth or fortieth days, as well as the anniversary of death, were designated as special memorial days for remembering the dead with requiem masses.[51]

Finally, Christian interment traditionally included farewell prayers expressing the belief that, instead of being the end of life, death was in reality only the beginning of a true existence. The rites sometimes ended with the anointing with oil and the "Kiss of Peace." Flowers were occasionally strewn on the grave.

Early Christian Cemeteries: O'Reilly points out the interest of the Christian Church, from earliest times, in the provision of suitable places of interment:

> For the burial of her dead, the church has always prescribed the setting apart and designation of places suitable for the tombs and graves. Regarding the bodies of the faithful departed as the habitations of the rational soul, like to the image of God — and the temple of the Holy Ghost — the law of the church demands that the place set aside for their interment should obtain a special religious significance. The ground, venerated by the relics of saints and martyrs, was always considered as sacred and was deputed so by suitable religious rites when such were possible. These designated locations were such as the customs and times preferred.[52]

While the earliest scattered converts to Christianity among the Jews were content to have their bodies interred without distinction among their Jewish brethren,[53] as soon as Christian colonies developed among non-Christians, a demand arose for special places of burial that could be the scene of a distinct ritual, as befitted a fundamental difference in viewpoint concerning the dead body. It was not possible for the small, struggling, persecuted early Christian Church to possess and maintain cemeteries such as we know today. The earliest Christian burials, from apostolic times to the persecution of Domitian, were in family vaults erected outside the walls, along the roads leading from great cities.

"Let there be no burial or cremation in the city" — so reads one of the original laws of the Twelve Tables. This sanitary rule was observed by the early Christians in Rome for several centuries, and only disregarded when persecution forced their successors to assemble for worship in cemeteries. Pagan Romans buried their dead along the highways and beyond their cities, and following both law and custom, the bodies of early martyrs were so interred. St. Peter was buried beyond the Tiber on the Via Triumphalis; and St. Paul, three miles beyond the city on the Via Ostiensis. Other saints were known to have been given burial outside the city walls. Only around the year 258 were the bodies of saints Peter and Paul transferred into the catacombs, lest they should be profaned during the persecution of the Church.

Thus, for three centuries, the early Christians in Rome and in many places in the empire were buried along public roads outside the walls of towns and cities, or in catacombs. Of the latter, there were some forty in Rome itself.[54] The tombs along the Appian Way constitute a notable instance of such extramural burial on privately owned lots.

Out of this tomb burial, and in response to an ever-increasing need for more room, the catacombs developed. (***See Plate 8***.) Originally these were galleries, chambers and passages, openly hewn out of soft rock, with public entrances; their enormous later extension was due to crypt enlargement for burial purposes. Leclercq[55] observes that the catacombs originated in the tombs of the wealthy Christians, who had them constructed in their gardens or villas, and, in place of reserving them to their household, permitted their use by their fellow Christians. This origin is clear from the inscriptions on the tombs in the more-ancient Roman cemeteries.

At the time they were commenced, the Roman government approved the construction of these excavated cemeteries and protected them against vandalism. Their secondary and accidental uses in sheltering and providing places of assembly for Christians driven by merciless persecution into such underground hideaways for the secret performance of their religious rites, and the resultant search and spoliation of the vast shelters, came later. Culminating in A.D. 253, the decree of the Emperor Valerian forbade Christians "either to hold assemblies or to enter those places, which they called their cemeteries."

Among other cities, there were catacombs at Naples, Palermo and Syracuse. Catacomb burial among the Christians is known to have been practiced in Greece, Persia, Egypt, Syria and in other places in Asia Minor. The catacombs at Paris are a series of charnel houses in which, by governmental decree, the contents of other cemeteries thought to be pestilential were dumped.[56]

When the great persecutions came to an end at the close of the fourth century, the Church

PLATE 8

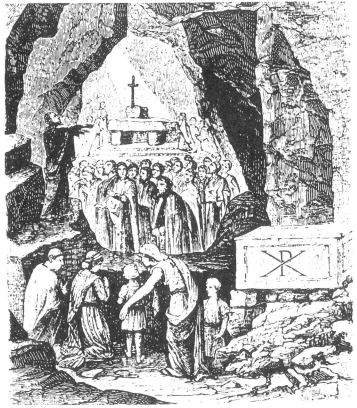

8A. Divine Service, Catacombs of St. Calixtus, A.D. 50.

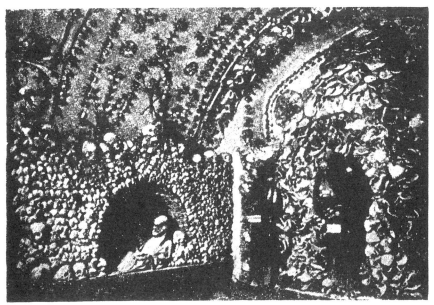

8B. Vault in Catacombs of Rome.

emerged from its long exile underground. A sign of its new freedom was the vogue for open-air cemeteries. Archaeological research indicates that these were established in Rome and North Africa before the reign of Constantine the Great. Although early Roman law had decreed that burial must be beyond the city walls, in the emergent Christian practice of open-air burial, cemeteries in most early instances were located mostly within the walls and in the vicinity of churches so that, by the time of Pope John III (560-575), most burials in Rome were intramural.[57]

Early Christian Burial Practices Grow More Complex: Concurrent with the growth and acceptance of Christianity in the early centuries after Christ was the pressure of pagan burial practices and the use of funeral ritual and display to indicate the importance, wealth or position of the dead in a more complex, urban form of society. The burial customs of the early Christians had been attuned to a community way of life; Christendom in the Empire period spread across many lands and included vast numbers of peoples. Consequently, the opportunity for infiltration of local customs was enhanced in the very process of its spread, and ritual and ceremony were perforce elaborated into the type of display, or spectacle, that could appeal to and socially define situations for the masses of people who were currently sharing in a new way of life.[58]

Around the 4th century, the Church established great religious feast days to commemorate publicly and solemnly the death anniversaries of the martyrs. Rush continues:

> At this time Christian life tended to center more and more about the Church. Not only were the death and the anniversaries of the martyrs celebrated in the Church, but the death of the faithful was linked in the Church service. Thus originated the practice of bringing the deceased to the Church, and there holding a wake over him. This became the usual practice throughout Christendom.[59]

O'Reilly notes that the formula of the funeral service of the Roman ritual, "is composed in three separate sections, the '*levatio corporis*,' or services in the house of death, and conveying the body to the church — the funeral services in the church — and the rites attendant upon the burial in the cemetery."[60]

From the standpoint of religion, he observes, the obligations of providing and obtaining the prescribed funeral rite is "not only suitable and becoming, but really urgent." The recognition of this obligation "has always been foremost in the history of the Church." The obligation included the Requiem or Mass for the dead. "However, no explicit law has been codified prior to the New Code, relative to this detail. Now a special canon states that, 'unless there is weighty reason to the contrary, the bodies of the faithful, prior to the funeral, must be transferred from the place where they repose, to the church, where the funeral services — the complete order of ceremonies and functions, which are completed in the approved liturgical books — shall be held.'"[61]

Early Christian Funeral Functionaries: Unlike the Roman funeral, which was conducted by paid secular functionaries and public officials, early Christian funeral functions were carried out by the brethren of the dead under the direction of the clergy. These early simple practices later gave way — in the funerals of saints, martyrs, and persons of civil and religious importance — to rites

PLATE 9

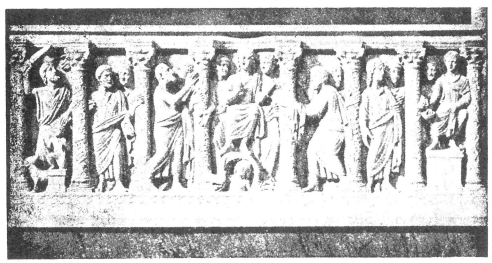
9A. Early Christian Sarcophagus.

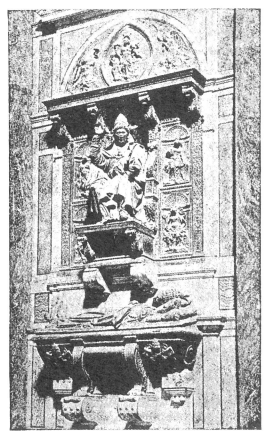
9B. Tomb of Innocent VIII.

as costly and elaborate as those that had marked the burial of Greeks and Romans of comparable position.[62]

Prior to the assumption by the state of the duty of burying the poor, the poor themselves tried to assure themselves of a decent interment by forming burial clubs. Some of these combined social with funeral functions and, at fixed times during the year, met for large-scale drinking parties.

But during the time of Constantine, as indicated earlier, the state assumed the responsibility of seeing that all who needed it received decent burial. Laws were made to prevent overcharge. Under the supervision of the Church, every person who required it was to have a free coffin. Even the poorest was to be borne to the grave in a procession that included a cross bearer, eight monks and three acolytes. Under the general supervision of overseers, called *decani*, burial parties worked in groups, some preparing for the religious procession, some carrying the body, others lifting the body and digging the grave.[63]

Stone indicates that, among the early Christians, friends carried the corpse to burial on their shoulders, and the highest clergy did not find such service beneath their dignity, although by rule, deacons were to carry deacons, and priests, priests. A dead bishop was commonly borne into several churches before being taken to the grave, the body usually resting on a bed of ivy, laurel or other evergreen.[64]

Burial of the poor was not left to indiscriminate care among the early Christians. Two classes of minor functionaries were assigned to visit the sick and bury the dead. The first were called *parabolani* because they risked their lives in caring for the sick with contagious diseases; the second were designated *laborantes, lectarii, fossarii, sandapilarii*, and *decanii*. As the names indicate, these had the responsibility of digging graves, carrying coffins, placing the remains in the ground, and performing other related services. The Church prescribed rigid rules for these operations and kept careful watch that they should be well performed.[65] While it has been suggested that these functionaries were the forerunners of the modern undertaker, it is more likely that, under different titles and management, they were the *libertinarii* and their assistants the *pollinctores* and *designatores* of pagan Rome.

After the 4th century, the Church itself built an elaborate set of religious and social controls over one of the most significant areas of human experience. In the process, the funeral service moved from the simple and reverential gestures of family and friends to a set of experiences and actions that were organized as part of the wider operation of an urban-type of society.

In summarizing Christian funerary beliefs and practices, it should be said that, while on the surface they might seem to have derived from the corresponding beliefs and practices of adjacent cultures, their basic pattern originated in Hebrew beliefs and customs, as adapted to the changing needs of the Christian viewpoint. Rites and ceremonies tend to follow accepted patterns of belief, as customs and usages tend to be drawn from or to give form to folkways already extant. By the year 400, the basic orientation toward death and the dead in the Western world was set. From this period through the next thousand years, death in Western culture will imply a "Christian" funeral, stylized and integrally a part of the panoply of religious behavior organized and controlled by the Roman Catholic Church. The Reformation will divide this traditional behavior into two main streams without changing the basic underlying death beliefs or modifying many of the practices.

FUNERAL BELIEFS AND CUSTOMS OF THE ANCIENT GERMANS AND SCANDINAVIANS
Cremation of the dead as a mode of burial held the attention of the Greeks and Romans for more than a millennium, yet fire disposition was practiced by early Scandinavians independent of the influence of classical civilization for more than 2,000 years. Since this custom has persisted in Western society, though with widely varying degrees of acceptance, it is quite likely that the beliefs and practices of ancient Northern Europe contributed an ideological thread to the tangled skein of modern mortuary behavior.

Cremation began in Scandinavia during the Middle Bronze Age, according to Hilda Ellis, having diffused slowly but with "startling thoroughness" from IndoEuropean areas northward through Germany.[66] It persisted through the Iron Age and was the predominant mode of disposal of the dead until the 10th century A.D. Evidently the practice of burning the dead went on in the North until Christianity was so firmly established that grave burial once more became the universal custom.[67]

Cremation as a Protection from the Dead: Although many minor burial customs or "folkways" continue to be practiced without foundation in basic belief concerning life and death, the introduction and acceptance of cremation in Northern Europe had its roots in the acceptance of new ideas about the afterlife. In this new belief, we can detect two important themes: one is to burn the body as a method of keeping the spirits of the dead from harming the living; the other, by the same method, "to free the spirit of the dead from the clogging prison of the body."[68]

Ancient Norse mythology contains many tales about the harmful spirits of the dead, who, improperly buried, return to plague the living. Ellis relates the gruesome story of the foster-brothers Aran and Asmundr as illustrative of these. The two agree that whichever of them shall survive the other will spend three nights with the corpse in the burial room. Aran drops dead one day, leaving Asmundr to fulfill the compact. Aran lies in the mound with his weapons, his hound and hawk, and his bridled and saddled horse, and Asmundr takes up the vigil beside him on a stool. On the first night, the dead man slew the hawk and hound, and devoured them. On the second night, he arose again, slew the horse and began to devour it so that the blood ran from his jaws, meanwhile inviting Asmundr to partake in the feast. On the third night, Aran rises again and attempts to eat Asmundr, but the foster-brother resists, draws his sword, overcomes the corpse, and escapes with no more damage than the loss of his ears.[69]

Cremation to Free the Spirit of the Dead: In the second theme, cremation to free the spirit of the dead from the clogging prison of the body, we can discern several contributing concepts. One of these is the belief that, in the afterlife, the dead may enter into the realm of the gods. Ellis notes that the practice of cremation, or suttee and certain kinds of sacrifice, are connected with this belief. Entrance into the Teutonic Valhall, or Valhalla, where the gods dwell, like the entrance into the Greek Elysian Plain, is not a democratic right but an aristocratic privilege.

Another concept is the belief that life or spirit continues to exist in the grave mound itself. From this belief sprang cults of the dead, with their fertility beliefs, ideas of rebirth, and inspiration by a deity, as well as the conception of the "everlasting battle" in which animated spiritual bodies engaged in fierce combat, devoured each other, and returned afresh each night to renew eternally the battle. To the latter belief are added the sub-themes of supernatural guardian women — the Valkyries — who give aid to certain heroes during life and, after death, bear them away to their abodes; and the use of the grave mound and its spiritual residents for magic, inspiration and wisdom.

Like almost all people of Northern Europe and Asia, the Scandinavians believed in the "journey to the land of the dead." Among the Scandinavians, this belief was reflected in the practice of ship burial, reserved for those of highest station. In the ship burials of the Viking Age in Norway,

> ...the dead man rests on a bed within the ship, surrounded by all the necessities of life and many choice possessions, with various animals sacrificed to accompany him, and the dead slave girl laid in the tent beside him.[70]

The ship was then set afire and drifted out to sea, a burning holocaust, carrying its precious cargo into the glorious afterlife. Yet other ship burials took place on land; and it is from the burial mounds of ships, some intact and some half burned, found in most North European sea-bordering countries that archaeologists and students of Scandinavian antiquity have found the richest materials for their reconstruction of the funeral customs and beliefs of these earlier peoples.

From the viewpoint of modern death beliefs, however, most significantly important has been the pre-Christian Scandinavian concept of the disembodied soul, which through ritualistic ceremonies performed by the living is liberated from the body so that it may enter into a spiritual afterlife. Even where this belief is found, however, the two worlds of the here and the hereafter were never completely separated, the nature and strength of the nexus varying with time and place.[71]

Another significant residue of belief incorporated into Western culture from the death customs of the ancient Scandinavian and German cultures was the notion of fire as a proper, perhaps ennobling, agent in the transforming of a bodily ridden soul into an incarnate spiritual entity. In the words of the historian Karl Blind:

> The twirling flame which rose from the pyre towards Heaven did not fill them with the idea of final destruction, but rather with that of enobling purification. They were easily brought to see in it a cleansing of what they conceived to be man's eternal being from mere earthly dross. They looked upon flame as true conductor of the dead, as the emancipator of the soul. The application of the fire to the corpse appeared to them to be a means even of appeasing and purifying the soul: a view we often find among the Greeks and Romans.[72]

Additionally, and perhaps equally as important, was the belief of the pre-Christian peoples of Northern Europe in the soul itself as potentially an incarnate entity that could be emancipated from the body through the agency of fire.

PLATE 10

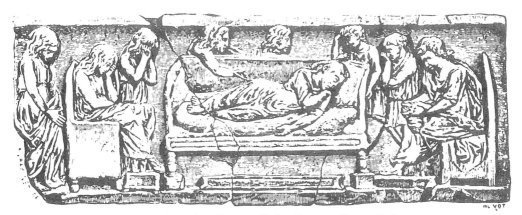

10A. Mourning Scene, Gallo-Roman Bas-relief.

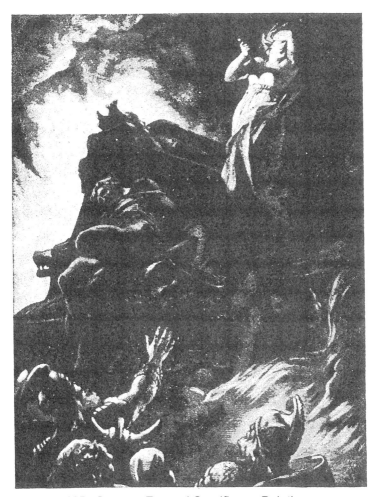

10B. German Funeral Sacrifice, a Painting.

Nevertheless, the worlds of the living and dead were not categorically separated; rather the evidence of archaeology and literature reveals a substantial and reciprocal relationship. Supernatural powers, for good or for evil, were potentially available to persons who could explain the mysteries of the other world. In the last analysis, the "cosmology of death" of these peoples turned the world of the dead back upon the world of the living, i.e., one's relations with the dead had more consequence for the living than one's relations with the living had for the dead.

For centuries, commerce and war kept contacts alive between the Teutonic and Mediterranean cultures. The great mingling came with the fall of Rome and the Western empire before the barbarian hordes. The beliefs and practices of the Germans and Scandinavians were brought into England chiefly through the Danish invasions. The Danes, who first appeared on the eastern and southern coasts of England in A.D. 787, made repeated invasions after 832, first wintered on the island in 851, and became firmly established there in 866. In 1016, Canute the Dane became soul monarch of England, and Danish or Norse rulers continued to reign until 1066. In that year, William the Conqueror defeated and slew Harold the Saxon at the Battle of Hastings, ushering in the Norman Conquest.

Strangely enough, though the Danes conquered the Romanized Celts, the burial customs of the defeated people prevailed. As Prente-Orton points out:

> The influence of the British population and of continental neighbors is best seen in the burial customs of the invaders. The Angles and the Saxons brought with them the custom of cremation, though the Jutes of Kent practiced the inhumation of the Roman Empire. In the heathen cemeteries of the North, however, there was a steady growth of inhumation instead of cremation, which lingered longest in East Anglia and Northumbria, where on the whole a Romanized population had been small.[73]

Some Common Elements in the Mortuary Beliefs of Early Peoples: As we examine the primary mortuary beliefs of the early peoples and cultures thus far considered, we are able to draw at least one solid conclusion: death does not end all relationship between the dead and the living but merely signals the transition from one form of relationship to another. Nock, perhaps better than any other, indicates the two broad orientations that define the continued relations of dead and living:

> Through the history of man's conduct in face of the mystery of death run two strands. On the one hand, there is the possibility that the departed one or some part or aspect or transformation of him may pass to a new place of spiritual existence, may enjoy new happiness or face new dangers; the happiness and the dangers are of course thought of in terms of earthly experience, but as subsisting under quite different conditions. This earthly expectation I have spoken of as a "possibility" because, except where a dogmatic religion is fully dominant, the expectation is normally tentative and hesitant; the individual does not and cannot hold it
>
> > As he believes in fire that it will burn
> > Or rain that it will drench him.
>
> On the other hand, there is the fact that the dead man's remains, whether buried or burned or exposed are actually localized in a particular spot. Hence that spot retains its importance, even when

it is dogmatically held that the essential element in the man whom we loved is elsewhere. Originally the belief in the practical necessity of the rites is strong. The dead man is thought of as an animated corpse, with natural need and natural vindictiveness. And he remains so, even in enlightened communities, in the eyes of many of the less educated. When this has faded, the grave remains the spot at which we took our leave of the dead man and at which his memory can appropriately be honored. This desire for honor remains strong, even after any idea of benefiting the dead man by tendance has disappeared. Epicurus denied the afterlife, but in his will he provided offerings in perpetuity to his father, mother, and brothers, for celebrations of his birthday and the anniversaries of others of his intimates. Hence funerary ritual is associated in the main with the tomb and not with the afterlife, as theoretically conceived, with things done and not with things held, and the variations of practice are normally conditioned by conveniences, safety, and economy or ostentation.[74]

CITATIONS AND REFERENCES FOR CHAPTER 2

1. For a comprehensive treatment of the death beliefs and customs of the Hebrews, see Lewis B. Paton, *Spiritism and the Cult of the Dead in Antiquity*, *op. cit.* Sepulture is well described in *The New Schaff-Herzog Encyclopedia of Religious Knowledge*, edited by Samuel Macaulay Jackson, D.D., L.L.D., with the assistance of Charles Colebrook Sherman and George William Gilmore (New York: Funk and Wagnalls Company, 1908) Vol. II, pp. 307-309.

2. Isaiah 59:10.

3. Paton, *op. cit.*, p. 250.

4. *Ibid.*

5. II Samuel 21:14.

6. Mitchell, *op. cit.*, p. 498.

7. Elizabeth Stone, *God's Acre* (London: John W. Parker & Son, 1858), pp. 10-11.

8. Luke 11:44.

9. Samuel M. Jackson, *The New Schaff-Herzog Encyclopedia of Religious Knowledge*, *op. cit.*, pp. 307-309.

10. Genesis 50:2, 26.

11. I Samuel 31:12, Amos 6:10, Joshua 7:25, Leviticus 20:14.

12. I Kings 14:11, Isaiah 23:12.

13. Joshua 7:26.

14. Jeremiah 26:23. See also Isaiah 4:9.

15. Matthew 27:7.

16. Paton, *op. cit.*, pp. 295-296.

17. *Ibid.*

18. Franz Cumont, *After Life in Roman Paganism* (New Haven: Yale University Press, 1922), pp. 68-69. Quoting Leblant.

19. I Cor. 15:54, 55.

20. William W. Buechel, "Christian Burial — What it Means," *The Ave Maria*, Vol. 80, No. 19, November 6, 1954, pp.8-9.

21. Nock, *op. cit.*, pp. 321-360.

22. Rush, *op. cit.*, pp. 247.

23. See Robert W. Habenstein, "The American Funeral Director" (University of Chicago: unpublished doctoral dissertation, Department of Sociology, 1954), p. 22 *seq*.

24. Rush, *op. cit.*, p. 2.

25. Habenstein, *op. cit.*, p. 4.

26. For a more detailed account of the genesis of the basic religious beliefs that underpin contemporary orientation to death and burial, see Robert W. Habenstein, "A Sociological Study of the Cremation Movement in America." (Unpublished M.A. Thesis, Department of Sociology, University of Chicago, 1949), pp. 6-21.

27. Rush, *op. cit.*, p. 15, pp. 27-43.

28. Puckle, *op. cit.*, pp. 32 *seq*.

29. Quoted in Rush, *op. cit.*, p. 203.

30. Rush, *op. cit.*, p. 206.

31. Graves, *op. cit.*, p. 23 ff.

32. Mitchell, *op. cit.*, p. 456.

33. Numbers 19:11-14.

34. Rush, *op. cit.*, pp. 101-105.

35. *Ibid.*, p. 19 ff.

36. *Ibid.*, p. 128.

37. St. John Chrysostom, *Eighty-Fourth Homily on St. John*, quoted in Puckle, *op. cit.*, p. 33 *seq*. Puckle stresses the simplicity of funerals during the Age of Faith.

38. Rush, *op. cit.*, pp. 112-117; also Graves, *op. cit.*, pp. 22-25. In this they were more courageous, or perhaps more indiscreet, than their 14th-century successors, lay and clerical, who, during the Great Plague, abandoned the dead. See Cardinal Francis Gasquet's work, *The Black Death* (London: George Bell and Sons, 1908), especially pp. 46-48.

39. Puckle, *op. cit.*, p. 36.

40. Mitchell, *op. cit.*, p. 456.

41. For an amply documented study of the mortuary practices of selected groups of pre-literates, see Effie Bendann, *Death Customs* (New York: Alfred Knopf, 1930).

42. Puckle, *op. cit.*, p. 61.

43. *Ibid.*, p. 62.

44. John C. Gebhart, *Funeral Costs* (New York: G.P. Putnam's Sons, 1928), p. 12.

45. Stone, *op. cit.*, pp. 550-561.

46. The Metropolitan Museum of New York contains numerous excellent examples of these ancient funeral processions, as found in friezes and paintings, and on pottery.

47. Rush, *op. cit.*, p. 160.

48. Mitchell, *op. cit.*, p. 456; Matthew 9:23, Luke 8:2; I Corinthians 15:54.

49. Acts 5:6.

50. Stone, *op. cit.*, pp. 550-556.

51. Jackson, *The New Schaff-Herzog Encyclopedia of Religious Knowledge*, Vol. II, *op. cit.*, p. 308 *seq*.

52. John A. O'Reilly, *Ecclesiastical Sepulture in the New Code of Canon Law* (Washington, D.C.: The Catholic University Press, 1923), p. 5.

53. Acts 5:6, 8:2, 9:37.

54. Stone, *op. cit.*, pp. 62-63.

55. Leclercq, *Manual d'Archeologie Chretienne*, quoted in O'Reilly, *op. cit.*, p. 5 *seq*.

56. O'Reilly, *op. cit.*, p. 11 *seq*.; J. Spence Northcote and W.R. Brownlow, *Roma Sotterranes, or Some of the Roman Catacombs* (London: Longmans, Green, Reader, Dyer, 1869), p. 54.

57. O'Reilly, *op. cit.*, p. 6 *seq*.

58. Mitchell, *op. cit.*, p. 457, makes an excellent summary of this reinfiltration of non-Christian burial practices and the corresponding reaction of the Church.

59. Rush, *op. cit.*, p. 160.

60. O'Reilly, p. 49 *seq*.

61. *Ibid*., pp. 47, 48.

62. Cf. Puckle, *op. cit.*, Chapter VI, pp. 99-129; Rush, *op. cit.*, pp. 193-235; Mitchell, *op. cit.*, pp. 467-478; and Friedlander, *op. cit.*

63. Puckle, *op. cit.*, p. 33.

64. Stone, *op. cit.*, pp. 56-57.

65. Wilson and Levy, *op. cit.*, p. 8.

66. Hilda Ellis, *The Road to Hel: A Study of the Conception of the Dead in Old Norse Literature* (Cambridge University Press, 1943), pp. 8 ff.

67. *Ibid*., p. 12.

68. *Ibid*., p. 13.

69. *Ibid*., pp 55-56.

70. *Ibid*., p. 47. An actual eyewitness of a Russian ship burial in the 10th century is reported by an Arabian observer, Ahmed lbn Foszian. See Carleton S. Coon, *A Reader in General Anthropology* (New York: Henry Holt & Co., 1948), pp. 414-416.

71. *Ibid*., pp. 198-201.

72. Karl Blind, *Fire Burial Among Our Germanic Forefathers: A Record of the Poetry and the History of Teutonic Cremation* (London: Longmans, 1875), p. 13.

73. C.W. Prente-Orton, *The Shorter Cambridge Medieval History* (London: Cambridge University Press, 1952), p. 173.

74. Nock, *op. cit.*, pp. 332-333.

Chapter 3

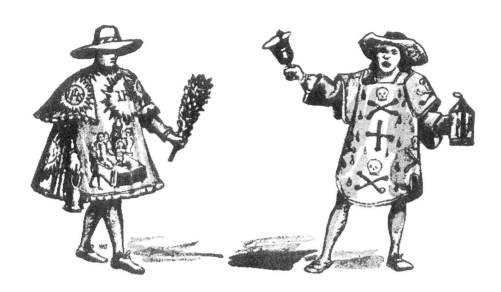

Death and Burial Through the Middle Ages & Renaissance

The defeat of the Emperor Romulus Augustulus, last of the western imperial Roman line, by the barbarian Odoacer in 476 marked the end of Roman power in the West, although the eastern empire, with Constantinople as its capital, did not fall until 1453, almost a thousand years later. In the first half of the 5th century, the Huns under Attila overran the greater part of Rome's empire and were followed by the Vandals, who swept down upon Italy and sacked Rome in 455.

 Without the stabilizing influence of Rome, western Europe was so transformed from what it had been under the *Pax Romana* that a new era in history began. In the ensuing chaos, civil society was broken up and new institutions were forcibly superimposed upon the ruins of older civilizations. Roman customs were preserved only in a few towns in southern Europe, in a few isolated localities sheltered by nature from the tidal wanderings of the barbarians, and in the eastern empire.

 The great migrations had many causes. The richness of Rome tempted the greedy; the weakness of the degenerated empire created a vacuum; and the pressures of Asiatic hordes behind them pushed the nearer barbarians across the Rhine and Danube boundaries. In England, as the Roman garrison withdrew, the wild tribes of the west and north descended upon their Romanized relations. Until the migrations subsided, the arts of peace had lean soil in which to thrive.

But if the barbarians conquered the Roman Empire, the Church conquered the barbarians, gave the new nations a pervasive common culture and a common second language, and provided within its walls — and through its monks and scholars — little islands of peace that served as a matrix for keeping alive the great tradition of Rome. This unsettled period is frequently referred to as the "Dark Ages."

While a case can be made in support of that title, care must be taken to apply it with reasonable limitations. Even at the worst of the long period of turmoil, as Castiglioni points out, the light did not entirely fail:

> The Christian idea... exercised a determining influence on the development of medicine: it gives a different valuation of human life, a fraternal concept of equality and charity which imposed on all the faithful the most severe sacrifices in order to lessen the suffering of others. The example of the early Christians who during the epidemics of the early centuries were tireless in caring for the sick at the peril of their own lives is an admirable proof of the value and the justifying force of those humanitarian ideas which... brought about the creation of a series of institutions designed to care for the aged and the sick.[1]

While quiet did not come all of a sudden all over the troubled Mediterranean area, by the 13th century, the descendants of migrant barbarians had built great cathedrals and would build even greater; had created literature in the new tongues, and would write more; and had speculated deeply and summarized their thinking into theological and philosophical treatises that we still study today.

CHRISTIAN INFLUENCE UPON FUNERAL BEHAVIOR DURING THE EARLY MIDDLE AGES

Funerals: With the emergence of the Christian Church from persecution, and the catacombs into daylight, the simplicity that characterized the Church's primitive burial practices gave way to an imposing dignity that better expressed its importance and that of certain of its members. The dead were brought to church, where a Requiem Mass was said or sung. By the late 5th century, the *Statuta Antiqua* assigned to penitents in Southern Gaul the duty of bringing the unattended dead to church for burial.[2]

In *The Penitentials of Theodore of Tarsus*, the Archbishop of Canterbury (A.D. 668-690), gives ten regulations for the burial of clerics, the first two of which provide:

> According to the Roman Church the custom is to carry dead monks or religious men to the church, to anoint their breast with the chrism, there to celebrate masses for them and then with chanting to carry them to their graves. When they have been placed in the tomb a prayer is offered for them; then they are covered with earth or stone.
>
> On the first, the third, the ninth and also on the thirtieth day a mass is celebrated for them; and, if they wished it, is observed a year later.[3]

Despite the invectives against it by the early fathers of the Church, ostentation gained ground, and the primitive custom of burying the dead in new white garments of linen to signify or prefigure the putting on of the "new clothing of incorruption" yielded by degrees to the practice of burying persons in the costumes by which, during life, they had indicated their positions, so that they continued "splendid in ashes, pompous in the grave." Kings were arrayed in royal finery, and emperors in imperial robes. Knights were shrouded in military garments. The dead bishop wore his episcopal garb, and priests their priestly vestments. Monks wore the habits of their several orders.

In A.D. 595, the last rites of the Empress Theodolinda, friend of Pope Gregory the Great, lasted for more than a week. After death, her body was brought to the Cathedral of Monza, the interior of which was hung with costly black drapes. There it was placed under a splendid "catafalque" (a decorated platform that supports a coffin) and lay in state, surrounded by lighted candles and tapers, so that patrons from all corners of Lombardy, Italy, might pay their respects.

Meanwhile, in hundreds of churches, Votive Masses (masses made in fulfillment of vows or promises) were offered for the repose of the soul of the empress, and bells were tolled. Finally, after the Requiem Mass, her body was interred under the high altar and surmounted with a magnificent shrine. The custom of building shrines, chapels and chanceries in churches was a pious practice by which the donors strove to remind those who survived and succeeded them of their demise, with a view to securing their prayers.[4]

Anglo-Saxon times in England began when invading Low German tribes conquered the country in the 5th century. When an Anglo-Saxon of importance died, the body was placed on a bier or in a hearse, and on it was laid the book of the Gospels as a symbol of faith, and the cross as a symbol of hope. For the journey to the grave, a pall of silk or linen was thrown over the corpse.

During the procession, priests bearing lighted candles and chanting psalms marched before and on either side of the dead and the bearers, while behind the bereaved there followed friends who had been summoned, and strangers who deemed it their duty as a corporal work of mercy to join the party. (***See Plate 11***.) If the procession reached the church in the evening, the night was spent in prayers. When morning came, mass was sung for the dead, the "soul shot" (a donation to the church) or mortuary fee was paid from the deceased's estate, the body was solemnly laid in the grave, and liberal alms were given to the poor.[5]

After the Norman Conquest in 1066, the funeral of a rich Englishman, from king down to squire, grew in pomp and length, and sometimes lasted a full week. It began with tolling of the bells at the moment of death and continued through the embalming of the body, or its anointing with fragrant herbs and spices. When the body had been wrapped in a winding sheet of fine linen — frequently included as a wedding present — it was carried from the death chamber into the great hall of the manor or palace, there to lie in state in the midst of black hangings and under the gleam of many waxen torches. The cost of this illuminating of the face of the dead during long watches was great. Wax was expensive, and as many as 400 large candles were burned at one burial.

At the end of three days' vigil, the corpse was sealed in a leaden coffin and brought to the church, where a Solemn Requiem Mass was sung, and the deceased's clothes were distributed to the poor.

Finally, after the body had been laid to rest, the principals at the funeral, including the officiating clergy, returned to the hall to eat of the "funeral baked meats."[6]

Church and Cemetery Burial in the Middle Ages: When Constantine's Edict of Toleration passed in A.D. 313, burial within the walls or limits of a city, rather than outside of them, was given tremendous impetus by a strange set of circumstances. Christians had long worshipped at altars in tombs and cemeteries, so it was now safe to transfer these altars and their relics to churches in towns and cities. Long accustomed to the association between the place of burial and the place of worship, Christians desired to be buried near their churches.

When, at his own request, Constantine was buried in the vestibule of the Church of the Holy Apostles, which he had built, he set a precedent not only for his successors, but also for church dignitaries and benefactors, and for many other people. He also greatly influenced the custom of burial within the walls and the development of churchyard burial to receive the overflow from the church building itself.

Although the spread of the custom of sepulture in church was at first neither general nor rapid within the first half-century after Constantine's death, it gained such wide and intense acceptance that it was common practice in Constantinople and other Roman cities. This occurred despite the fact that Roman emperors, whether pagan or Christian, had long manifested concern for community health in the making of burial laws — all had feared contagion from the pollution of earth, water and air by the decomposition of corpses. But sentiment winked at sanitation.[7]

The Emperor Theodosius in A.D. 381, renewing the edicts of his predecessors, forbade interment in cities and decreed that, to prevent infections, coffins, urns and sarcophagi within the walls of Rome should be removed to a distance. The law that no cemetery was allowed in or near the city of Rome was soon extended to other cities of the Roman empire, and it was subsequently embodied in the legal code of Justinian the Lawgiver (A.D. 534), the greatest of the emperors of the eastern empire.

Ecclesiastical prohibitions united with civil law in condemning the practice of mixing the dwellings of the living and the dead. Gregory the Great, pope from 590 to 604, restored the disregarded ban on intramural burial.

Oddly enough, Christian religious belief became part of the obstacle to the abolition of the practice. It was not difficult to persuade pagan Romans, who regarded a corpse with disgust, to bury it at a distance and outside the walls. But Christians did not look upon their dead with loathing and as a result, and in spite of emperors and popes, "tyrannical custom overcame the law" so that that which had been the "prerogative of emperors had at last become the common right of all."[8]

At the end of the 5th century, and during the whole of the 6th, burials within cities were very common and continued so in spite of the fact that synods and councils of the Church tried to enforce the ancient codes. Charlemagne (742-814) attempted to stamp out the practice by first prohibiting the burial of the laity within churches; then extending the prohibition to all persons; and finally ordering the destruction of tombs and forbidding that they should rise above the ground in the future.

PLATE 11

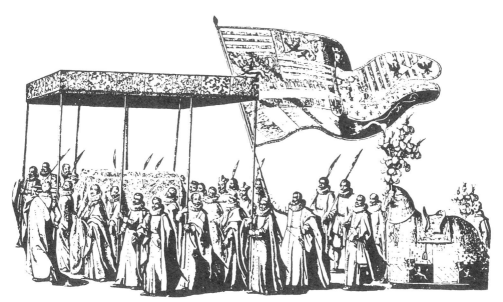

11A. Funeral of Archduke of Brussels, 1622.

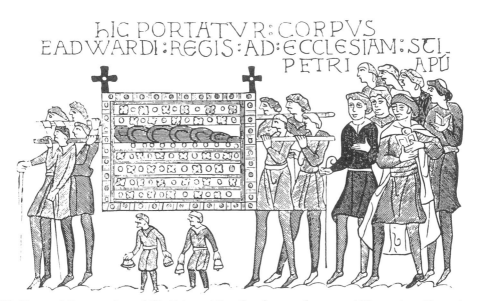

11B. Funeral Procession of St. Edward the Confessor, from an 11th-century Tapestry.

So tenaciously did people cling to the outlawed practice, however, that, at the end of the 9th century, in codifying and publishing Church canons, the pope himself accepted the established fact and, in one canon, erased the old prohibition against church burial. The pope gave as his reasons the fact that it distressed relatives to see their dead carried far from them, and that transportation involved heavy expense to the poor.

Such occasional permission notwithstanding, intramural burial proved so great a nuisance and menace that, from the 10th to the 18th century, councils and synods in various parts of the Catholic world made vigorous efforts to abate or prohibit the practice. As Wickes points out, no matter how modes of interment were affected by superstition or religion, the belief was universally accepted, from the beginning of history to the 9th century, that it was injurious to the living to expose them to the corruption of the dead, and that, in crowded communities, the dead became a source of disease and pestilence. It was paradoxical, he notes, that intramural burial should have been permitted just when "nature's laws began to be better understood."[9]

Reference has already been made to the practice of using the church building itself for sepulture. From the 6th century on, as a result of the efforts to prevent earth burials within the walls of towns and cities, burial within church buildings themselves became increasingly common, until the churches, too, found themselves involved in a most serious problem.[10]

Whether graves were placed under altars, in walls or under floors, the amount of space available for sepulture within a church was severely limited. In recognition of this fact, a 10th-century English canon titled *De Non Sepeliendo in Ecclesiis* ("About Not Being Buried in Churches") calls burial in churches a "privilege" to be granted in the future to priests and to such persons as merited such special recognition by the eminence of their lives.

When the archbishop of Canterbury rebuilt his cathedral in 1075, he provided vaults in the chancel and even beneath the altar. These were reserved for important personages while the great majority of people continued to be buried in the churchyard.

Burial within the church itself had its nuisance aspects. The conditions mentioned by Ramazzini, who wrote much later, must have been better, if anything, than in earlier days when preparation of the body was more primitive. "There are so many tombs in the church, and they are so often opened that this abominable smell is too often unmistakable. However much they fumigate the sacred edifices with incense, myrrh, and other aromatic odors, it is obviously very injurious to those present." Ramazzini quotes Lilio Giraldi of Ferrara (1479-1552) as — very properly censuring the custom of interring the dead indiscriminately in churches — being contrary to the practice that, in remote times and in the earliest days of Christianity, limited burial within the church itself to martyrs.[11]

Although religious orders once restricted church burial to their own members, they came to accept the corpses of persons of rank and of benefactors, until abuses of such hospitality of sepulture caused the church-going public to become incensed and the clergy to grow indignant. In 1581, Cardinal Bourbon, archbishop of Rouen, decreed in council, "...not even the rich should be buried in churches."

There was some logic in the effort people made to be buried in church precincts. Berner believes that in pagan days, the burial place was considered, if not sacred, at least religious through the *illatio mortui*. The early Christian Church at first upheld this view, but later rejected it by ecclesiastical decree, maintaining that, "among Catholics the place itself is not made holy simply by the burial of the human body." Instead of the body consecrating the soil in which it lay, the body was made sacred by being buried in soil that had been consecrated. Because it was believed that evil spirits were powerless in consecrated ground, the term "God's acre" was applied to churchyards.

Fear of vampires and ghouls, which in some places was strong during the Middle Ages, made a churchyard or, at least, intramural burial a much sought-after privilege. Christian tradition supported this practice. The concern of the Church for the remains and souls of the dead produced regulations concerning burial, and the concept of a consecrated place brought with it a decisive break with the past as communal (rather than individual or local) places of interment became the rule.

The same Church that consecrated the soil of the graveyard also took measures lest it be profaned. In England from the time of King Egbert (A.D. 740), Christian burial was denied those who "lay violent hands upon themselves," although this severe deprivation was not extended to those whose suicide came in a fit of madness or frenzy. Those found guilty of *felo de se* ("murder of one's self") were sometimes buried at a crossroads with a stake driven through the body; sometimes in unconsecrated ground, in a ditch or on the heath; or sometimes in the churchyard by night.[12]

It was common practice throughout Europe until the time of the Black Plague, which swept over the continent in the 14th century, for each church or town to maintain a small churchyard burial ground sufficient for the needs of its parishioners. When, during a brief period in the second half of the 14th century, the Black Death carried off an estimated two-thirds to three-quarters of the population of England, such churchyards proved wholly inadequate. In London, for example, the 120 small churchyard plots had to be supplemented by three "extramural" cemeteries — two in Smithfield and one at Aldgate. These soon passed into the hands of friars and eventually became monastery grounds.[13]

But extramural burial was the exception, not the rule. Although churches were erected near existing centers of population and became foci for greater concentration during normal times, the ground could be used repeatedly for returning the dead to the earth because of the natural spacing of births and deaths. Thus, for example, the church of St. John the Baptist in Widford, Hertfordshire, with less than half an acre available for a graveyard, interred no fewer than 5,000 people in the beautiful small plot that looks down upon the wide ford of the Ash. This was uncoffined burial, however, with no effort made to preserve the remains of the dead. Only in relatively recent times, as coffined burial became the universal practice, have the old churchyards proved too small.[14]

Do not interpret the prior statement, however, to mean that the ability to provide minimum space for disintegration was wholly acceptable then, or a standard to be imitated now.

In 1552, Archbishop Latimer denounced the state of St. Paul's churchyard in London as productive of "much sickness and disease" and made reference to its all-too-familiar odors. That these should have arisen is not surprising. For some years prior to 1582, as many as 23 of the parishes of London that had given up their own burial grounds were using St. Paul's churchyard for their dead. In 1582, this number was reduced to 13, when 10 of the parishes joined in seeking their burial needs in a new cemetery laid out near Bishopsgate.

Even with this relief, it is difficult to see how 13 parishes could find burial facilities in St. Paul's churchyard, which, by 1584, was so crowded, with former burials made so shallow, "that scarcely any grave could be made without corpses being laid open."[15]

Disposal and Contagion: "Rightly or wrongly," Creighton comments, "taught by experience or misled by fancy, the medieval world firmly believed that the formal and elaborate disposal of the dead had a sanitary aspect as well as a pious."[16]

An illustration in point is the use of the interdict, a spiritual weapon employed on rare occasions by the pope to enforce discipline on rebellious rulers or peoples. This punishment took the form of a prohibition restraining the faithful from ecclesiastical functions. Stone remarks, "The most fearful part of an interdict has always been felt to be not allowing the rites of sepulture, and the burying of the dead in unconsecrated ground."[17]

Writing of the last years of the reign of Richard I (1157-1199) and John II (1167-1216), the chronicler Ralph of Coggeshall in Essex bewails the decree of Pope Innocent III in interdicting all Christian rites save only baptism by the clergy of France: "Oh how horrible... to refuse the Christian rite of burial to the bodies of the dead, so that they infected the air by their foetor [*a strong, foul smell*] and struck horror into the souls of the living by their ghastly looks."[18]

The same interdict was extended to England in 1208 during the reign of King John. The belief that the dead infected the air was current in England for several centuries before the Black Death. Creighton calls this belief an "instinct" as wide as human nature and observes that, among early writers, there is a clear perception of the relation between the disposal of the dead and sanitation and contagion, with concern growing acute particularly after a battle, massacre or natural catastrophe.

When the Welsh raided as far as Shrewsbury in 1234, strewing the country with naked corpses for the birds and animals to feed upon, "the foetor of so much corruption infected the air on all sides so that even the dead slew the living."[19]

To prevent contagion, as early as 1348 the Venetian Doge Dandolo appointed a commission entrusted with such precautions as the "special removal of corpses, the depth of graves, prohibition of exposing the dead on the streets, a guard against visiting ships, and so on."[20]

The theory of the origin of the plague virus from the corruption of the dead was commonly held in the 16th century and for a long time thereafter. Ambrose Pare (1510-1590), the father of French surgery, held it. Discussing the causes of plague, Dr. Gilbert Skene wrote in the 16th century about "dead carrions unburied... which by similitude of nature, is most indecent, as every brute is most infectant and pestilential to their own kind."[21]

Creighton well-summarizes the whole matter of the disposal of the dead and the spread of contagion during the Middle Ages:

But even if these truths had been generally apprehended, religious prescription and usage would have been too strong to allow any radical measures being adopted. The grand provocative of plague was no obvious nuisance above ground, but the loading of the soil generation after generation, with an immense quantity of cadaveric matters, which were diffused in the pores of the ground under the feet of the living, to rise in emanations, more deadly in one season than in another, according as the level of the ground-water and the heat of the earth determined the degree of oxidation, or the formation of the more dangerous half-way products of decomposition... The skirts of the city were used also to deposit the soil (sewage) upon. Thus it happened that the ground outside the walls, which came in time to be the densely populated liberties and out-parishes, and the chief seat of all later plagues, had for generations before received the refuse of the city, and a large proportion of the bodies of the dead.[22]

The Purgatorial Doctrine and the Formation of Leagues of Prayer and Other Pious Practice: The Catholic doctrine of "purgatory" — the belief in a state of purgation in which "those whose souls are not perfectly cleansed undergo a process of cleansing" before they can enter heaven — was in part responsible during the Middle Ages for the formation of numerous confraternities, guilds, brotherhoods or leagues of prayer devoted to burying the dead and praying for the souls of the faithful departed.

Do not confuse these lay organizations with the religious orders living in communities and bound together by vows. In Medieval England, such lay burial-organizations were common. Typical of all of them were the regulations of the Guild of Abbotsbury that, among other matters, provided: "If anyone belonging to this association chance to die, each member shall pay a penny for the good of the soul, before the body be laid in the grave." The Steward of the Guild made the necessary funeral arrangements, which included a Requiem Mass, burial with solemnity, the payment of the soul shot or mortuary fee, and a liberal distribution of alms.

Davey found the inscriptions on the earliest English tombs "pathetic" — "Of your charity pray for me." When a member of the Guild of All Souls in London died, the survivors were wont to give the poor a loaf of bread for the repose of his soul. The custom survived into the 19th century.[23]

In an age that lacked newspapers and printed death notices, the announcement of a death was made by human voice. Originally, this function was bound up with the purgatorial doctrine. The crier — later named the "Death Crier" and, in some parts of England, "The Death Watch," and, still later, dressed in black with a death's head and crossbones painted on the front and back of his gown or tabard, and with a bell in hand — after the death of a person of distinction or a member of the League of Prayer, a crier went the rounds crying: "Of a charity, good people, pray for the soul of our dear brother or sister" [here naming the dead] "who departed this life at such and such an hour" [stating the time]. (***See Plate 12***.)

At this clamor and the ringing of the bell, the town or city folk on the crier's itinerary threw open their sash and doors and murmured an *Ave* or a *Pater Noster*.

In London, when royalty died, the death watch was no ordinary public servant paid as an official by the civic corporation, but instead a nobleman, attended by a procession consisting of a cross bearer and the entire Guild of the Holy Souls, each bearing a lighted candle.

Prior to the Reformation, as the funeral procession bore the corpse to the grave, passers-by and bystanders uncovered and stood in reverence until it had moved beyond them. When they met a procession, the pious even turned about and joined it, walking with the mourners part of the way to the grave.

Vestiges of the old processional dress still survived into the 19th century in the scarf and hood of black silk occasionally worn by ladies, and in the "weepers" — bands of black for a dead man, and white for a dead woman, worn on the arms of gentlemen in mourning.[24]

The burial guilds survived the Reformation. Wilson and Levy, making special pleading for funeral reform in England, write of these guilds:

> Burial in the early and later Middle Ages was largely defrayed and — apart from the functions of the church — administered and assisted by gilds and corporations in order that the attendant expenses should not bear heavily upon the estate of the dead or the purses of their living relations.[25]

Puckle enumerates some of the equipment paraphernalia provided by the guild:

> The guild supplied a hearse... also a pall, bier, candles, etc. These articles were collectively owned, and held always at the disposal of those of the fraternity who might have need of them; they might, moreover, be borrowed by members for the use of friends, in which case a toll was taken of a certain quantity of wax, which would be made up into candles as required.[26]

Many of the same items were also made available through the church.

The Wake During the Middle Ages: During the Middle Ages the vigil for the dead, originating out of the Hebrew practice as an act of precaution against premature burial, was continued as an act of piety. One of the canons enacted under King Edgar in England in the 10th century reads: "Let him (the parish priest) shrive him, give him Housel, and Extreme Unction, and, after death, carefully order, and not allow any absurdity with the corpse, but with the fear of God bury it wisely."[27] (To "shrive" is to give absolution; "Housel" is an old word for the Eucharist.)

In the Irish canons, a woman was given a penance of 50 days on bread and water for wailing after the death of a layman or laywoman.[28]

The learned monk Regino, who became an abbot in Lorraine, France, in 892, compiled in 906 his work *Of Synodical Cases and Ecclesiastical Discipline*. In this book, among other matters, he warned that:

> Diabolical Songs be not sung at night hours over the bodies of the dead. Laymen who keep watch at funerals shall do so with fear and trembling, and with reverence. Let no one there presume to sing diabolical songs nor make jests and perform dances which pagans have invited by the devil's teaching. For who does not know that it is diabolical, and not only alien from the Christian religion, but even contrary to human nature, that there should be singing, rejoicing, drunkenness, and that the mouth be loosed with laughter, and that all piety and feeling of

PLATE 12

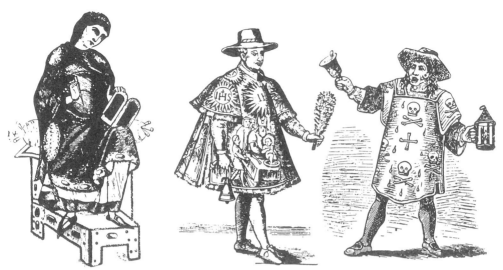

12A. (Left) Anglo-Saxon Widow, 9th Century.
12B. Death Criers, French Costumes, 17th Century.

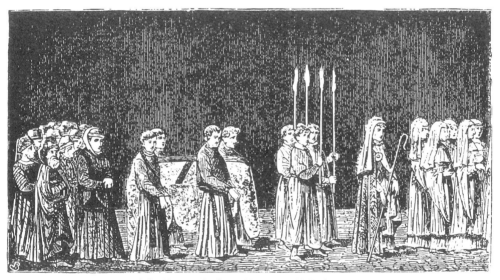

12C. Funeral of an Abbess, 10th Century.

charity be set aside... But if any one wishes to sing, let him sing the *Kyrie Eleison*. But if he does otherwise, let him be quite silent. If, however, he will not be silent, he shall be forthwith denounced by all, or adjured that he no longer has God's permission to stay there, but is to withdraw and go to his own house. On the morrow, moreover, he shall be so punished that others may fear.[29]

That the custom of behaving riotously at wakes became widespread is evident from the *Corrector* of Burchard of Worms, written a hundred years later between 1008 and 1012. Burchard asks: "Hast thou observed funeral wakes... when the bodies of Christians are guarded by a ritual of pagans; and hast thou sung diabolical songs there and performed dances which the pagans have invited by the teaching of the devil; and hast thou drunk there and relaxed thy countenance with laughter... as if rejoicing over a brother's death"[30]

By the 14th century, disorder at wakes had progressed beyond rioting and drunkenness with the addition of a new custom: "rousing the ghost." While some have sought to explain this irreverent custom as originating in an effort to bring back (through necromancy or black magic) the spirit of the departed, it would seem less strained to account for it as a grim kind of horseplay.

Aristotle has defined humor as incongruity intellectually perceived. Not all onlookers at a funeral bear an equal burden of grief. To persons lightly concerned, the heavy solemnity and deep dolor is a startling backdrop for the ludicrous. The dead were "raised" during the 14th century by playing practical jokes on superstitious relatives to frighten them, and by taking liberties with the corpse. The extent to which this grisly roughhouse was practiced is apparent from the fact that the Council of York (1367) condemned "those guilty games and follies, and all those perverse customs which transformed a house of tears and prayers into a house of laughing and excess."

In the same vein, the Guild of Palmers — pilgrims returned from the Holy Land, who also wore two palms crosswise in token of their pilgrimage — permitted its members to join in waking the dead only if they abstained from "raising apparitions and from indecent games."

In the south of Ireland, the vigil keepers entertained themselves with a sham battle. Their Scottish brethren fought mock duels that frequently ended in real fights and bloodshed. Everywhere, the families of the dead plied the wakers with intoxicants and food, of which latter pancakes were a favorite item.[31]

Funeral Feasts: In addition to serving as an occasion for praying for the dead, the wake filled several secondary functions, among which was the opportunity for those present at the death to clear themselves of any suspicion of foul play; for those not present at the death to see that no foul play had taken place; and, for all who might inherit from the deceased, the chance to witness whether an equitable distribution of property was being made.

As a further function, the wake served as a feast to welcome the principal heir to his new estate. Etymology reveals the story: the old word for the funeral feast was "averil" or "arvel," meaning "heir ale" or "succession ale." A common practice in Medieval England that persisted even as late as the Stuart kings (James I, the first of the line, ascended the throne in 1603) was to place a cup of wine in the coffin next to the corpse. By drinking of it, the mourners felt that they had established some kind of communion with the dead.[32]

Funerals of State During the Middle Ages and the Use of the Effigy: The funeral of a great personage often lasted a week, from the time a tolling bell announced the death, through the washing and embalming of the body, the exposition in state, the Requiem Mass, burial, and the banquet of the "funeral baked meats."

Waxed death masks were often made of the nobility as soon as possible after expiration. It was not uncommon for a waxen presentment to be exhibited in church upon the catafalque in place of the real body — a practice originating, no doubt, in hygienic and aesthetic necessity, especially during hot weather, since the funeral might have lasted many days. The custom persisted in England until the reign of William and Mary (1689-1702), and in France until the middle of the 17th century. It is last mentioned in connection with the death of Anne of Austria (1666): "The Queen-mother died today. She was immediately embalmed, and by noon her waxen effigy was on view at the Louvre. Thousands are pressing in to see it."[33]

The funeral of Henry V (reigned 1413-1422), king of England and victor of Agincourt, illustrates not only the elaborate and prolonged funeral rites given to monarchs and great dignitaries, but also shows the physical need that these produced for some method of keeping the corpse from becoming offensive. It also displays a quaint refinement of the process of bone burial described in detail below. After the king's death in France, his body was boiled to obtain a perfect skeleton for transportation to England. Before leaving France, the bones were taken to the church of Notre Dame, where a fitting funeral service was conducted over them. Above them, in the coffin, was placed an effigy of boiled leather, robed in purple and shaped to represent the king "as well as might be desired." In its hand the figure carried the royal scepter, and on its brow it wore the kingly diadem.

After the services, the coffin containing the effigy and bones was placed in a splendid chariot or hearse and draped with a covering of red velvet, sprinkled with gold leaf. Accompanied by the king of Scotland as chief mourner, and all the princes, lords and knights of his house, the funeral procession moved from town to town until it reached the port of Calais, France. From there, it was taken by boat to London, where it was finally laid to rest in Westminster Abbey. Henry's widow caused a silver-plated effigy of her husband, with a solid-silver-gilt head, to be placed on the tomb. This effigy was destroyed during the Reformation.[34]

Sepulchral Monuments: The beginnings of Christian sepulchral monuments in England are found in stone coffins, whose lids formed a continuous portion of the pavement of churches. At an early date, it became customary to mark these with a carved symbol, such as a cross, to express piety, or some emblem to convey the occupation or position of the deceased.

This simple incising was succeeded by the practice of carving an effigy of the dead person in the stone, or even a representation showing the coffin opened, with the dead displayed wholly or partially within. Little by little, the tops of the tombs were raised above the level of the pavement, until they could no longer be walked upon.

Next, the custom grew of surmounting them with a festoon or canopy. As these grew in size and magnificence, they encumbered the church and were placed at the east end, parallel with the chancel (the part of the church reserved for the clergy), or were erected in chapels especially constructed to shelter them and opening from the side aisles.

The beauty, magnificence and cost of some of these monuments were great. Some were enriched with semi-precious and precious stones and adorned with lifelike figures of solid brass. The finest on record is that of Henry III (reigned 1207-1272), who had provided for the body of Edward the Confessor (reigned 1042-1066) a coffin of solid gold and precious stones — the workmanship of which was so fine that it surpassed the material in cost.

The first tomb effigies were made of wood, plated over with bronze or copper, plain or gilt. Later, brass was used, and some monumental effigies were made of silver. One of the earliest of the latter was placed on the tomb of Catherine, the daughter of Henry III, who died in 1251.

These monumental effigies, however rich and elaborate, consistently display a humble attitude in the presence of death, despite some identification showing status and occupation. Crusaders, and even those prevented from fulfilling their vows to visit the Holy Land, were represented with crossed legs; prelates, with their right hand raised, as if in benediction; bishops carried a crozier in their left hands and abbots in their right; priests held a chalice; warriors bore arms; kings were crowned — and so on through a long list of ranks, titles and functions.

Other symbols represented the virtues of the deceased. Thus, stone lions at the feet of the effigy told of the dead man's courage, industry or vigilance. Emblems represented achievement, and dragons pierced by the staves of the abbots of Peterborough gave a clue to their triumph, and the Church's, over the devil. These representations were more in keeping with the Christian tradition than the skull and crossbones of later medieval monumentary art.[35]

The Plagues: Beginning in the 6th century, during the reign of the Emperor Justinian and as a part of the great cycle of pestilence that periodically swept across the world since the dawn of history, the bubonic plague entered Europe. In 542, it carried off in one day 10,000 people in Constantinople.

Repeatedly, the plague swept over England — the cycle of epidemics of the 14th century, known as the Black Death, proving most severe. Plague, although showing some signs of decline, recurred in the 15th, 16th and 17th centuries. The years 1664 and 1665 were dismally remembered as marking the Great Plague of London. In 1665, out of a population estimated at 460,000, bills of mortality for the city showed 68,596 deaths.[36]

The successive waves of plague did much to change the economic and social structure of Europe. In England, for example, the earlier visitation wiped out a high percentage of serfs, forced freedom from the land upon those who were left, and did much to end the system of semi-slavery.

Because funeral customs and practices depend in part upon what people are able to earn and provide for the dead, a social revolution of this kind is significant for the present consideration. Apart from this, the plagues produced burial crises that fascinate us by their sheer magnitude. One visitation must have been much like any other.

Shakespeare's contemporary, the poet-playwright Thomas Dekker, described London and its "sinfully polluted suburbs" during the plague of 1603. While walking the streets at night, he hears from every house the loud groans and ravings of the sick, the death struggles of the dying, the shrieks of the bereaved, the cries of alarm, and servants crying out for masters, wives for husbands, parents for children, children for their mothers. Here, a distraught man runs to look for a sexton; there, a group sweats as it carries a coffin. Persons push bodies from their houses into the street by stealth lest the officers of the law seal up their houses with the mark of death.

During the plague of 1547, an order was issued prohibiting burial between six in the evening and six in the morning. In 1665, when the times were reversed, the 12 hours of darkness proved too short to bury the dead. In his imaginary *Journal of the Plague Year*, the eminent novelist Daniel Defoe (1661-1731) tells of the Aldgate plague pit at midnight, with seven or eight lanterns set on the heaps of earth round the edge, and of the constant journeying to and fro of the dead-carts. Defoe probably got his story from eyewitnesses. Certainly this was a case in which truth could be given no heightening by the art of fiction,[37] and fact must have transcended fancy. (***See Plate 13***.)

The Plagues Overload the Cemeteries: Turner of Boulogne, preaching at St. Paul's Cross, London, on August 8th, 1563, when 5,000 a week were dying in London alone of the plague, besought the lord mayor to bury the dead in a field beyond the city, and to halt the tolling of the funeral bell, "for that the tolling of the bell did the party departing no good, neither afore their death nor after."[38]

The story was repeated of the pilgrim on the road to Bagdad who was overtaken by a special traveler. "Who are you, and to where do you hurry?" the pilgrim asked. "I am Plague," the figure shouted across his shoulder, "and I go to Bagdad to slay a thousand people." On his flight from the city, the pilgrim overtook the grisly traveler. "You told me that you would slay a thousand in Bagdad," he chided, "and yet I found ten thousand slain." "I spoke accurately," answered Plague, "I slew but a thousand. The other nine thousand died from fright."[39]

So great were the numbers dying that Christian burial rites could not be provided. After the consecrated ground was filled, great trenches were dug and into them bodies were placed, layer upon layer, with a sprinkling of earth between layers, until they were filled. On the site of the present Charter House in London, it is estimated that more than 50,000 burials were made.

Great difficulty was experienced in finding persons who would risk contagion by burying the dead and, as the sexton's bell tolled the passing, people shut themselves within their houses, lest they be infected by the corpses being carted or borne to the charnal pit.[40] Yet, as Puckle points out, although new cemeteries were hastily constructed as old churchyards were filled, "In all this stress of circumstances... no thought was given to the cremation of bodies; surely proof enough that the practice was repugnant to the people, who even in such circumstances as these refused to adopt the pagan practice as being against the usage of the Christian Church."[41]

Various laws were passed in an effort to reduce contagion. The Act of 1547, forbidding burial between six in the evening and six in the morning, doubtless was based upon the belief that people were less susceptible to the foul vapors of contagion during the day than they were at night — a belief that popularly persisted far into the 19th century. The curfew also had the effect of forcing plague deaths into the public eye, and of making prowling at night in a cemetery conspicuous, thus rendering it more difficult for ghouls to ply their trade.[42]

Coffined Burial Becomes the Custom: Although the use of coffins appears in many cultures and even antedates written history, the modern American prevalence of coffined burial is a development of recent centuries. The word itself is derived from the Greek *kofinos*, meaning basket, coffer or chest. In the Old Testament, there is only one record of coffined burial: When Joseph, the Hebrew patriarch and son of Jacob, died, he was embalmed and "put in a coffin in Egypt."[43]

Herodotus tells how when Cambyses, king of the Medes and Persians (died 522 B.C.), set forth to conquer Egypt, he sent spies ahead. These reported back how they had seen Ethiopian bodies coffined in hollow pillars of transparent crystal. This was probably glass, the manufacture of which was known to the Egyptians as early as 2000 B.C.[44]

Baked clay or earthenware coffins were most common among the Greeks, although they used other substances, too. The Roman coffin, called *arca* or *loculus*, was generally made of stone. The Romans used coffins of many kinds, among them bricks covered with tiles; coffins of lead and glass; and stone coffins with urns, *paterae* and *lachrymatories* in them. (A *patera* is a "saucer-like dish of earthenware or metal used for drinking or libations," and a *lachrymatory* is a "small vessel" found in ancient tombs once believed to have contained the tears of mourners.)

But they preferred a particular kind of stone that was quarried in Assos, in Troas, the territory of ancient Troy, lying in northwest Asia Minor, south of the Dardanelles. They believed that this stone possessed the power of consuming the body, except for the teeth, in a few weeks. Strangely enough, from this supposed power came the Greek word "sarcophagus" or "body eating," which was applied first to the stone itself and then to the principal object made from it, the sarcophagus.

Many early stone coffins have been discovered among Roman antiquities in England. The Celts left simple coffins made of unhewn flat stones set on edge to form the sides, with a crowning flat stone for the lid. These were succeeded by the stone coffin, cut from a solid block, tapering from the upper end in rough resemblance to the body outline, with a hewn recess and a special widening, to receive the body, extending into another recess for the head, and a hole in the bottom to permit drainage of the fluids of decomposition.

Such coffins first appeared among the Anglo-Saxons about A.D. 695 and were common for higher-class burials for the period through the reign of Henry VIII (died 1547). These solid-block coffins, when buried outside, frequently were in excavations so shallow that their tops were clear of the ground while, in churches their lids formed a portion of the pavement. Lead coffins were sometimes used during the Middle Ages.[45]

The earliest known wooden coffin was that of Arthur, the half-mythical king of England who reigned in the 5th or 6th century. In large English *tumuli* or burial mounds, coffins made out of hollow logs have been unearthed, holding skeletons and charred bones. Other coffins made of elm logs with the bark clinging to them, and with fittings of small riveted brass strips, have been discovered.[46]

PLATE 13

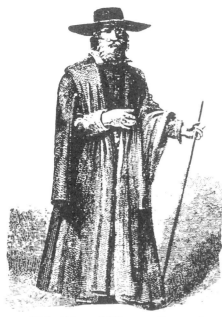
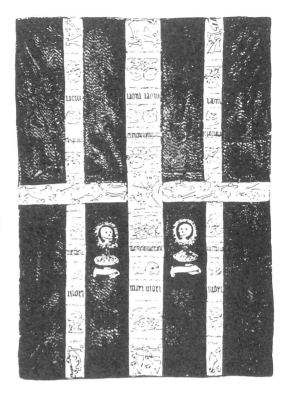

13A. (Above) "Corpse Bearer," 18th Century, England.
13B. Coffin Pall, Church of Folleville, France, Late Renaissance.

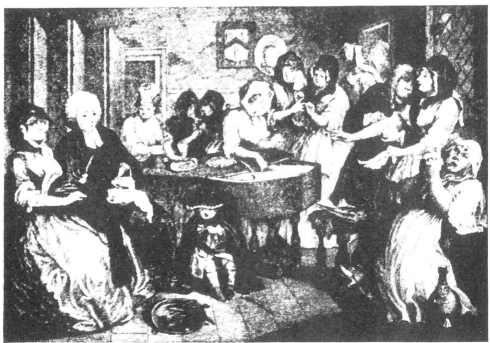

13C. Funeral Scene in Hogarth's "The Harlot's Progress" Showing Rosemary Sprigs.

A custom of briefer duration, lasting for about a century from the time of the Norman Conquest (1066), was that of wrapping the corpse for burial in the strongest leather or in a bull's hide. Henry I of England (died 1135), his son Prince Henry, King John (died 1216), and James III of Scotland were among notables shrouded in a bull's hide.[47]

All these practices, however, represent exceptions to the general rule that the dead were laid uncoffined in their graves. During the Norman dynasty, (1066-1154), and for a long while afterward, many persons of distinction preferred to be buried in the plain earth. Such was the general custom during the reigns of Edward II (reigned 1307-1327) and Edward III (1327-1377). Knights were sometimes laid to rest uncoffined but clad in full armor. In excavating for repairs to the choir of the Cathedral of Gloucester, workmen discovered the remains of three abbots who had been buried uncoffined in shallow graves, but wearing gloves and garments. Even during the reign of Queen Elizabeth I (reigned 1558-1603) it was customary to bury the dead wrapped only in winding sheets.

The practice is further indicated by the implications of a statement found in the minutes of the vestry of St. Helen's Church, Bishopsgate, March 5th, 1564, "that none should be buried within the church unless the dead corpse be coffined in wood." Presumably, even some of those who qualified by wealth and position for church burial still preferred to be carried to their graves on biers, and there to be removed and placed uncoffined in their sepulchers.[48]

But coffining or shrouding, whether in stone, wood, lead, leather or hide, was reserved for the wealthy and important. The shroud and the shrift (absolution) of the poor and unimportant were simple and short. In England, the humble were usually sewed up in sheets or wrapped in a linen shroud and carried to their graves in the parish shell, a coarser kind of temporary coffin with a movable lid that was used only for conveyance and saw duty for many years. The simple burial service recited, the body of the poor was placed in the earth, covered only with the winding sheet, and the clods were shoveled upon it. Charitable friends paid for masses for the dead, while guilds defrayed the small expense originating in this simple funeral.[49]

In some places in England, coffined burial was not permitted even to some who could afford it, and only certain of the prosperous were allowed a coffin or chest — "to be chested" is the old phrase. In 1580, the city fathers of Rye in Sussex forbade coffined burial to all but the mayor, the councilmen and their wives, and to such as were licensed by the mayor.[50] By implication, the service book of the Anglican Communion, the *Book of Common Prayer*, the burial portions of which date from 1546-1547, indicates the frequency of uncoffined burial in England at the middle of the 15th century. It does not mention a coffin, making reference only to the corpse or body, as when it says "the earth shall be cast upon the body."

In 1563, the General Assembly of Scotland decreed that a bier should be made in every county parish "to carry the *dead corpse* of the poor to the burial place, and that those of the villages or houses next adjacent to the house where the *dead corpse* lieth, or a certain number out of every house, shall convey the *dead corpse* to the burial place and bury it six feet under the earth."[51]

As commerce and industry enriched England, and the standards of living for all classes rose, coffined burials, hitherto the privilege of the rich, became increasingly the common practice of all. In 1603, the dramatist Thomas Dekker stated that the coffin-makers of London were busily employed and growing rich. Yet, Sir Henry Spelman observed that, as late as 1650, interments without coffins were common among the humbler classes, decent covering fulfilling the full need for burial.

In London, 15 years later at the worst of the last great visitation of the plague, most burials were in coffins,[52] although registers and churchwardens' accounts bear frequent witness to uncoffined burials through the 16th and 17th centuries.[53]

SOCIAL DEVELOPMENTS AND FUNERAL PRACTICE

Funeral Ostentation Grows Among the English Middle Classes: As the Middle Ages closed in England, ostentatious public funerals for the rising middle class were the order of the day. Speaking of merchants, Sylvia Thrupp, social historian of medieval England, says: "The final problem in expenditure that perplexed the merchant arose out of the question as to how he should be buried, the size of the torches and tapers to be placed about his body in the hearse, the number of persons to attend the rites and the funeral baked meats at his house, the number, quality and cost of the mourning clothes to be distributed, the month's mind, and other stipends to be paid, and so on at length."[54]

> For any man who cared about his social position it was therefore logical to wish for as splendid a funeral as could be arranged without working hardship to his heirs. On the other hand, the priest would tell him that worldly standards should at this point give way before humility and piety; he should spend his money on alms, not on vain display. Torn between the habits of a lifetime and a fear that his priest might be right, the merchant either compromised or left the problem to his executors.[55]

This tendency toward ostentation intensified in the 15th century, and costs mounted as more wax torches were carried, more shields of arms displayed, more mourning gowns distributed, and more lavish entertainments provided.

Whether a funeral should be costly or inexpensive, however, was a matter of free choice to a man before his death, and to his heirs after it. As Thrupp puts it: "No commercial organization of the funeral as a whole developed to force expenses up."[56]

A merchant could still provide a funeral for his son for half a mark during the reign of Edward IV (reigned 1461-1470, 1471-1483) — a mark was the equivalent of thirteen shillings and four pence — and, for less than nine shillings, the Grovers Company gave respectable burial to an almsman.

Wills afford some indication of funeral costs. Of surviving 14th-century wills, that of William Thorneye, an alderman of London, drawn in 1348, provided that 80 pounds, the highest amount so to be set aside, should be spent on his funeral and for the repose of his soul. For 20, 30 and 40 pounds, respectively, three other aldermen purchased funerals, masses and other memorial works. Some wealthy men firmly set a limit of four pounds, or ten or twenty marks, for expenditures for funerals and for the alms to be distributed to the poor attending them. In 1403, John Doget ordered

25 torches for his hearse, in addition to 20 marks to be spent on other items, and requested that no one wear black except his wife, executors, servants and debtors. This provision suggests that it might have been customary for all of a dead man's friends to be robed in mourning.

There is some evidence that while wealthy merchants gave lip service to a distaste for worldly show as bringing no profit to the soul, they were nonetheless willing to make compromise with it. Thus, although Nicholas Wyfold made testamentary provision that he should be buried "without any grete hers, poni ponis, cost or other vaine glorie of the worlde," he set aside the substantial sum of 100 marks to defray costs. "Excess," Thrupp observes, "brought common sense reaction in its train. Not every merchant was gratified to think of his company brethren descending like locusts on the family larder after his memorial services."[57]

Custom, social pressures and the desire to maintain status or personal and social importance — not to seem, even in death, unworthy of one's occupation — militated against penuriousness or apparent stinginess in the funerals of important people. It would probably be unfair to ascribe all ostentation or lavish expenditure to the vanity of the dead, however. The surviving family or occupational group, too, had its position to maintain.

The Development of Burial Clubs: To help people of the working classes, particularly guild members, defray the heavy expenses of a funeral, and to perpetuate the memory of dead friends, burial clubs were formed. Throughout the Middle Ages, great importance was attached to the religious ceremonies attending burial. Guilds provided prayers, masses, yearly reminders, and palls or "mort" cloths. (***See Plate 13***.) To defray the cost of these services, a small regular contribution called "quarterage" was levied among the living. It became customary for the guild to pay for the services of a chaplain, as well as for candles and other equipment and supplies.[58] Guild members were expected to attend the funerals of departed members, and to pray regularly for the repose of their souls.

While the burial clubs were most common among guild members, they were to be found among other groups of the laboring classes, as well. The activities they sponsored ultimately gave rise to several new full-time occupations. One of these functionaries did nothing but invite people to funerals by rapping on their doors with the key to the house of the departed. Another, the bell ringer, marched through the streets, calling out the names of the deceased on the first anniversaries of their deaths and requesting prayers for them.[59]

The Shroud in England Changes from Linen to Wool: Shrouding the corpse presents interesting and significant considerations. Throughout most of the Middle Ages, when the corpse was shrouded at all, the shroud was of linen and often loosened at the feet and hands to permit easy escape on the day of resurrection.

Up to the middle of the 16th century, the Church provided that an infant dying within a month of baptism was to be interred in his or her "chrisom," a primitive baptismal robe constructed to permit the priest to anoint the child on the back and breast, and normally worn by the child for seven days afterward to protect these places, or until the mother was "Churched," that is, blessed in church after childbirth. For burial, the infant wearing the chrisom was swathed with bandages, or "swaddled."[60]

PLATE 14

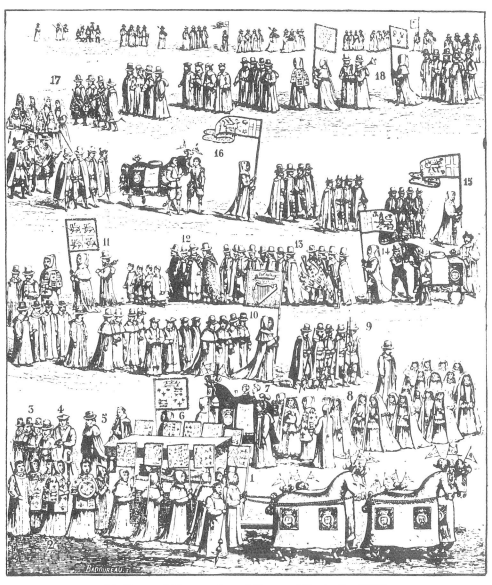

14. Funeral Procession of Queen Elizabeth, 1603.

No. 1 represents the wax effigy of the queen; 2. Kings at Arms; 3. Noblemen; 4. Archbishop of Canterbury; 5. French ambassador and train bearer; 6. Great standard of England; 7. Master of the Horse; 8. Lady Marchioness of Northampton; 9. Captain of the guard; 10. Great standard of Ireland; 11. Standard of Wales; 12. Gentlemen of the Chapels Royal; 13. Trumpeters; 14. Standard of the Lion; 15. Standard of the Greyhound; 16. The queen's horse; 17. Poor women; and 18. Banner of Cornwall, and the alderman, recorders, town clerks, etc.

For some unaccountable reason, the priors of Durham went to their graves in their boots. Such burial in robe of office marked an unconscious return to Roman ways, during which magistrates and military men were shrouded in their purple robes of honor or other rich raiment, while persons of rank or wealth were cremated in their official garments.[61]

Creighton could not say when the custom of burial in a sheet or "cerecloth" (a cloth treated with wax, alum or gummy matter) was no longer followed in England, although it is certain that it was decreasingly observed by the poorer classes during the 17th century.

As the population increased and funerals became more elaborate, note was taken of the fact that linen of great value was being buried each year in the form of cerecloths for the dead. Linen was imported, and England's expanding paper industry wanted all the used linen it could obtain for the production of high-grade paper. At the same time, the woolen industry wanted customers. Thus, paper manufacturers joined woolen manufacturers in securing passage of the "Burial in Woolen Act" of 1666. This act provided that woolen cloth should be substituted for linen in the shroud and in the lining of the coffin, but that no penalty should be enacted for burying a plague victim in linen.

Because this act was frequently disregarded, amending statutes were added in 1678 and 1670 providing that a relative of the deceased must swear to an affidavit attesting to the use of a woolen shroud. (*See Figure 1*.) A heavy fine, part of which was given to the informer, was assessed for violation of this law. In spite of these sanctions, many people disobeyed the law, preferring to pay the penalty rather than bury their relatives in wool. Sometimes the law was successfully violated by covering the body with flowers or hay. Not until 1814 were these peculiar acts, passed to aid manufacturers rather than to improve funerals, repealed.[62]

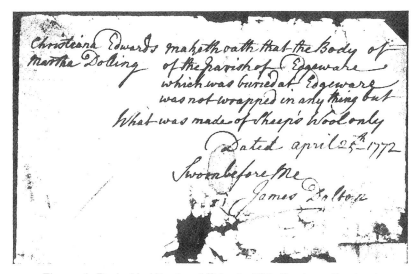

Figure 1: Buried in Woolen Affidavit, 18th Century, England.

The Free Distribution of Mourning Clothes: A curious medieval custom was that of distributing ceremonial robes to mourners. Originally, the mourning garment — called a "weed," although the term is now restricted to "widow's weeds" or a "doole," something given away in dolour, a double etymological pun — was a long black cloak similar to those worn by nuns. It was designed as an outer garment; large enough to fit many sizes of people since, obviously, it could not at short notice be prepared in carefully personalized and tailored fashion; and to completely cover ordinary attire.

Garments of this type were provided by close relatives of the dead for other relatives, the clergyman conducting the services, intimate friends and poor retainers (to the last, as an act of charity). At the funeral of the Earl of Oxford, more than 900 black gowns were distributed in spite of the fact that the deceased had been heavily fined during life by Henry VII (1457-1509) for excessive display of wealth.

Such extravagance led to sumptuary regulations in England in the 16th century "restricting the use of mourning as to quantity and dictating also the quality of materials, and the exact manner in which the garments were to be fashioned."[63]

As funerals grew in elaborateness, it was to be expected that establishments would develop devoted exclusively to the sale of mourning garments and other funeral paraphernalia. Such business in France, called a *Magasin de Deuil*, was long antedated in Italy by the *Mercerie de lutto*, from which Italians could buy or rent in a few hours all that was needed to conduct a respectable funeral in a country in which climate made speedy burial a necessity.[64]

English Burial Fees During the Waning Middle Ages: In a large parish like Cripplegate, there was an obvious gradation of dignity of burial according to the importance of the dead. A few, such as the poet John Milton (died 1674), were buried within the church in leaden coffins; others, who paid full burial fees, received like interment in the churchyard; but the majority for whom burial dues were remitted were laid to rest in a sheet, uncoffined, in a part of the graveyard set aside for the poor.[65]

The nature of the burial fees in England can be seen from those set up for the parish of St. Saviour's Southwark: "In any churchyard next the church, with a coffin, two shillings, eight pence; without a coffin, twenty pence; for a child with a coffin, eight pence; without a coffin, four pence; the College Churchyard, with a coffin, twelve pence; without a coffin, eight pence."[66]

Mourning Colors: Mourning colors owe their choice partly to resemblance, real or imaginary, between the facts of death and burial and certain colors, and partly to the operation of that whimsical thing called fashion. How much of fashion there is in funerary color selection can be seen in the fact the ancient Egyptian and Burmese adopted yellow; the Persians and Abyssinians, brown; and the Armenians and Syrians, light blue. White, symbolizing hope, is the mourning color of the Chinese, as it is, for a different reason, among certain aborigines, who smear their bodies with white clay as a sign of bereavement. The choice of color in this case might originally have been accidental.[67]

Although, in modern times, black is the generally approved color for mourning, white coffins for children are still customary, and purple is used to designate death and mourning for royalty and many Christian groups. These conventional uses represent changes from the earlier practices of the Roman Empire, in which white became the mourning color for women, and from the general practice of the Middle Ages throughout western Europe, when white was the color of mourning worn by all.

The vogue of black was given a powerful impetus in 1498 when black was substituted for white by Anne, the widow of Charles VIII of France,[68] even though Mary Queen of Scots, as late as 1560, mourned the death of her second husband, Lord Darnley, in white.

The French King Louis XI (reigned 1461-1483) forsook purple, the customary mourning color of the French court, for a hunting suit, half red and half white, pleading that he did so "for the sake of simplicity."[69] He did not set a new fashion thereby. Mortuary custom is in part based on an intrinsic seemliness in things in which frivolity has small place.

The Widow During the Middle Ages — Her Lot and Her Raiment: Special conventions governed the conduct and clothes of the widow during the long period when marriage was universally regarded as indissoluble and sacramental, and remarriage was considered with disfavor, except in the case of a very young woman. For the widow of an important man, it was customary to retire to a convent, or to live in strict seclusion in the "dower house" garbed as a nun, honoring the virtues of her late spouse in retrospective contemplation by the practice of spiritual and corporal works of mercy.

Puckle sees in this self-immolation and lifelong imprisonment the shadow, at least, of the earlier practice that required the widow actually to be sacrificed and buried with her husband so that he might enjoy her comforts in the afterlife.[70]

Curious customs of dress were also associated with widowhood. One of these was the wearing of the *barbe*, a long pleated arrangement of fine linen, so called because it resembled a beard (*barba* in Latin). The position of the *barbe* was determined by rank. Lower orders wore it beneath the chin; those above the rank of baroness, above it.

The widow's bonnet, now seldom seen, was derived from the nun's habit, its streamers a survival of the veil, now thrown back and reduced in size, but originally covering the face.

The widow's cap represents the ancient custom of cutting off the hair as a sign of mourning or renunciation. While the widow "admitted the principle, she was no longer prepared to part with her hair," Puckle comments.

The white cuffs worn by a widow as a symbol of mourning also stemmed from the convent.

The higher their rank, the more rigidly were women bound by the mourning etiquette of their times and position. Prior to the 15th century, a widowed queen kept to her black draped apartment for a year after her husband's death.[71]

Local Customs Add Color: Within the framework of the general cultural beliefs and practices, much latitude existed in the Middle Ages, as now, for the development of local customs. The list of these is long. It is a widespread custom among Protestants, for instance, to sprinkle a handful of dirt on the corpse, an act reminiscent of the Roman custom of covering a body found unburied with at least three handfuls of earth while reciting the ceremonious farewell.

The custom of sprinkling earth on the coffin was formally instituted for the Church of England by a rubric, or rule for conducting the liturgical service, as an assigned part of the duty of the officiating clergy. Later, any bystander could make the gesture.

The Jews placed a bag of earth in the coffin, and each mourner helped fill the grave with earth.

Among the Irish, it was an old custom that the priest should bless and sprinkle a handful of earth upon the corpse before burial. The pious construed this deed as appeasement of the other occupants of the churchyard.[72]

Possibly as a disinfectant against the plague, at all English funerals a sprig of rosemary was handed to all who attended the burial rites. The sprig was later thrown into the open grave. This custom was still found in England past the middle of the 19th century.[73] A similar custom, substituting carnations and other flowers pulled from floral pieces, was long observed in America. (***See Plate 13***.)

It was long customary in various parts of Christendom to bury the clergy with their feet extending toward the east, in the belief that Christ would there appear to summon the world to judgment. Thus, the clergy would be first to arise and lead their flocks to the great tribunal. From this practice, the east wind in Wales is called the "Wind of the Dead Men's Feet."[74]

A nod should be given to customs that disappeared. Puckle tells of a curious functionary, a sort of male scapegoat called the "sin-eater." It was believed in some places that by eating a loaf of bread and drinking a bowl of beer over a corpse, and by accepting a six-pence, a man was able to take unto himself the sins of the deceased, whose ghost thereafter would no longer wander.[75]

Customs that were local, or general customs that have ceased to be followed, should be distinguished from mere individual eccentricities, such as the upside-down burial of Richard Hull. In accordance with a notion once popular that, on the day of judgment, the world would be turned around, Hull is buried upside down on his horse beneath a stone tower on Leith Hill in Surrey, England.[76]

Medieval Preoccupation With the Physical Side of Death: Funeral practices in part depend on the *zeitgeist*, the spirit of the time shaping the view men take of death. For whatever reason — could it have been the fact and threat of periodic plague, or the inevitable reaction of individuals who lived with dangerous zest? — the Middle Ages manifested an intense preoccupation with the physical side of death. "Charnal houses" (structures in which human skeletons were stored) were a common sight. The bodies of executed prisoners were suspended from trees so that others might profit from the lesson. Poets sang of death as robbing the body of beauty, power or sensuality. Statues and woodcuts displayed death at its most horrible — as ugliness, putrefaction, filth.

The cry, "Memento mori" — "Remember that thou wilt die" — wails through the long period and is characteristic of it. The great Dutch historian Johan Huizinga points out that the imploration to remember death reached poor and great alike. The poor heard it through the preaching of the mendicant orders, the tolling of the funeral bell, and the cry in the streets, "Bury your dead." The rich heard the message in the sermons of men like Denis the Carthusian, who reminded his audience that when a nobleman lay down in bed at night, "he should consider how, in the same manner as he now lies down himself, strange hands will soon lay his body in the grave."[77]

The greatest of the didactic plays of the Middle Ages, called "morality plays," is *Everyman*, which comes out of the early 15th century. The plot concerns Everyman, who, as his name indicates, represents the human race. In the play, God calls on his servant, Death, to summon

Everyman to judgment. But Everyman is "full unready his reckoning to make" and, when Death proves obdurate, Everyman pleads with Fellowship, Kindred, Cousin, Goods, Knowledge, Beauty, and other companions to enter the grave with him. They refuse, and so he turns to Good Deeds, unbinds him by being shriven, and enters the grave, while the Doctor tells the audience that, at the last, all things forsake Everyman save Good Deeds. It is a grim "sermon on the boards" (a grave play), but quite characteristic of the age that gave it birth.[78]

More terrible than this stately drama was the death dance, which came into vogue during the Middle Ages as a result of popular, morbid preoccupation. To the men and women of these times, death was a commonplace fact to be stared at, and because few bodies were properly preserved, people became engrossed with the disposition of the body rather than with the afterlife of the soul.

It is easy to understand how the theme of the dance macabre, once conceived, planted itself in the popular imagination and there found fertile soil for growth. This grisly theme was expounded by the woodcuts of Guyat Marchant, the poetry of Jean LeFevre, the murals of the church of LaChaise-Dieu, the frescoes of the cloister of the churchyard of the Innocents at Paris. The theme later led to Holbein's dancing skeleton, and, much later, to Goethe's *Totendanz*.

As people grew obsessed with it, the spiritual side of death seemed less engrossing and less important. The note of promise, the "sleeping in Christ" that characterized the Christian viewpoint, is drowned out in fearsome noises from the grave for those who are caught up in the cult of the gruesome. One is enveloped and preoccupied with the fear of one's own death; not the fear of living no more, or of being punished for one's sins, but the fear of dying and decaying with other corpses, naked, with clenched hands and rigid feet, mouth agape and bowels crawling with worms. Here was death graphically and symbolically represented without sentimentality, spoken of without euphemism, lived with starkly and morbidly.

Even funeral decoration was influenced. It was not uncommon in the 14th century for painters to picture the dead as rising from their graves to join in the dance macabre in search of new members for their fellowship. Even tombs were decorated with images of decaying corpses.[79] (***See Plate 15***.)

The Sexton Emerges: With the growth of the practice of churchyard burial, the Church of the early Middle Ages naturally extended its authority over the burial processes and, at the same time, burials began to lose their domestic or neighborhood character. The desire to be interred near the church and near some saint, martyr or holy person brought revolutionary changes in burial practices. As Wilson and Levy point out:

> The rise of the church as an expression of organized Christianity and Christian worship changed the whole aspect of the burial problem. A new epoch opened with public burial in churches and in churchyards, which brought with it profound changes in the popular attitude towards burial and the disposal of the dead. The religious outlook on death began to assume importance: the solicitude of the living for the bodies and spirits or souls of the dead was invested with religious sanctions and brought about, ere long, the first decisive break with the past by prescribing communal instead of local places of sepulture, sanctified by their associations with Christian worship.[80]

PLATE 15

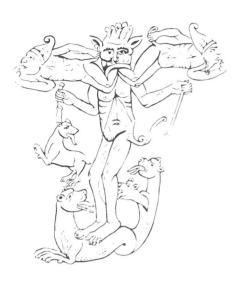 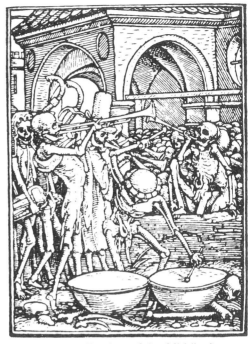

15A. (Left) Death Devouring Man and Beast, Tapestry Design of the Middle Ages.
15B. Bones of All Men, an Early Woodcut by Holbein.

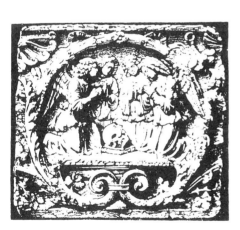 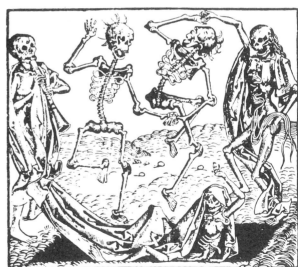

15C. (Left) Angels Praying Over a Skull, 16th-century Bas-relief.
15D. "Danse of Death," Nohl.

During the early Middle Ages, there apparently was no secularized person to whom were entrusted any, several or all of the burial tasks, as they had been entrusted to the *libitinarii* and *pollinctores* among the pagan Romans. The occupation of sexton emerged at this time. The sexton was originally an under officer of the church, to whom were delegated the care of church property, the ringing of bells, and, frequently, the digging of graves. This absence of mention of other functionaries makes it apparent that, until the early Renaissance, the tasks of undertaking, earlier assigned to secular officials, were undermined, proscribed or absorbed by the officials of the church.

An exception to the foregoing statement is found in embalming for mortuary purposes. An infrequent practice at the beginning of the Middle Ages, it grew to be far more common by the close of the Renaissance.

We have seen that the Hebrews limited their preservative techniques to the application of oils, perfumes and spices to the surface of the body, seeking to preserve it not for eternity but only until the sepulcher should be closed at the end of the three-day vigil.

The early Christians, as previously noted, regarded the body as the temple of the Holy Spirit and generally looked with disfavor upon Egyptian embalming methods as involving mutilation. In spite of this attitude, however, there is well-established evidence that some primitive Christians were embalmed, and that some had their organs removed for independent burial.

Such development is not surprising in view of two facts. The first is the continued use of Egyptian embalming methods by the pagan Romans. While only a small minority, even among the rich and powerful, continued to be embalmed, the practice was widespread throughout the Roman Empire during the three centuries after Christ. Thus, in A.D. 66, the body of Poppaea, wife of Emperor Nero, was embalmed in Egyptian fashion before interment in the Mausoleum of Augustus; and in A.D. 95, the body of Annia Priscilla, wife of Flavius Abascantus, freedman secretary of the Emperor Domitian, was mummified and laid in a marble sarcophagus.[81] In this case, there was a literal tendency even for Christians to do as the Romans did "when in Rome."

The second circumstance tending to break the prejudice of the early Christians against embalming was the close association of their primitive places of meeting and worship with their cemeteries and with the relics of the saints and martyrs. Bradford points out: "Early Christians primarily disfavoured the mutilation of the body, but subsequently, as a consequence of their churches being built over the tombs of the martyrs and their altars hallowed with their relics, they came to look at things in a new perspective."[82]

Independent Heart Burial: This new embalming perspective gave rise to the preservation of dismembered bodily fragments of saints and martyrs, which were regarded as holy relics. While Bradford dates the beginning of the practice of independent heart burial with the enshrinement in 1117 of the heart of D'Arbrissel, founder of the Order of Fontevrault, he asserts that, in essence, such separation of parts was ancient and could be traced to evisceration, "which had been in vogue from the later Stone Age and elaborated by the Egyptians with a highly developed ceremonial, of which the embalming of the dead became a leading feature — special prominence being given to the heart."[83]

The heart of St. Ignatius (died 107) has been preserved as a relic. The Emperor Sigismund is reputed to have brought to England the heart of St. George (died 303) when he was made Knight of the Garter in 1416. The crypt of the church of St. Benoit-on-the-Loire exhibits a reliquary said to contain the heart of St. Benoit (died 547). The heart of St. Catherine of Sienna is said to be interred beneath the high altar of the Church of St. Mary Supra Minerva in Rome.

Whether these separations of the heart from the body were made immediately after death or later is not clear, but some 700 years after the death of St. Benoit, the body of Peter, Bishop Poitiers, was entombed at Fontevrault, while his viscera were given burial at St. Cyprian's Church in Poitiers. Two years after this, the remains of D'Arbrissel, to whom reference has just been made, were separated and his heart was buried at Orsan Monastery while the remainder of the body was buried in the town of Fontevrault itself.

Other instances of the ceremonial interment of the heart apart from the body have been recorded. In 1235, for example, the heart of Abbot William of St. Albans was buried apart, near the altar of St. Stephens. Royal prestige was lent to the custom by Jeanne, Queen of Navarre, who kept the heart of her husband, King Philip, apart from his body until her death, when, by her orders, it was enshrined in the same urn as her own in the church of the Jacobins in Paris.

In 1480, Rene, King of Sicily, directed in his will that the day after his death, his heart should be borne to the church of the Friars Minor of Angersto to be buried in the Chapel of St. Bernardine.

In 1514, the heart of Anne of Brittany was buried with great pomp at the Carthusian Church at Nantes; in 1621, the heart of Louis of Lorraine, Cardinal de Guise, was buried in pompous ceremony at the Cathedral of Notre Dame of Paris.

In medieval visceral embalming, it was the practice to remove the viscera, together with the brain, eyes and sometimes the tongue, and to place these in a cask that was often buried later with the embalmed body. Such division of the organs made multiple burials easy. English King Edward I (reigned 1272-1307) took advantage of it to have parts of Queen Eleanore's body deposited in three tombs erected in her honor.[84]

Gannal describes how M. Regner, apothecary to the king of France and to Madame la Dauphine, assisted by his eldest son, prepared Madame's heart for independent burial:

> The heart, after having been emptied, washed in spirits of wine and dried, was placed in a glass vessel with its liquor (embalming fluid); and this same organ, having been filled with a balm made of corrella, cloves, myrrh, styrax, and benzoin, was put into a sack of cere-cloth of its own shape, which was again enclosed in a box of lead, cordiform, which was immediately soldered.[85]

Not even a papal decree was able to stamp out this practice of dividing the body for burial, with separate graves for the several portions, and separate funeral rites. Bradford finds that divided burial was "far from rare" in the 17th century, and that there were many instances of it in the 18th and even in the 19th centuries, among which the heart burials of the French statesman Gambetta (1838-1882) and the English novelist Thomas Hardy (1840-1928) were conspicuous.

As much as anything, the development of arterial embalming has served to eliminate the practice today so that evisceration and divided burial are now extremely rare.[86]

Independent Bone Burial: Although much importance was attached to being buried in one's native soil, lack of embalming and refrigeration, together with slow transportation, made it virtually impossible to return home the bodies of those who died in foreign countries. Faced with a similar problem, the Macedonians did not embalm the body of Alexander the Great to return it to his native Macedonia, but preserved it in honey for transit. The Spartans used the same material to conserve the corpse of King Agesipolis I during its conveyance to Sparta for burial.[87]

The Middle Ages developed another practice to facilitate transportation. The poor and the unimportant who met death at a distance from their homes presumably were disposed of where they fell or died. The noble, the rich and the important were sometimes brought back in part — their bodies being cut up and boiled to extract the bones. These were placed in a chest and returned home, while the juices and soft portions were buried not without ceremony near the place of death.

The crusaders considered human remains sacred, and the bodies of many knights who lost their lives in the East were boiled so that the bones could be packed in a chest for Christian burial at home. Pope Boniface III outlawed this practice and pronounced it "an abuse of abominable savagery, practiced by some of the faithful in a horrible and inconsiderate manner."

Despite this, many Englishmen who died in France during the Hundred Years War (1337-1453), including Edward of York and the Earl of Suffolk, both of whom died at Agincourt (1415), were so boiled and buried divided, after a dispensation granted by one of the successors of Boniface.[88]

Embalming in the Middle Ages: While actual funeral or other embalming was not common during the Middle Ages, records show that the art, as derived ultimately from the practices of the Egyptians, was not lost, though actual embalmings were few and far between. As we have seen, the rise of Christianity gradually pushed aside the older pagan burial beliefs and customs and substituted new practices. In this shift, while there is some evidence that a small minority of early Christians in Rome, and particularly in Egypt, were embalmed, embalming itself, whether because of its intimate associations with pagan religions, its costliness, or its attendant mutilation of the body, fell under some ecclesiastical disapproval.

In the 3rd century, St. Anthony, the father of monasticism, denounced the practice as sinful, intimating that the ancient Egyptian rites were out of harmony with Christian doctrine.[89] He probably was protesting, too, against Egyptian death and afterlife beliefs associated with embalming, and attacking the excessive expense of Egyptian funerals. It is not likely that most people of his time regarded embalming as sinful, in and of itself, even though it had extremely limited vogue because only the very wealthy could afford it, or royalty was felt to deserve it.

A few illustrations must suffice. The body of Charlemagne (died A.D. 814), embalmed and dressed in imperial robes, was placed in sitting position in his tomb at Aachen. The body of Edward I of England, buried in Westminster Abbey in 1307, was found intact in 1770.[90] The preserved remains of Canute (died 1035) were discovered in Winchester Cathedral 500 years after his death while, in the 16th century, the body of William the Conqueror was related to be well preserved at Caen.[91]

The corpse of Henry I was embalmed and brought to England in 1135 for burial in the Church of Reading Monastery. The process employed in his case consisted in the removal of the brain, tongue, heart, eyes, etc., by means of incisions, and embalming with various drugs. The viscera were interred in the Church of St. Mary de Pre at Emandriville. The salted, eviscerated body was later shipped, wrapped in a tanned bull's hide,[92] according to the custom of the time.

In 1281, Cecily Talmache of Hamstead, Suffolk, was embalmed at a charge of six pounds, five shillings and four pence, a total made up of the following itemized costs: for wax and spices, four pounds, four shillings and two pence; for fine linen and silk, one pound, twelve shillings; for the chandler, nine shillings and two pence. Sir John Cullum commented that this sum would purchase 28 quarters of wheat.[93]

Although, as Bradford points out, "Sanitary reasons dictated evisceration and embalming as a corollary to the practice of intramural interment, and was in active operation in the early twelfth century," it must be concluded that embalming could not have been widespread in the medieval period, as descriptions of medieval cemeteries indicate.[94]

Moreover, as will be seen, the shortage of persons capable of embalming would have prevented the practice from becoming other than highly infrequent. But even had skilled practitioners been available in large numbers, the cost of their services, and of the rare spices, chemicals, unguents and wrappings, all of which were considered necessary, would have put the process far beyond the means of all except the very wealthy. Yet not even these were commonly embalmed. When, for example, Princess Mary died in 1481, her unembalmed body was wrapped tightly in a long cerecloth and placed in a leaden coffin. When the coffin was opened in 1810, the body was in an excellent state of preservation due to the very secure wrapping that had excluded the air.[95]

Although embalming was not commonly practiced in England during the Middle Ages, it was reported in *Gentleman's Magazine* in 1789 that there was discovered in the village church in Danbury, Essex, a preserved body, sheeted in lead and boxed in an elm coffin. When the lead was opened, the body was revealed lying wholly perfect in a "liquor or pickle resembling mushroom catchup." Someone tasted the preservative and found it like "catchup, and of the pickle of Spanish olives."[96]

Great interest in embalming was aroused by the fact that the bodies of certain saints, such as that of St. Rose of Viterbo, were said never to have decayed. Such resistance to decomposition appeared the more remarkable in view of the fact that, in certain Paris cemeteries, flesh disappeared from the bones in as little as nine days.[97]

Distressing experiences with unembalmed or poorly embalmed corpses could not but help but point to the need for better methods of preservation. When Queen Elizabeth I died, although her wish was respected that she should not be embalmed, Chancellor Lord Burleigh gave orders to her surgeon to "open her."

Lady Southwell gives an account of the sequel to this dramatic episode: "Now the Queen's body being cered up, was brought by water to Whitehall, where being watched every night by several ladies, myself that night watching as one [of] them, and being all in our places about the corpse, which was fast nailed up in a board coffin, with leaves of lead covered with velvet, her body burst with such a crack that it splitted the wood, lead and cere cloth; whereupon the next day she was fain to be new trimmed up."[98]

The Surgeon and the Anatomist Take Over: While the Middle Ages carried over the Egyptian practice of cavity embalming, this era did not carry with it the highly skilled Egyptian embalming team. Yet, during this period, the task was assigned for funerary purposes to a group already experimenting with it for other ends.

Until the rise and development of the craft guild produced the barber-surgeon, medieval embalming was more or less a secondary function of the surgeon and anatomist. Whether they sought this function or not, it was theirs by reason of the fact that their normal occupations gave them an acquaintance with the body — albeit extremely limited, it is true, in many regards.

Further, they had access to surgical texts that contained instructions on embalming, such as Pietro d'Argellata's, and they were probably inquisitive enough to welcome the chance to work with a body before it had deteriorated and become obnoxious with decay.

Cadavers, moreover, were hard to obtain and, unless they were preserved, the effort to dissect them became a race against putrefaction. Hence, the anatomist and the surgeon had strong motivation for experimenting with embalming. In the early 14th century, the practice was established in Italy of acquiring the bodies of executed criminals for the purpose of performing "anatomies." Due to the lack of embalming, it was necessary to eviscerate the corpse and then hurriedly dissect it before the odor of putrefaction made further work impossible.[99]

Quite possibly, too, when the medieval surgeons and anatomists turned their anatomical and embalming skills to the preparation of the corpse of an important person in burial, they exacted a substantial fee for their services.

The art of the medieval medical embalmer closely resembled that of his Egyptian prototype. The most obvious, and therefore often the first step, was to remove those parts of the body most susceptible to rapid decomposition: the intestines, stomach, liver, pancreas, kidneys and esophagus. On occasion, as an added precaution, the tongue, eyes and brain were also removed.

The opened and eviscerated body cavities were then washed with water, alcohol and a pleasant-smelling substance, such as rose water. After the cavities were dried, they were filled with a variety of spices, chemicals and an absorbent, such as cotton. This filling served a three-fold purpose. It aided in drying out the body, gave it a pleasing odor, and helped preserve its natural shape.

The body openings themselves were filled with tar or oakum (loose fibers picked from old hemp ropes) to prevent the entry of insects. Finally, the body was securely wrapped in many layers of cloth to reduce contact with the air and to check decay.

It is most likely that Galen of Pergamon (A.D. 130-200), whose autocratic influence dominated medicine for almost 1,300 years, left some account of embalming in his works. His was the voice that carried early medicine from A.D. 200 through the Middle Ages, until the publication of *De Corpora Humani Fabrica* by Vesalius in 1453.

The excellent description of Egyptian cavity embalming left by the Greek Herodotus (about 484-424 B.C.) should be compared with Pietro d'Argellata's of the embalming of Pope Alexander V, who died at Bonnea in 1410.

In his *Chirurgia*, a treatise on surgery in six books not published until 1480, Pietro d'Argellata (died 1423), professor of anatomy at the University of Padua, gave the earliest complete account of medieval embalming, describing three variants of the basic cavity method. (***See Plate 16***.) He was the pupil of Guy de Chauliac (1300-1368), whose works bear a strong resemblance to the writings of Paul of Aegina, a Byzantine Greek of the 7th century who wrote *Epitome of Medicine* in seven books, practiced in Alexandria, and might be regarded as the last representative of Greek medicine before the Arabian conquest.[100]

Says d'Argellata:

> Nevertheless I relate this method to you as it is the same one used to embalm the highest pontiff, Pope Alexander V. His doctor opened up the abdomen to the pubis, making a straight line incision without injuring the viscera, tying up the colon in two places, cutting it between the two ligatures, leaving out the waste. The rest of the intestines were then removed together with all the viscera. He then used a sponge and washed everything clean with alcohol, and proceeded to pour alcohol into the body. He then used a sponge to dry up any moisture that was left. He then filled the whole abdominal cavity with one pound of aloes, caballainies, succatrinol, acaciae, nucis xuperuni, Galluae, and muscatae. Then he covered the abdomen with cotton, powder, and more cotton, repeating this until the whole cavity was filled, after which the domestic appeared and sewed the body up in the same manner in which a furrier would sew up furs. They then put powder into the cavity of the esophagus and larnyx, filled it with cotton adding balsam. They put egg white into the rectum. They then made a few more tufts of cotton and put them into the mouth, nostrils, and ears. After all this they covered the entire body with waxed linen to which a little turpentine was added. They also put his thighs and arms close to the body and covered them with linen. When finished they put his ornate Papal cloak on him because he had to lay for eight days without giving offensive odor. This method of embalming the Doctors of that era liked best. In this way the putrefaction of the dead body was prevented. The face of the Pope was washed with thoroughly salted rosewater.[101]

In the same work, d'Argellata is the first to mention the use of low temperatures to retard decomposition, a physiological innovation that remains useful to the present time.

In an early treatise on embalming written subsequent to the Middle Ages (1605), Peter Forestus, a Dutch physician, describes the embalming experiences of other physicians in some detail:

A renowned doctor from Spirigio embalmed the princess Joan from Burgundy. In 1582 the Countess of Hautekermaken was embalmed by the writer before he knew that the task had been assigned Professor Heurnie of Leyden, Holland. He likewise embalmed Prince Auraici, who died July 10, 1584, in collaboration with a colleague, Dr. Cornelius Busenius.[102]

In the first thousand years of the Christian era, there had been considerable retreat in the practice of medicine and surgery, and in the study of anatomy.[103] To explain, in part, this lack of progress, Park, the medical historian, points out that "dissection was forbidden by the clergy in the Middle Ages on the ground that it was impious to mutilate a form made in the image of God."[104]

While agreeing generally with Park's argument, Riesman says in extenuation of this viewpoint of the Middle Ages that, earlier, there had been little dissection; that Egyptian physicians had not practiced it; and that while it might have been carried on to some extent in the Alexandrian school, it was not a common practice among the Greeks and was definitely forbidden to the Arabs by the *Koran*; so that all through the era of Arabian domination in medicine and surgery, the science of human anatomy lay dormant. And this in spite of the fact that without dissection, no medical advance could be made beyond Galen, whose own work had not been based on dissection.[105]

The first serious anatomist of the Middle Ages was Mondino de'Luzzi ("Mundinus," 1270-1326), who served as professor at the University of Bologna from 1314-1324 and had the advantage of dissection, even though his actual experience was limited to two cadavers and he did not emancipate himself from the authority of the ancients.[106]

The limitations under which anatomists worked can be seen in the decree of the enlightened Hohenstaufen Emperor Frederick II (1194-1250), making it lawful for each anatomist to dissect the human body at least once in every ten years.[107]

By and large, the European anatomists of the early Middle Ages were persecuted and hindered in their studies; and, finding it difficult to secure corpses, sought means to preserve those they had as long as possible.[108]

Perhaps the closest alliance between medicine and religion during the Middle Ages took place in and around cloisters during the period of monastic medicine. Certain monks and churchmen practiced medicine, perhaps out of necessity, as intelligent, educated men with access to most of the learning of the day and much collective experience fortified by common sense. They spent a great deal of time translating older medical texts — Greek, Arabic, Latin, etc. — into colloquial Latin.[109]

From the close resemblance between the techniques of medieval embalming and the practices of the Egyptians, it is reasonable to assume a direct link between the two. Beyond exceptional cases, however, there is little evidence of any extensive use of visceral embalming during this period. The knowledge, more than the practice, was preserved.

The Reformation and Christian Funeral Beliefs and Practices: The question of indulgences, or remission of part of the temporal punishment due to sin, was tied up with the doctrine of purgatory, and was a major point at issue in the dispute between Martin Luther (1483-1546) and the Roman Catholic Church. With the rejection of the doctrine of purgatory

16. Portion of a Treatise on Embalming, d'Argellata, 15th Century.

by the reformers of the 16th century, and of the mass and the mediation of the priesthood, the groundwork was laid for changes in funeral customs and practices based on these beliefs.

Full change did not come instantly, so ingrained are habits. While the final result in England, for example, was "so radical that little of the ancient ritual remained," Davey observes that it took much longer to penetrate the habits and customs of people than is usually imagined.[110]

The new service of the Church of England, compiled in 1546-1547, consisted of scriptural passages in conformity with a religion that rejected belief in purgatory, and therefore in the validity of prayers for the dead. Little by little, older practices disappeared.

Down through the reign of Queen Mary Tudor (died 1558), a lying-in-state period was common practice, even for the poor, as it gave an opportunity for relatives and friends to gather and to pray for the departed soul. The Reformation ended this custom in England, except for those of high rank who lay in state chiefly for purpose of review and ceremony.

With the abolition of monastic orders, and burial and purgatorial brotherhoods, guilds and leagues, the funeral street processions that once followed the bier lost much solemnity. The solemnity of the Requiem Mass went with the Reformation, as did vestments, candles, incense and holy water. Growing puritanism found an outlet in the Vestiarian Controversy, in which a group within the English Church sought further to strip away the residuum of Roman Catholic externals of worship.

Thus, in successive steps, pageantry yielded to plainness. With the Counter-Reformation in Catholic countries on the continent, the ceremonial of the Church moved in an opposite direction so that, as Davey observes, "nothing can be imagined more theatrically splendid than the church decorations and ceremonies on occasions of funerals of eminence."[111]

The Reformation did not change the fundamental Christian doctrine that the body, no matter what its decay, is not worthless. The reformers kept the belief in the resurrection of the dead. Christians should therefore be fittingly buried, and burial places should be properly maintained.

Burial was a concern of the Church, to be attended by the congregation, even, if possible, when the poor were buried. The tolling of bells summoned the congregation to a burial, and if all did not come, the minister and schoolchildren, or at very least the sexton and the gravedigger, represented it. On the way to the cemetery, children and mourners sang Christian burial hymns. At the grave itself, prayers were recited, appropriate scriptural passages read, and the passing of alms boxes or collection plates encouraged almsgiving for the poor. Custom in some countries provided that, after the closing prayer, the Creed was pronounced. Burial services in the Reformed Church were very similar to these.[112]

Manifest on every occasion when the congregation gathered was the desire to provide pious instruction and exhortation. A Protestant funeral was no exception. The reading of scripture and the singing of hymns, lessons in themselves, were supplemented by a brief discourse on death and resurrection, which was given in the home, in the church or at the grave. For a fee, the minister prepared and delivered a special sermon, making particular reference to the life and death of the deceased.

Out of this early practice, which joined consideration of the last things — death, judgment, and heaven or hell with the memory of the departed — emerged the Protestant funeral sermon of today. Occasionally, even among the early Protestants, the pious were fond of carrying the cross in the procession and of thrice casting earth upon the body at the grave. Although they were then generally regarded with distrust, these practices have since been widely accepted as additions to the funeral rites.

The benediction of the dead was and is even more mooted. Luther and the Augsburg Confession permitted the blessing of the dead, while the Reformed Church rejected prayers for the dead unconditionally, the blessing among them.[113]

CITATIONS AND REFERENCES FOR CHAPTER 3

1. Arturo Castiglioni, *A History of Medicine* (New York: Alfred A. Knopf, 1947), pp. 245-246.
2. John T. McNeil and Helena M. Gamer, *Medieval Handbooks of Penance* (New York: Columbia University Press, 1938), p. 21.
3. *Ibid.*, p. 202 *seq.*
4. Richard Davey, *A History of Mourning* (London: Jay's, Regent St. W., 1890), pp. 22-23.
5. *Ibid.*, pp. 23-24.
6. *Ibid.*, p. 34.
7. Stephen Wickes, *Sepulture: Its History, Methods and Sanitary Requisites* (Philadelphia: P. Blakiston Son & Co., 1884), p. 44 *seq.*
8. *Ibid.*, p. 46.
9. *Ibid.*, p. 48.
10. J.F.A. Adams, *Cremation and Burial* (1875) A reprint of a review, the name of which is not given. The article is to be found in the pamphlet collection of the Cremation Society, Vol. II, p. 267. Quoted in Wilson and Levy, *op. cit.*, p. 12.
11. Bernardini Ramazzini, *De Moribus Artificum*, trans. Wilmer C. Wright (Chicago: University of Chicago Press, 1940), pp. 153-155.
12. Wilson and Levy, *op. cit.*, p. 14.
13. Creighton, *op. cit.*, p. 332.
14. Wilson and Levy, *op. cit.*, p. 13.
15. Creighton, *op. cit.*, p. 334. Quoting *Remembrancia*.
16. *Ibid.*, p. 11.
17. Stone, *op. cit.*, p. 17.
18. Ralph of Coggeshall, Rolls series, No. 66, p. 112. Quoted in Creighton, *op. cit.*, p. 11.
19. Creighton, *op. cit.*, p. 12.
20. Castiglioni, *op. cit.*, p. 361.
21. Quoted in Creighton, *op. cit.*, p. 156.
22. *Ibid.*, p. 336.

23. Davey, *op. cit.*, p. 63.

24. *Ibid.*, p. 54.

25. Wilson and Levy, *op. cit.*, p. 82.

26. Puckle, *op. cit.*, pp. 34-35.

27. Quoted in Stone, *op. cit.*, p. 68.

28. McNeil and Gamer, *op. cit.*, p. 121.

29. *Ibid.*, pp. 318-319.

30. *Ibid.*, p. 333.

31. Puckle, *op. cit.*, p. 64.

32. *Ibid.*, pp. 102-104.

33. Davey, *op. cit.*, p. 34.

34. *Ibid.*, p. 38.

35. Stone, *op. cit.*, pp. 174-176.

36. *Encyclopedia Britannica*, 1890, Vol XIX, p. 164 *seq*.

37. Creighton, *op. cit.*, p. 649 *seq*.

38. Stow's *Memoranda*. Camden Society, New Series, XXVIII (1880) p. 125. Quoted in Creighton, *op. cit.*, p. 336.

39. After Puckle, *op. cit.*, p. 184.

40. *Ibid.*, p. 185.

41. *Ibid.*, p. 185.

42. See also C.J. Polson, ed., *The Disposal of the Dead* (London: English Universities Press, 1953), pp. 299-300.

43. See Genesis 50:26.

44. Herodutus, *History of the Persian Wars*, Book III. Quoted in Wickes, *op. cit.*, pp. 134-135.

45. Wickes, *op. cit.*, pp. 134-136.

46. *Ibid.*, p. 135.

47. *Ibid.*, p. 136.

48. Davey, *op. cit.*, pp. 137-138.

49. *Ibid.*, pp. 34-39.

50. Puckle, *op. cit.*, p. 42.

51. *Ibid.*, p. 116. Quoted from William Andrews.

52. Creighton, *op. cit.*, Vol. II, pp. 36-37; Davey, *op. cit.*, p. 139.

53. Charles Cox, *The Parish Registers of England* (London: Methuen & Co., 1910), p. 120.

54. Sylvia Thrupp, *The Merchant Class of Medieval London* (Chicago: University of Chicago Press, 1948). p. 152.

55. *Ibid.*

56. *Ibid.*, p. 153.

57. *Ibid.*, p. 154.

58. Sir Ernest Pooley, *The Guilds of the City of London* (London: Collins, 1947), p. 8.

59. Puckle, *op. cit.*, p. 84 *seq.*

60. *Ibid.*, pp. 40-42.

61. Stone, *op. cit.*, p. 55.

62. Polson, *op. cit.*, p. 8; Creighton, *op. cit.*, p. 37; Davey, *op. cit.*, p. 139.

63. Puckle, *op. cit.*, p. 65.

64. Davey, *op. cit.*, pp. 86-90.

65. Baddeley, *Parish of St. Giles, Cripplegate* (London, 1888), quoted in Creighton, *op. cit.*, Vol. I, p. 335.

66. *Old Southwark and Its People* (London 1878), quoted in Creighton, *op. cit.*, Vol. I, p. 335.

67. Polson, *op. cit.*, p. 10; Puckle, *op. cit.*, p. 162.

68. Polson, *op. cit.*, p. 10; Puckle, *op. cit.*, p. 93.

69. Puckle, *op. cit.*, p. 93.

70. *Ibid.*, p. 90.

71. *Ibid.*, pp. 91-94.

72. *Ibid.*, pp. 162.

73. Davey, *op. cit.*, p. 55.

74. *Ibid.*, p. 138.

75. Puckle, *op. cit.*, pp. 69-70.

76. *Ibid.*, p. 161.

77. J. Huizinga, *The Waning of the Middle Ages* (London: Edward Arnold Company, 1924), pp. 124-135.

78. J.S. Tatlock and R.G. Martin, *Representative English Plays* (New York: The Century Co., 1924), "Everyman," pp. 31-44.

79. Huizinga, *op. cit.*, pp. 124-135.

80. Wilson and Levy, *op. cit.*, pp. 9-10.

81. Friedlander, *op. cit.*, Vol. II, p. 212.

82. Charles A. Bradford, *Heart Burial* (London: George Allen & Unwin, 1933), p. 5.

83. *Ibid.*

84. *Ibid.*, pp. 5, 6, 14, 56, 58.

85. J.N. Gannal, *History of Embalming (and of Preparations in Anatomy, Pathology, and Natural History)* (Paris, 1838), trans. R. Harlan, M.D. (Philadelphia: Judah Dobson, 1840), pp. 113-115.

86. Bradford, *op. cit.*, pp. 5, 6, 14, 19.

87. Friedlander, *op. cit.*, Vol. II, p. 212.

88. Huizinga, *op. cit.*, pp. 128-129, 333.

89. Creighton, *op. cit.*, Vol. I, p. 159.

90. *Encyclopedia Americana* (1932) Vol. X, p. 273.

91. *Encyclopedia Britannica* (1929) Vol. VIII, p. 384.

92. Bradford, *op. cit.*, p. 23; Puckle, *op. cit.*, p. 41.

93. p. 31.

94. Simon Mendelsohn, *Embalming Fluids* (New York: Chemical Publishing Company), pp. 10-12.

95. Bradford, *op. cit.*, p. 133.

96. *Gentleman's Magazine*, 1789, quoted in Polson, *op. cit.*, p. 217.

97. Huizinga, *op. cit.*, p. 133.

98. Davey, *op. cit.*, p. 45.

99. David Riesman, *The Story of Medicine in the Middle Ages* (New York: Paul B. Hoeber, 1935), pp. 3-8 *passim*. Charles Joseph Singer, *A Short History of Medicine* (London: Oxford, 1928).

100. Richard A. Leonardo, *History of Surgery* (New York: Froben, 1943), pp. 118-120.

101. Quoted by Thomas Greenhill in the *Art and Knowledge of Embalming* (London: 1705) from the account of the embalming of Pope Alexander V in the 29th book of Peter Forestus, who in turn drew directly upon Pietro d'Argellata's *Chirurgia*. See also Fielding H. Garrison, *An Introduction to the History of Medicine* (Philadelphia: W.B. Saunders, 1929).

102. Peter Forestus, "On the Art of How to Embalm the Dead Human Body," in *A New Medical Treatise, Embracing the External and Internal Pathological Ulceration of the Whole Human Body*, edited by Petrum Offenback, M.D. (Frankfort am Main: Printed by Zachariane Palthemium, 1605), translator unknown. In the collection of the National Foundation for Funeral Service Library in Evanston, Illinois.

103. Riesman, *op. cit.*, pp. 3-8 *passim*.

104. Roswell Park, *An Epitome of the History of Medicine* (Philadelphia: F.A. Davis, 1908), p. 3.

105. Riesman, *op. cit.*, p. 173 *seq*.

106. Leonardo, *op. cit.*, p. 114.

107. *Ibid.*, p. 120.

108. Bradford, *op. cit.*, p. 27.

109. Castiglioni, *op. cit.*, pp. 292-294.

110. Davey, *op. cit.*, p. 54.

110. *Ibid.*, pp. 50, 54.

112. Jackson, *op. cit.*, pp. 307-309.

113. *Ibid.*

Chapter 4

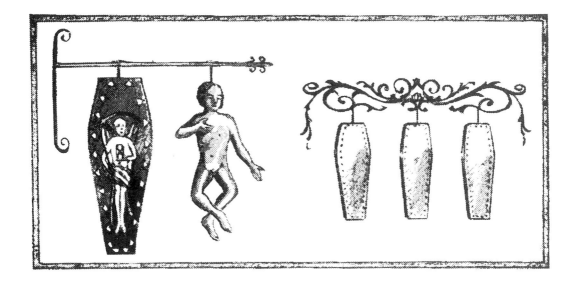

Medical Embalmers and the Rise of English Undertakers

We have seen thus far that while, at various times and in various places, there have been persons set aside by custom, law or both to carry out the several procedures required for the burial of the dead, there is no unbroken line extending from the modern funeral director back to the ancient Egyptian team of funeral functionaries.

Only in embalming can we discover some kind of continuity. And even in this specialty, while the link between today and ancient Egypt is unbroken, there were almost 1,500 years during which funeral embalming was rarely practiced — and even then it was carried on only incidentally and secondarily by someone primarily engaged in an occupation other than the burial of the dead.

This chapter will continue to follow the development of embalming from the late Middle Ages to relatively modern times, and it will trace the beginnings and growth of a new, lay occupational group: the English tradesman undertaker. It will also show how this new group gradually took unto itself a number of functions relating to the burial of the dead — among them funeral embalming.

With the development of the English funeral undertaker and his American counterpart, we are well on the road that leads to the emergence of the modern American funeral director.

Embalming and the Growth of Medical Science: From the 9th century on, a slow breaking away from Egyptian practices is to be noted in the writings of physicians and surgeons on the subject of embalming. Rhazes (9th and early 10th century), d'Argellata (15th century), Forestus (16th century), and Clauderus (17th century) all suggest some breaking with the past.[1]

If, by the 15th century, decomposition was a morbid preoccupation, it was also something of a challenge, and with the revival of interest in anatomy and surgery, correlative with the rebirth of secular or lay medicine, physicians began to show a professional interest in the preservation of the corpse by other-than-traditional Egyptian methods. In two cases varying widely as to purpose, Huizinga records how, in an effort to keep them intact until burial, the features of Pierre of Luxembourg were touched up with paint; and how, when a heretical preacher of the sect of the Turlupins died in prison before sentence could be passed, the body was preserved in quicklime for a fortnight so it could be burned in public with a living heretical woman.[2]

The artists who drew anatomical plates seconded the demand for better methods of preservation. Most prominent of these was that supreme genius, Leonardo da Vinci (1452-1519). During the course of his anatomical studies, which he eventually summarized in 750 magnificent plates, da Vinci dissected more than 50 cadavers — an unusually large number for the time. While so engaged, he developed a system of venous injection that, years later, might have served as an inspiration to Ruysch and Hunter.

It is not known whether da Vinci ever injected a preservative solution into any of his cadavers, but the mere fact that he anticipated Harvey's injection of the veins by more than 200 years is proof of his anatomical and physiological genius.[3] In any event, regardless of whether da Vinci's techniques were immediately utilized to their full extent for funerary embalming, this proved a precursor of modern embalming procedures.

Although the early counterpart of the modern undertaker did not appear until the 17th century, it is evident that by the 15th, most of the principles of embalming in vogue today were known to medical practitioners. After that time, there remained only the discovery of the circulation of the blood in the early 17th century to stimulate the use of arterial embalming.

At least two centuries before, cavity injection with compounds of metallic salts had been employed. In 1866, the remains of John of Lancaster, Duke of Bedford (died 1435), consisting of a lock of hair and 50 grams of a blackish substance interspersed with globules of metallic mercury, were transferred from a grave in the Cathedral of Rouen to the Museum on Antiquities of that city. LeRoy in 1918 published the results of an analysis of what he supposed was the mercurial embalming preservative employed — the "balsamic mercurial unguent." He was able to identify metallic mercury, phosphates, sulphites, aluminum oxide, ferrous oxide, lime, silicon dioxide, and the oxides of magnesium, sodium, and potassium.[4]

Injection techniques to inflate portions of the body for purposes of tracing the continuity of the blood vessels were practiced by such early anatomists as Jacob Sylvius, Carpi, Eustachius, Stephanus, Malphigi, Gleason, De Graff and Swammerdon. The work of these men was carried on from the mid-15th to the mid-17th century.[5] A 17th-century Florentine physician, Girolamo Segato, is known to have turned the human body into stone by injecting the tissues with a solution of silicate of potash. As a second step, he immersed the body in a weak acid solution.

From these and other instances, it is clear that by the end of the 17th century, the medical world understood the possibilities of injection embalming, even though some physicians, surgeons and anatomists kept their precise techniques a secret. The Dutch professor Fredrick R. Ruysch (1638-1731), while searching for a means of inhibiting putrefaction in anatomical specimens, devised a technique for arterial embalming, but he did not divulge its media and operative details, although it is known that the injection was followed by evisceration.

Credit for first taking this step belongs to Gabriel Clauderus, a German physician who described the process in a work titled *Methodus Balsamundi Corpora Humani, Aliaqua Majora Sine Evisceratione*. Meanwhile, in England, William Harvey (1578-1657), physician, anatomist and greatest of physiologists, injected colored solutions into the arteries to support his theories concerning the circulation of blood. He announced his discovery to his pupils in 1618. Although his researches are basic to modern embalming techniques, their full utilization for this purpose was not immediately made.[6]

The 18th century witnessed further great advances in both arterial and cavity embalming. In his lectures, Dr. William Hunter (1718-1783), the great Scottish anatomist, included directions for the use of arterial and cavity embalming for preserving the human body not only for laboratory use but also for burial. Because Hunter was the first to report fully and openly the fluid and method to be used, he is generally considered the originator of the injection technique of preserving human remains.

Utilizing his brother's methods, John Hunter, younger brother of William, continued to prepare anatomical specimens and, in 1775, embalmed the body of the wife of Martin Van Butchell, the eccentric London dentist, employing both cavity and injection techniques. During this celebrated embalming, Hunter, assisted by Cruickshank the surgeon, employed oil of turpentine and camphorated spirits of wine for arterial injection, and camphor for cavity packing.

Van Butchell subsequently kept the body on display, attired in fine garments, in a glass-lidded case in his sitting room. "The dear departed," he called his wife when introducing her to guests.

As news of the exhibit spread, Van Butchell was so besieged by curiosity seekers that he was compelled to announce, "no stranger can see his embalmed wife unless... at any day between nine and one, Sunday excepted." When Van Butchell remarried after some years, his second wife objected to her predecessor's remains, and they were removed to the Museum of the Royal College of Surgeons in London.[7]

By 1800, physicians, surgeons and anatomists in many parts of Europe were improving old embalming processes or experimenting with new ones. Leaders in the field during the 19th century included Dr. Matthew Baillie; the Neapolitan, Dr. Tranchini; the Frenchman, Dr. Falconry; the Irishman, Dr. Morgan; the Englishmen, Drs. Marshall and Pettigrew, the latter an authority on Egyptian mummies, as well as a physician; and the Russian, Dr. Tschniernoff.

While the medical profession was improving embalming techniques, a new specialist, the chemist, was providing better fluids with which to work. Of the earlier chemists to be concerned with embalming, the best known was the Frenchman Jean Nicholas Gannal, whose *History of Embalming* remains one of the few classics dealing with the subject.

The Role of the Barber-Surgeons in Embalming: Leonardo da Vinci tells us in his *History of Surgery* that the barbers of monasteries were called "Barbers and Reducers." The latter title referred to the fact that, among other methods of healing, they reduced the quantity of blood in their patients; that is, they were bloodletters. Monks were obliged to have the crowns of their heads shaved regularly for the tonsure and, in some monasteries, were bled five times a year.

From the early 12th to the late-13th century, in seven councils, the Church forbade the clergy to practice medicine on the grounds that men who had taken religious vows should have concern for the care of the soul rather than for that of the body; that the Church abhorred the shedding of blood; and that churchmen should not touch matters that could not openly be talked about.

But the practice of bloodletting was still the vogue and, since it was forbidden to the monks, medieval barbers, who already had some experience with it, took up the process.

For the barber, bloodletting led into more general surgery and, from this humble beginning, ultimately arose the trade of the barber-surgeons, or "Surgeons of the Short Robe," as distinguished from the latter day surgeons of the College de St. Come, who wore long robes. Lay though they were, the barber-surgeons thus traced their origins to the days of monastic medicine.

With the rise of guilds in the late Middle Ages, theirs became a powerful craft, united by corporate bonds. As such, they possessed group organization and solidarity; restricted admission to their ranks; exercised strict domain over the right to embalm; took measures to see that their members were fit to carry out the practice of surgery, of which embalming was an important subordinate skill; and addressed the law with the voice of authority.[8]

Although from Egyptian times to the present there had always been embalmers, until the rise of the guild system in Europe and the assumption of authority by the barber-surgeons, there existed no single group that exercised strict control over the embalming process and perpetuated the tradition through generations. The success of Ambrose Pare, a barber-surgeon and the father of modern surgery, elevated the prestige of the barber-surgeons to the detriment of the Surgeons of the Long Robe.[9]

In 1550, Pare described the embalming practice of his time:

> Our countrymen the French embalm the bodies of their Kings and nobles with spices and sweet ointments... *but the bodie which is to bee embalmed with spices for very long continuance, must first be embowelled, keeping the heart apart that it may be embalmed and kept as the kinsfolk think fit*: also the brain shall be taken out. Then you shall make deep incisions along the arms, thighs, etc., to let out the blood and give space for putting in the aromatic powders. The whole body should be washed over with aqua vitae and strong vinegar, wherein shall be boiled wormwood, aloes, coloquintidi, common salt, and alum. Then the spices... shall be stuffed in

and the incisions sewn up, and then let the whole bodie bee anointed with turpentine dissolved with oil of roses and camomile, adding if you think fit, some chymical oils of spices, then let it be strewed over again with the forementioned powder, then wrap in a linen cloth and then in searcloths. Lastly let it be put in a coffin of lead and filled up with dry sweet herbs.[10]

A document dated 1389, found in a bundle of papers dealing with the fraternities and guilds of the city of London, delineates the purposes of the Fraternity of Barbers of that place, and provides some indication of the antiquity of the guild and its significant funeral practices:

ITEM. That when any brother of the said Fraternity dies the brethren of the said Fraternity shall go on to the Vigil to the dirge, and on the day (of the funeral) to the Mass, and to the dirge and to the mass of the month's obit, and that each such brother dead have thirty masses from their common box and that each brother who is absent without reasonable excuse at any of the said four times, shall put into their common box in place of his offerings and expenses, as he ought to have done if he had been present, three pence.[11]

On October 20, 1604, the barber-surgeons of London decided to apply for a new charter enumerating 27 clauses that they desired to have included. The sixteenth clause declared:

...openinge searinge and imbalmeinge of the dead corpes to be pply belongeinge to the science of Barbery and Surgery, And the same intruded into by Butchers Taylors Smythes Chaundlors and others of mecanicall trades unskillfull in Barbery or Surgery, And unseemely and unchristian lyke defaceinge disfiguringe and dismembringe the dead Corpes, And so that by theire unskillfull searinge and imbalmeinge, the corpes corrupteth and groweth... pntlie contagious and ofensive to the place and psons approachinge.[12]

Although the barber-surgeons had been embalming in England for more than two hundred years, only at the beginning of the 17th century did they find it necessary to obtain a formal decree that, of all men, they alone possessed the right "to open, seare and imbalm" the corpse. Thus, in addition to the sixteenth, the twenty-fifth clause of the new charter, obtained within three months, read:

No butcher, tailor, waxchandler or other persons (are) to cut, dissect, or embalm any dead body, but the same (is) to be done by members of the Company approved and appointed by the Masters or Governors of the Barber-Surgeons.[13]

On January 7, 1646, the barber-surgeons of London invoked their charter rights against a Mr. Michael Makeland. *The Annals* recount the incident:

Mr. Michaell Makeland appearing to this Court at the request of our Mr (Master) he was here complayned of to have embalmed severall humane Bodyes within this City against the Ordinance of this Company in that behalf being an Apothecary and not a Surgeon approved according to Law.[14]

Makeland's appearance marks a step forward in the history of funeral undertaking. He is the first person known by name to take positive action to break the prerogative of embalming legally assigned to medical and surgical practitioners.

Again in 1652, the company of barber-surgeons rose to defend their exclusive chartered right to embalm. The entry of October 26th reads:

> This daie it is ordered that at the chardge of the howse the pnte... Masters wth the Clark shall seeke in the Rowles for the charter of the wax chaundlers and to tak a coppie of that pte of the charter touchinge the libertie gyven unto them for the imbaulmynge of dead bodyes And as they shall finde the same soe to take the advice of my lord cheife Justice about the same at the chardge of the howse.[15]

How they fared in the matter was not recorded.

The Emergence of the Funeral Undertaker: It bears repeating that by the middle of the 17th century, the barber-surgeons of London invoked the law in an effort to defend their exclusive right to embalm. Such action to prevent infringement is indication that, by accident or design, other occupational groups — butchers, tailors and wax chandlers among them — were being called upon to give a service that, for one reason or another, the chartered group was not giving in the manner or, more likely, at a cost the customer desired.

Two conclusions present themselves from the foregoing material. The first is that funeral undertaking as a clear-cut, distinct secular occupation had not appeared in Europe before the 17th century. The second is that embalming developed as a medical specialty long before, and independent of, undertaking.

The appearance of facts and ideas can sometimes be roughly dated by the appearance of names for them in the language. The words "embalmer" and "undertaker" offer an interesting case in point. "Embalm" as an English word is of the 14th century. Its first written English use on record, according to the *Oxford Dictionary*, was in 1340 in the phrase, "They... with oynements the body embawnyd." Its immediate origin was in the French word "enbaume," which, in turn, had been derived from the Latin "balsamum," "balsam," and, farther back, from the Greek "balsomon." To embalm was to preserve with a balsamic resin or aromatic oil.

Prior to 1340, it is likely that any printed reference made to the process in England would have been in Old French or Latin. The use of the word in Middle English in 1340 merely indicates that funerary embalming in England antedated Chaucer (1340-1400), who himself used the phrase, "Let the corse embalm" in 1385.

In 1587, De Mornay speaks of "lmbalmers... of dead bodies," and Bacon in 1626 remarks that, "The Romans... were not so good embalmers as the Egyptians." By 1600, the terms "embalm" and "embalmer" probably had a standardized, if not wide, usage, in England.[16]

Significantly, for the present consideration, the word "undertaker," in the sense of one who prepares the dead for burial and takes charge of and manages funerals, has no history of comparable length in English usage. As early as 1400, the term "undertaker" can be found, but it describes one who "undertakes" a task or enterprise with no reservation as to the nature of this task. Through the 17th century, it also carried the same meaning as "underwriter," that is, one who provides the financial backing for an enterprise.

The first suggestion that the word might have been used in its present, highly circumscribed sense is found at the end of the 16th century in connection with the duties of heralds. Heralds were chartered in 1483, with their duties elaborately defined in 1600 by the solicitor-general Sir John Doddridge, as being concerned with the granting of coats of arms, the recording of pedigrees, and the supervision of funerals.[17]

In discussing the heralds, Barron speaks of Garter King Sir William Dethick, who served from 1586 to 1605. Barron describes Dethick as irascible, so much so that he would "brawl at funerals with the minister or the undertaker."[18] This statement contains the suggestion that, while the herald supervised funerals, someone else — an "undertaker" — undertook to provide some of the funerary paraphernalia.

If such a functionary existed at this time, his services were probably not made available to ordinary folk or used by them. Homans' study, "English Villagers of the Thirteenth Century," shows that the Church controlled all aspects of the burial of the dead except the "lychweake" or death watch ("lich" or "lych" is a Scottish- or English-dialect word meaning "corpse"), a folk custom according to which neighbors and friends sat up with the dead, meanwhile eating and drinking.[19]

Feudal Funerals: Long after the feudal period passed in England, and after its rigmarole, paraphernalia, machinery and titles ceased to have much real meaning in describing the actual social, political, economic and military relations of people, the pageantry persisted. Strangely enough, after it ceased to have real uses during the later feudal period on through the Renaissance, heraldry and pomp reached its peak development.

Significantly included in the conspicuous display that underlined and emphasized a highly stratified social order was the elaborate funeral to which the title "feudal" has since been attached. Even in a country in which social control has been perpetuated as much by ceremony as by law, and in which the age-old deposit of social dramaturgy is carefully husbanded for constant reuse, the elaborate feudal funeral seems inordinately lavish when compared to the ceremonies marking other human events, such as marriage and birth.

Originally, the trappings of a feudal funeral were family owned — yards upon yards of black drapery for the chief rooms and the staircase; an elaborate black mourning bed; funeral carriages; a velvet pall; a hearse with "hatchment" (a panel upon which the deceased's coat of arms were temporarily displayed); mourning clothes and mourning gifts... enough somber materials to change the usual hearty feudal home atmosphere to one of blackest gloom.

The purchase of these goods and this equipment was enormously expensive and, as a result, the cost of an upper-class funeral in England, especially the funeral of a noble person, was an excessive drain upon his estate.

With this fact in mind, Bradford surmises that the trade of undertaker, "unknown in England before 1688," arose that year "from a desire to retrench the enormous expense incurred by the less wealthy families in providing their own coaches, hangings, and other furniture for every funeral."[20]

The term "undertaker" in its modern sense goes back at least to 1698, at which date its present usage was recorded in a parish register: "The furnishing of funerals by a small number of men called undertakers."

Mencken notes that "it ["undertaker"] once had a formidable rival in *upholder*, the original meaning of which was a dealer and repairer of old furniture... traced by N E D (*New English Dictionary*) to 1333, but it does not seem to have come into use to designate a funeral contractor until the beginning of the 18th century."[21]

At least one unidentified 17th-century poet referred to the "upholder":

> Th' upholder, rueful harbinger of death,
> Waits with impatience for the dying breath;
> As vultures o'er a camp, with hovering flight,
> Snuff up the future carnage of the fight.[22]

As late as 1938, an undertaking firm in the Kensington district of London still clung to the quaint title of "funeral upholders,"[23] although the term had long since lost currency.

The first appearance of "undertaker" in American Colonial newspapers to designate one who undertakes to supply the funerary paraphernalia and services seems to have been in 1768.[24] However, it might have had ordinary verbal usage somewhat earlier.

Coffins, Funeral Goods and the Early Undertaker: We have seen that, while the use of coffins for persons of importance extends into antiquity, the popular practice of coffined burial developed only in the last several hundred years. As late as 1820, Lord Stowell's decision in "Gilbert vs. Buzzard" established the point that, while it is an offense to the body "to be carried in a state of naked exposure to the grave" a coffin is not "of the same necessity."[25]

"Friendly Societies," descendants of the earlier Leagues of Prayer and burial guilds, continued to arrange for the burial of the lower classes.[26] Part of the manner of operation of a burial society toward the end of the 17th century is revealed in an unidentified public notice quoted by Ashton:

> This is to give Notice that the Office of Society for Burials, by mutual Contribution of a Halfpenny or Farthing towards a Burial, erected upon Wapping Wall, is now removed into Katherine Wheel Alley in White Chappel, near Justice Smiths, where subscriptions are taken to compleat the number, as also at the Ram in Crucifix lane in Barnaby Street, Southwark; to which places notice is to be given of the death of any Member, and where any Person may have the Printed Articles after Monday next. And this Thursday about 7 o'clock Evening will be Buried by the Undertakers the Corpse of J.S., a Glover over against the Sun Brewhouse, in Golden Lane; as also a child from the Corner of Acorn Alley in Bishopsgate Street, and another Child from the Great Maze Pond, Southwark.[27]

Ashton also lists an early 18th-century undertaker's advertisement. From it, clues can be gathered as to the service he and his kind rendered and the goods they provided during the reign of Queen Anne:

PLATE 17

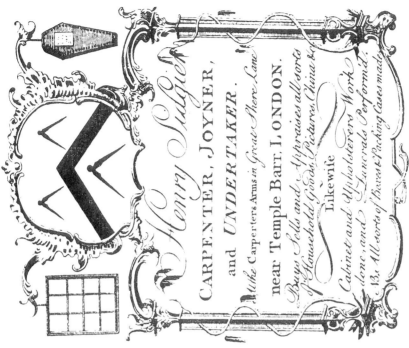

17C. Part-time Undertaker, 18th-century English Tradesman's Card.

17A. Early 18th-century English Funeral Invitation.

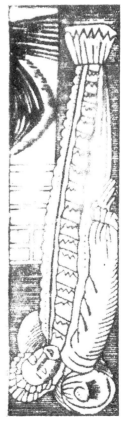

17B. Corpse Lying in State, 18th-century Drawing.

> For the good of the Publick, I Edward Evans, at the Four Coffins in the Strand, over against Somerset House; Furnish all Necessaries for all sorts of Funerals both great and small. And all sorts of set Mourning both Black and Gray and all other furniture suitable to it, fit for any person of Quality. Which I promise to perform 2s. in the Pound cheaper than any other of the Undertakers in Town or elsewhere.[28]

The handbills of undertakers of this period were filled with decorative details indicating a morbid preoccupation with the grisly side of death — "grinning skulls and shroud clad corpses, thigh bones, mattocks and pickaxes, hearses and what not."

If some undertakers made a sideline of upholstery, some drapers made a sideline of furnishing funerary goods. A late-17th- or early 18th-century notice informed the public that:

> ...Mr. John Elphick, Wollen Draper, over against St. Michael's Church in Lewes, hath a good Hearse, a Velvet Pall, Mourning Cloaks, and Black hangings for Rooms to be Lett at Reasonable Rates. He also Sells all sorts of Mourning and Half Mourning, all sorts of Black Cyprus for Scarfs and Hatbands, and White silks for Scarfs and Hoods at Funerals; Gloves of all sorts, and Burying Cloaths for the Dead... Prices of the Newest Fashions, and all sorts of Ribbons, Bodies and Hose, very good Penny worths.[29]

Coffined burial involved the making of wooden coffins, a skill already possessed by carpenters, cabinetmakers, joiners and other workers in wood; thus, these artisans found themselves drawn into the new and vaguely defined occupation of undertaking:

> Eleazar Malory, Joiner at the coffin White Chapel, near Red Lion Street end, maketh Coffins, Shrouds, letteth Palls, Cloaks, and Furnisheth with all other things necessary for Funeral at Reasonable Rates.[30]

Eighteenth-century tradesmen's cards provide additional information concerning the emerging undertaker's trade. A collection of these by Ambrose Heal[31] shows cabinet-makers, carpenters, upholsterers and undertakers — using such titles as the "Arms of the Carpenters' Company," "Chair and Tea Chest," "Four Coffins," "Royal Bed," and "Three Covered Chairs and Walnut Tree" — advertised their goods and services in language sometimes quaint, sometimes amusing, but always revealing:

> YOU MAY BE FURNISHED WITH ALL SORTS AND SIZES OF COFFINS AND SHROUDS READY MADE AND ALL OTHER CONVENIENCES BELONGING TO FUNERALS.
>
> SAFETY FOR THE DEAD. SIR WILLIAM SCOTT HAS DECIDED THE RIGHT TO INTER IN IRON.
>
> FUNERALS DECENTLY PERFORMED.
>
> VELVET PALLS, HANGINGS FOR ROOMS, LARGE SILVER'D CANDLESTICK AND SCONCES, TAPERS FOR WAX LIGHTS, HERALDRY FEATHERS AND VELVETS, FINE CLOTH CLOAKS AND MIDLING DO. RICH SILK SCARVES, ALLAMODE AND SARSNETT HAT BANDS, BURYING CRAPES OF ALL SORTS.[32]

It is worth noting that this advertising emphasizes two points: the wide range of funerary goods made available, and the protection of the corpse.

Heal has also assembled shop signs of the late-17th and most of the 18th centuries. In them, the preoccupation with the physical and gruesome side of death is apparent. The undertaker's favorite insignia is the coffin, usually hanging vertically, and often inscribed or decorated with skeletons, skulls, crossbones or other grim emblems. The earliest of such signboards, dating from about 1680, identified the business establishment of William Boyce, "at ye Whight Hart & Coffin in ye Grate Ould Bayley, near Newgate."

Others, mostly in the early 18th century, include such grim designations as the "Naked Boy and Coffin," "Four Coffins," "Crown and Coffin," "The First and Last" and the "Three Coffins." (*See Plate 18*.)

Other signboards told of the coffin-plate makers and the coffin-plate chasers or engravers.

Carpenters also announced their shops, which might have been undertaking establishments. It was not beyond possibility that undertakers hired cabinetmakers to make coffins in connection with their lines of furniture. An early 18th-century signboard (*see Plate 18*) directs attention to:

> George Smithson, Broker, Undertaker and Sworn Appraiser. Opposite the Bull and Gate, Holbourn, London Buys and sells all sorts of Household Goods and at Reasonable Rates. NB. Funerals Performed.[33]

The curious assortment of vaguely related tasks joined in one establishment under the versatile George Smithson is, in itself, clear indication that, as of date given, the occupation of funeral undertaker had not emerged in England as a well-defined, highly specialized trade, even though the undertaker was a recognized tradesman, at least by the end of the 17th century.

If, on the one hand, his occupational role grew simpler by the gradual elimination of certain tasks, such as brokerage and appraisal, it also grew more complex, on the other hand, by assimilating new and closely related tasks, such as embalming.

Among the round of activities of the modern funeral establishment, embalming is so universally regarded as a legitimate function of the establishment itself, to be performed by the staff of the establishment, and so uniquely the occupational prerogative of that staff, that it is difficult even to imagine today how another occupational group once could have claimed this function to itself and attempted to deny it to the tradesman undertaker. Yet, as we have seen, such was the strange fact.

Tradesman Undertaker and Medical Embalmer: With the renaissance of lay medicine, surgery and anatomy in the 15th, 16th and early 17th centuries, embalming became, as we have seen, one of the prerogatives of the surgeon or barber-surgeon, even though its funerary use was limited to the wealthy or important (and not all of these were embalmed).

Whatever the reason — it might have been cost, or it might have been the lack of surgeons and anatomists to carry the load of business, or their unwillingness to give the necessary time to increased demands for their services, although this is not likely in view of their complaints

— at the opening of the 18th century, the undertaker himself was practicing a crude form of embalming.

In his earliest comedy, published in 1702, *The Funeral, or Grief a la Mode*, Sir Richard Steele, better known for his *Spectator Papers*, has the undertaker ask his hired assistants:

"Have you brought the Sawdust and Tar for embalming? Have you the hangings and the Sixpenny nails for my Lord's Coat of Arms"? (The hatchment must be put up, and mutes must be stationed at intervals from the hall door to the top of the stairs.) "Come, you that are to be Mourners in the House, put on your Sad Looks, and walk by Me that I may sort you. Ha you! a little more upon the Dismal. This fellow has a good Mortal look, place him near the Corpse; that Wanscoat face must be o' top of the Stairs: That Fellow's almost in a fright (i.e., full of some strange misery) at the Entrance of the Hall. So! but I'll fix you all myself. Let's have no laughing now on any Provocation; Look Yonder, at that Hale, Well looking Puppy! You ungrateful scoundrel, Did not I pity you, take you out of a Great Man's Service, and show you the Pleasure of receiving Wages? Did I not give you Ten, then Fifteen and Twenty Shillings a Week to be Sorrowful? and the more I give you, I think the glader you are."[34]

This quotation goes beyond demonstrating the absorption of the task of embalming into the undertaker's routine — "Sawdust and Tar" embalming, it is true. It also emphasizes another role coming into the undertaker's bundle of tasks — the dramaturgic role, in which the undertaker becomes a stage manager to create an appropriate atmosphere and to move the funeral party through a drama in which social relationships are stressed and an emotional catharsis or release is provided through ceremony.[35]

The feudal period dramatized death with high ritual, it is true, but the ceremonies were an integral part of the life of English aristocracy. In the centuries that followed, others of lesser rank who had become prosperous, or those who felt it proper to do better by the dead than had been their lot when alive, sought to imitate the aristocratic funeral of the earlier period.

To meet these demands, undertakers who had previously provided a limited portion of the funeral were forced to do more. They found it necessary to hire functionaries — mutes, mourners, liverymen and the like — to stage or organize the funeral. Such undertakers assembled the "cast" — the quick and the dead — supplied the trappings to form the proper setting and create the proper atmosphere of heavy gloom, and sought to coordinate the actions of all involved. In brief, as the funeral became more of a performance, with new roles to be played, the undertaker, in taking charge of these activities, was shaping a new occupation, independent in its own right.

In view of the fact that surgeons and anatomists were an older occupational group, with that of the barber-surgeons a well-organized craft, it is not surprising to find that these entrenched interests regarded the first crude efforts of the funeral undertaker to embalm as an invasion of their occupational domain. Thomas Greenhill's *Treatise on the Art of Embalming* (**see Plate 19**), printed for the author in 1705, is partly dedicated to the cause of rescuing this art from the "tar and sawdust" competition of the undertaker. In this jurisdictional dispute, Greenhill pleads rigorously:

PLATE 18

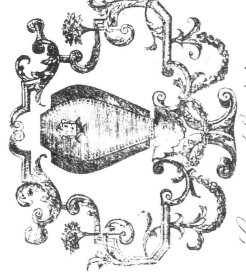

18C. Precursor to Furnishing Undertaker, Tradesman's Card of 1740.

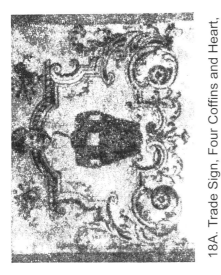

18A. Trade Sign, Four Coffins and Heart, c. 1720.

18B. Whight Hart and Coffin.

>...to see our Profession over-run by *Quacks* and *Mountebanks* and that *Valet de Chambres* are suffer'd to Bleed, dress Wounds, cut Fontanells, and perform the like Operations, is what has reduc'd *Surgery* to so low an ebb. In like manner the noble *Art of Embalming* has been intirely ruin'd by the Undertaker...
>
>...They (the Egyptians) had these several Persons belonging to and employ'd in *Embalming* each performing a distinct and separate Office, *viz.* A *Designer* or *Painter*, a *Dissector* or *Anatomist*, a *Pollinctor* or *Apothecary*, an *Embalmer* or *Surgeon*, and a *Physician* or *Priest*, which last was a great Philosopher, and taught and instructed the others in these Ceremonies, as we shall shew in its proper Place.
>
>By this means, not only the Art of *Embalming* but likewise every branch of Physic, flourish'd and came to the greatest perfection, whereas, in our Age, every Art grows the more imperfect as it encroaches on another, and the civil Wars now a Days between *Physicians*, *Surgeons*, and *Apothecaries* have been the chief occasions of reducing Physic to so low an ebb; for whilst these have been fighting for each others Countries the Monarchy was usurp'd by *Quacks* and *Undertakers*, who are the only Vultures that attend such battles, in order to prey immediately on the vanquish'd Enemy.
>
>Is it not therefore a shame for us, who, no doubt, esteem ourselves a much more polite People than these Heathens were, to suffer a sort of Men call'd *Undertakers* to monopolize the several Trades of *Glovers*, *Milliners*, *Drapers*, *Wax Chandlers*, *Coffin-Makers*, *Herald-Painters*, *Surgeons*, *Apothecaries*, and the like... and 'till such Time as *Quacks* and *Undertakers*, *Hawkers*, *Pedlers* and Interlopers, and all such persons, as were not brought up in the Emploiment they profess, be remov'd we can think no otherwise but that *Art* must sink...
>
>We may as well expect one, that has never seen a Campaign, should understand Military Discipline... as that an *Upholsterer*, a *Taylor*, a *Joyner*, or the like *Undertaker*, should be well skill'd in the misterious *Art of Embalming*.[36]

In addition to single voices of protest such as Greenhill's, the surgeons and barber-surgeons collectively protested against what they considered an invasion of their prerogatives. We have seen that, as early as 1604, in making application for a new charter, the barber-surgeons of London asserted their right to embalm, as against butchers, tailors and wax chandlers; and that, in 1646, they defended that right against an apothecary.

The abortive entrance of the wax chandler into the field of embalming through the field of funeral undertaking merits a word of explanation. During the later Middle Ages, wax chandlers (a "chandler" originally was a maker or seller of candles, in spite of the more common present use of the word to describe a person who deals in groceries, provisions and small wares) had a role in the preparations for funerals, insofar as they furnished the wax candles. The volume of this business was considerable due to the fact that many funeral processions were held at night, candles were used at the wake, wax was needed to seal shrouds and coffins, and pitch was sometimes required to make the coffin watertight, or for crude embalming.

PLATE 19

NEKPOKHΔEIA:
OR, THE
Art of Embalming;
Wherein is shewn
The Right of Burial,
THE
FUNERAL CEREMONIES,
And the several Ways of
Preserving Dead Bodies
IN
Most Nations of the WORLD.

With an Account of

The particular Opinions, Experiments and Inventions of modern Physicians, Surgeons, Chymists and Anatomists.

ALSO

Some new Matter propos'd concerning a better Method of *Embalming* than hath hitherto been discover'd.

AND

A *Pharmacopœia Galeno-Chymica, Anatomia sicca sive incruenta*, &c.

In Three PARTS.

The whole Work adorn'd with variety of Sculptures.

By THOMAS GREENHILL, *Surgeon.*

LONDON: Printed for the Author.

19. Title Page of Early Work on Embalming, Published 1705.

Perhaps it was the chandler's immediate contact with pitch or "tar and sawdust" that motivated him to enter into competition with the surgeon and anatomist, and thus made him the special target for their less-than-successful protests.

In any event, there seems to have been no stopping of cheaper embalming practices offered by various kinds of special tradesmen who, in one way or another, by supplying goods and services, participated in the funeralization and burial of the dead.

Because Europeans accepted embalming half-heartedly, we must turn to America to gain a clearer picture of the manner of the absorption of this and other tasks into the normal round of work now called "funeral directing." Before leaving England, however, we should examine the relationship of the undertaker to workers in two related occupational areas: the clergy and the sanitarians.

Clergy and the Undertaker: While the 17th-century surgeon and anatomist regarded the crude embalming of the funeral undertaker, chandler and others as wholly unacceptable from the standpoint of a decent practice in preservation, as well as an encroachment on their prerogatives, opposition to the growing number and organization of burial functions taken over by the tradesman undertaker came from another group, and for a different reason.

Among the clergy, religious reformers with a social bent were wont to use the churchyard elegy not only to point out the solemn lesson of the equality of all men in the grave, but also to make strictures against specific evils of society. In his poem "The Grave," Robert Blair, an Edinburgh clergyman, summarized the mood of such pronouncements[37] by interspersing his remarks on the vanity of man's pursuits with a section in which he makes a very critical address to undertakers:

> But see! the well-plum'd HEARSE comes nodding on
> Stately and slow: and properly attended
> By the whole sable tribe, that painful watch
> The sick man's door, and live upon the dead,
> By letting out their persons by the hour,
> To mimic sorrow, where the heart's not sad...
> ...But tell us, why this waste,
> Why this ado in earthing up a carcase
> That'h fall'n into disgrace, and in the nostril
> Smells horrible? — Ye UNDERTAKERS, tell us,
> 'Midst all the gorgeous figures you exhibit,
> Why is the *principal* conceal'd for which
> You make this mighty stir? — 'Tis wisely done:
> What would offend the eye in a good picture,
> The painter casts discretely into shades.[38]

To echo the poet's strictures, the editor felt impelled to comment:

> *Pompous funerals* are as *ridiculous* as they are *unnecessary*: *Ridiculous* in respect to the *living*, except in the views of those who reap *pecuniary* advantage from them, and unnecessary respecting the *dead*, who are the principal subject and occasions of them.[39]

From the Reformation to the present, representatives of various denominations have sometimes criticized funeral customs, funeral expenses and the behavior of undertakers, comparing the funerals of more-recent dates with the funerals of primitive Christianity, and alleging that some of the pomp and majesty of the traditional feudal funeral represented a reversion to pagan worldliness and was therefore unbefitting to Christians.

The sable false-front of the post-feudal funeral, with its mummers, hired-by-the-job retainers, and its plumes and paraphernalia, could not help but lend logic to such strictures, particularly when these goods and services were bought, rented or hired with the "widow's mite" (a very small monetary contribution by a poor person). Yet, at worst, 17th-, 18th- and 19th-century undertakers, like any other tradesmen, sold people what they demanded.

Burial and Sanitary Reform: While a segment of the clergy, from the early 17th century on, demanded funeral simplicity in the name of religion, equally vigorous voices demanded it in the name of sanitation. For centuries, intramural burial in England had been accumulating the dead on small plots of ground within cities, until finally resulting in a sanitary problem that could no longer be ignored.

During the cholera years of 1831-1833, some 31,000 deaths in England, and 21,000 in Ireland, compelled the establishment of a public-health agency, which provided an opportunity for the use of the remarkable sanitation research abilities of Edwin Chadwick.[40]

In 1839, under the auspices of the Poor Law Commissioners, Chadwick began to investigate the conditions under which the urban English worker lived, worked and died. In 1842, he summarized the findings in his famous report on the *Sanitary Condition of the Laboring Population of Great Britain*,[41] the supplement to which, *The Practice of Interments in Towns*, describes the burial customs of working people and the conditions of the interment of the dead.

Summing up this report, Finer writes:

> *The Report on Intra-Mural Interments*, published at the end of 1843 was of all Chadwick's Reports the most grisly and revolting. There were descriptions of such places as Russell Court, near Drury Lane, where the ground, raised several feet by continuous burials was "a mass of corruption" which poisoned air and water alike; or that place in Rotherhithe where "the interments were so numerous that the half-decomposed organic matter was often thrown up to make way for fresh graves, exposing sights disgusting, and emitting foul effluvia." There were horrible descriptions of corpse wakes; of dead bodies remaining days and days before burial in the one room which served the family for dining and sleeping alike; of children sleeping, or trying to sleep, under the eyes of the dead man. There were descriptions of child murders committed to realize the moneys invested in the burial club. Chadwick had also to describe the burial of corpses under the flags of the churches, so that however well-coffined, "sooner or later

every corpse buried in the vault of the church spreads the products of decomposition through the air which is breathed, as readily as if it had never been enclosed."[42]

Chadwick's recommendations were far in advance of his time. He wanted all cemeteries "municipalized," and all "trading cemeteries" abolished. Religious rites were to be simplified and standardized. To prevent child murder for insurance — all too common at the time — he recommended that a medical officer should be required to certify before burial as to the fact and cause of death. In 1848, five years after Chadwick made them, many of his recommendations were incorporated into the Public Health Bill.

But his strictures did not go unchallenged. Churchyard burial was not unprofitable to the Church, and some of the clergy objected to his efforts to set up a nationalized cemetery in London. The large cemetery companies that had been burying up to 20,000 dead per acre led the opposition.

Moreover, the mid-century English undertaker took umbrage at his damaging bill of particulars.[43] The charges Chadwick made against the London undertakers were chiefly two: In the first place, although there was intense competition for dead bodies, there was no corresponding decrease in funeral costs. Quite the contrary, costs were so high that a death in the family was a virtual economic disaster. As a result, in greater London, more than 200 burial clubs flourished, a clear indication of the need felt by the poor to spread the cost of burial over a wide number of persons. These "Friendly Societies," as they became more formally organized, were the forerunners of modern "industrial" insurance. The rates charged were relatively excessive, but on the weekly collection basis, the overhead was high. Yet it was the best that the poor could afford.

Not only were undertakers competing with one another to the small advantage of their clients, but, as Lewis points out, there were in and about London "at least a thousand, and perhaps as many as three thousand, lesser tradesmen — drapers, tailors, publicans (tavern keepers), carpenters, cabinet-makers, upholsterers, auctioneers — who displayed the undertaker's insignia in hope of catching one or two orders a year."[44]

Wherever these casual undertakers found a case, they were supplied by one of the principals of the trade, and in "the last analysis it was some sixty of the leading undertakers who performed the real service, the inferior agents merely interposing their unnecessary offices and stepping up the charges to allow for their own remuneration."[45]

Undertakers also sought to work in close cooperation with the operators of burial clubs; worse, it was not exceptional for an undertaker to be president of a club.

If the sanitation movement produced no direct, significant changes in the operation of funeral establishments in England during the second half of the 19th century, it made its influence felt in reforms relating to existing burial grounds and the prohibition of new cemeteries within cities. It was impossible, moreover, to apply stringent regulation to the place of burial without involving undertakers. In passing, it should be noted that, in both England and America, the sanitation movement was in part responsible for the increased practice of cremation.[46]

Yet, before the 19th century ended, in spite of the failure of the sanitation movement directly and immediately to check the excesses of the feudal funeral among the poor, and to put an end to disorganized and duplicative services among the trades engaged in preparing and burying the dead, burial custom and usage gave evidence of bringing order into the funeral trades and of sloughing off some of the pompous display and ceremonial inherited from the previous epoch.

In his *Life and Labor of the People of London*, Booth suggests the degree to which the changes had taken place by the end of the century. In discussing the trades of London, he points out that under the general category of "Funeral Furnishers and Undertakers," there were the subdivisions: "Coffin and Coffin Furniture Makers," "Funeral Furniture" and "Plume Makers." An employer might be either an "Undertaker," or "Funeral Furnisher" or both.[47]

Booth makes it clear that the trade of undertaker was shaping itself into definite form, with subdivisions appearing as a consequence of the need for specialization and division of labor:

> The Undertaker measures the dead body (though there are some who like to be measured while still alive), makes the coffin, or has it made, arranges with the cemetery authorities, provides the carriages and men, and accompanies the funeral to the grave. In all cases it is he who is the director of the funeral.
>
> The funeral furnisher, on the other hand, where he is not also an undertaker, has no personal connection with the conduct of the burial. He may be a wholesale manufacturer, or a job master, providing the undertaker with coffins, carriages, and all the appurtenances of a funeral, or he may be a funeral-carriage master only. In London, the usual practice seems to be for those undertakers who have not enough business to keep a stable fully employed, to make or furnish the coffins and then to apply to the carriage master, known to the trade as a "Black Master," for the hearse, etc.
>
> Coffins are made by "coffin-makers" who belong to this industry only, and do not overlap with either carpenters or cabinet makers. A carpenter might soon learn to make coffins, but a coffin maker could not turn to general carpentry.[48]

While coffin-making in England has broken cleanly with cabinet-making and carpentry on the one hand, and with undertaking on the other, and has become an independent trade, it has also ceased to be the central symbol of the group of tasks related to burial, as it was formerly. In its place is undertaking, emerging likewise into a distinct occupational type in which the personality of the undertaker, who is the director of the death ritual, weighs heavily.

Booth also notes:

> It is more important to have a strong, presentable man, with a good suit of black clothes of his own, than a highly skilled workman. And further, respectful, and if possible, sympathetic manners, are especially necessary; for future orders depend much on the satisfaction of present customers and their consequent recommendations.[49]

In summary, the evidence points to the development in England of a specific trade of undertaking far removed and different from its dispersed beginnings in the 17th century among lay "Jacks of all Trades" who sold funeral goods and services.

At the close of the 19th century, the rise of the undertaker, who gathered functions formerly scattered over several trades into a unified single occupational task, was partly to be accounted for by the inability of the Church to keep authority over all aspects of the burial of the dead; partly by the development of new techniques of preservation by the anatomist, the surgeon and the chemist, together with the inability of these workers to retain complete control over the funerary uses of their discoveries; and partly by a changing social order, in which urbanization threw aside the funerary vestiges of the feudal system, but retained the "decent funeral" as a social axiom.

This new type of funeral involved the erection of a "front," usually suggestive of a social status somewhat above the actual life position of the deceased or the bereaved, and increasingly required ceremonies of disposal directed by a person who could not only take charge of other funeral tasks but, with skills beyond the competence of the average person, also organize and direct the funeral. In answer to popular demand, the funeral undertaker made such services available for a fee.

Thus, the modern undertaker emerged in England in the shape of a competitive occupational service specialty engaging in a trade primarily for pecuniary purposes.

In turning from this consideration of the development of the English undertaker to that of the American funeral director, we should remember that there are, as we shall see, many good reasons for asserting that, while there has been considerable cultural interchange between the two English-speaking countries, there also has been much independent development. The American counterpart to the English undertaker developed against a social, economic, geographical, cultural and occupational background quite different in pertinent regards from that of England. To understand the differences in the end product, it is necessary to understand the differences in the development processes.

For this reason, the next several chapters will move to the American scene and trace the history of funeral service in America, from Colonial times to the present day.

CITATIONS AND REFERENCES FOR CHAPTER 4

1. See Johnson, *op. cit.*, Chapter II.

2. Huizinga, *op. cit.*, p. 128.

3. See Leonardo, *op. cit.*, pp. 126-127; Mendelsohn, *Embalming Fluids*, *op. cit.*, p. 12.

4. Simon Mendelsohn, "Embalming from the Medieval Period to the Present Time," *Ciba Symposia* (Published by Ciba Pharmaceutical Products, Inc., Summit, N.J., May, 1944), pp. 1805-1812.

5. Mendelsohn, *Embalming Fluids*, *op. cit.*, p. 12.

6. *Ibid*.

7. C.J.S. Thompson, *The Quacks of Old London* (Philadelphia: J.B. Lippincott Co., 1929), pp. 322-324.

8. Sidney Young, *Annals of the Barber-Surgeons of London* (London: Blades, East and Blades, 1890), p. 112.

9. Leonardo, *op. cit.*, pp. 118-119.

10. Bradford, *op. cit.*, p. 27 *seq.*

11. Young, *op. cit.*, p. 33.

12. *Ibid.*, pp. 111-112.

13. *Ibid.*, p. 114.

14. *Ibid.*, p. 218. Bradford states that the act of 1511 forbade anyone to practice as a surgeon in London without the approval of the Bishop of London or the Dean of St. Paul's. See Bradford, *op. cit.*, p. 29.

15. Young, *op. cit.*, p. 331. Spelling in the above four references varies due to editor Young's decision to use modern English or the language of the period.

16. Note its use in Greenhill, *op. cit.*

17. Oswald Barron, *Shakespeare's England* (Oxford: At the Clarendon Press, 1916), p. 80 *passim.*

18. *Ibid.*, p. 81.

19. George C. Homans, *English Villagers of the Thirteenth Century* (Cambridge, Mass: Harvard University Press, 1941), pp. 391-393.

20. Bradford, *op. cit.*, p. 13.

21. H.L. Mencken, *The American Language*, Supplement I (New York: Alfred A. Knopf, 1945), p. 571.

22. Quoted from *Trivia* in John Ashton, *Social Life in the Reign of Queen Anne* (New York: Charles Scribner's Sons, 1925), p. 35.

23. Mencken, *loc. cit.*

24. See Chapter 6.

25. See Wilson and Levy, *op. cit.*, pp. 80-82.

26. See J.L. and Barbara Hammond, *The Bleak Age* (New York: Penguin Books, 1934), p. 226 ff.

27. Ashton, *op. cit.*, p. 38.

28. *Ibid.*

29. *Ibid.*, p. 36.

30. *Ibid.*

31. Ambrose Heal, *London Tradesmen's Cards of the XVIII Century* (London: B.T. Batsford, Ltd., 1925).

32. *Ibid.*, pp. 22, 61-62.

33. Ambrose Heal, *The Signboards of Old London Shops* (London: B.T. Batsford, Ltd., 1947), pp. 174-175, Plate XVCVI.

34. Quoted in Ashton, *op. cit.*, pp. 35-36.

35. For a further discussion of this function of the funeral director, see Chapters 10 and 13 of this book.

36. Greenhill, *op. cit.*, pp. vi, 177-179.

37. Robert Blair, *The Grave: To which is added Gray's Elegy* [*written*] *In a Country Church Yard. With Notes Moral, Critical, and Explanatory*, by G. Wright (London: Scatcherd & Whitaker, 1785).

38. *Ibid.*, pp. 14-15.

39. *Ibid.*, p. 15.

40. R.A. Lewis, *Edwin Chadwick and the Public Health Movement 1832-1854* (London: Longmans, Green & Co. 1952).

41. Sir Edwin Chadwick, *Report on the Sanitary Conditions of the Labouring Population of Great Britain* (London: W. Clowes and Sons, 1843).

42. Samuel E. Finer, *The Life and Times of Sir Edwin Chadwick* (London: Methuen & Co., 1952), pp. 230-231.

43. *Ibid.*

44. Lewis, *op. cit.*, pp. 70-71.

45. *Ibid.*, p. 71.

46. For a detailed account of the relation of the sanitation movement to the practice of cremation in contemporary England and America, see Robert W. Habenstein, "A Sociological Study of the Cremation Movement in America," *op. cit.*, Chapters I-IV.

47. Charles Booth (ed.), *Life and Labor of the People of London*, 9 vols. (London: Macmillan and Co., 1895), vol. V, p. 205.

48. *Ibid.*, pp. 205-206.

49. *Ibid.*, p. 206.

PART TWO:
The Rise of American Funeral Undertaking

Chapter 5

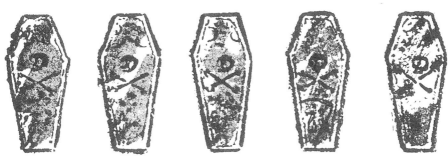

American Colonial Funeral Behavior

American Colonial settlements were founded, in the main, by English-speaking people seeking fortune, fame, freedom of religious organization or, simply, the chance to acquire a decent human existence. To this country they brought a body of beliefs and institutions, skills, arts and crafts — a social heritage that remains a basic substructure to the distinctive American mode of living.

Yet, for many reasons, not the least of which was the impact of non-English-speaking peoples on an emergent American culture, the New World society cannot be represented as a simple extension of the Old. This is particularly true with regard to funeral behavior for, although there are basic similarities, the modifications and developments in the organization of American funeral practices led to a vastly different response to the problems of death and the disposal of the dead.

Part of the task of developing a history of funeral service in America consists, then, in sketching out some of the more basically relevant ideological elements, whether socially inherited or acquired by new experience, which lie behind Colonial funeral customs.

Ideological Framework for Colonial Funeral Practices: The Virginia Colony, founded in 1607 at Jamestown, had as its underpinning a distinctly commercial motif. The impulse behind the Massachusetts Bay Colony, on the other hand, was primarily religious, although its charter was obtained from and underwritten by commercial interests. Interestingly enough, the underwriters, in common language usage, were called "undertakers," and the commercial referent continued through most of the 17th century.

Having no quarrel with the established Church of England, the Virginia colonists incorporated it into their government, where it remained, along integrated church-state lines, until after the Revolution. The pilgrim fathers, conversely, rejecting not only the Anglican but also all other denominations and sects except their own creed, set up a theocracy that continued for more than a century.

In neither case, however, was there any reason compelling the disassociation of death and the disposal of the dead from a sacred or religious context. On the contrary, as will be seen, death became one of the prime occasions for pulpit exhortations on the essential mortality of mankind and the need for more exemplary ways of living.

Although it can scarcely be argued that American funeral behavior took on distinctive characteristics through secularization (i.e., a disassociation of religious belief from the phenomenon of death), there were, nevertheless, certain developments in the organization of religious beliefs that had either an immediate or eventual effect on the funeral practices of the colonists.

One of these was the early Puritan removal of the clergy from certain ceremonial functions, including funerals. The Old World source of this usage is illustrated, for example, by a section of *The Directory for the Publick Worship of God, agreed upon by the Assembly of Divines, at Westminster; examined and approved anno 1645, by the General Assembly of the Church of Scotland*, etc., presenting the following rule:

> Concerning Burial of the Dead: When any person departeth this life, let the dead body, upon the day of burial, be decently attended from the house to the place appointed for public burial, and there immediately interred without any ceremony.[1]

And, in an earlier instance, the Independents in 1604 published at Amsterdam in *An Apologie or Defense of such true Christians as are commonly (but unjustly) called Brownists*:

> ...the celebration of marriage and burial of the dead, be not ecclesiastical actions appertaining to the ministry, but civil, and so to be performed.[2]

The general inclination of the ministry of the early New England Colonies was to avoid the "popish" error of saying prayers over the dead. Nevertheless, funeral sermons eventually were preached in church, starting about 1700, and, later, prayers were said in graveside ceremonies.

A broader and more far-reaching development was the attempt by the colonists to shed their *legal* system of ecclesiastical law and to formalize the controls of the New World society by recourse only to common law, tempered by the inference that "if it isn't reasonable, it can't be good law."[3]

In England, the story remained different. The ecclesiastical regulation of interment went unchallenged throughout the Middle Ages, and the law of the clergy controlled burials and cemeteries in England without serious lay interference until the adoption of the English Burial Acts of 1855.[4]

Thus, despite the fact that America had an English church for its first 14 years, and that, until the Revolution, the established church was incorporated into the Virginia Colony, American courts-at-law have looked to 1607 for precedent in common law regarding matters involving burial of the dead.

Although the impulse of the colonists was generally to reject ecclesiastical law on principle, or because it did not fit all the exigencies of Colonial existence, many canons specifically were brought into usage. This was the case with funeral practices. "Early American burial was in the churchyard," notes Jackson, "and though always yielding to temporal sovereignty, through the Colonial adherence to the equitable principles of the English common law, the commands of the church found their way into our law of burial."[5]

If ecclesiastical law was not, in fact, totally rejected by the colonists, neither was it embraced in any organized, codified or integrated form. The consequence of this avoidance seems to have been a lack of clear-cut definitions for mortuary behavior, and it is certain that the Church controls of burial that existed in England were not mirrored in the Colonies. The effect of this development on the rise of the American funeral undertaker will be noted later.

Two other large-scale elements of Colonial ideology need to be pointed out that both have a general reference to the rise of Protestantism: one looked to the realm of human action and was reflected in the special way of regarding one's work; the other centered around human reflection and found expression in theology and philosophy.

The terms "Protestantism" and "industriousness" share a close affinity. Traditionally, *hard* work, as well as good deeds, has been an avenue of salvation for the Protestant; this is particularly true in the teachings of Calvin, who interjected a commercial rationale into the theology he espoused.[6]

Undoubtedly, industriousness that had something more than a simple common-sense basis was part of the English heritage of the early colonists. The almost compulsive nature of the industriousness of the colonists has since become legend. Hardship, disaster, decimation by plague, malaria, smallpox, or Indians — all or each of these could not keep the work of settling the New World from going on apace.

Idleness was not only looked upon as a cardinal sin, but it also became a breach of law. For example, when the situation demanded it, Captain John Smith, the founder of Virginia, might put men of noble birth to work in the cornfields with the humble but not ignoble hoe. The colonist was impelled by a moral, almost sacred, sense of obligation to apply himself to his work.

On the other hand, such application yielded returns that could never be hoped for in the Old World. Three to five years of bondage seems, today, a high cost of indenture, but to the colonist-to-be — in light of the potential *substantial* basis to the freedom gained — those years in bondage might seem almost negligible. Work, ownership, substance and salvation all became parts of a unity of existence that made up life in the Colonies, founded, as it were, upon the principle that considered hard work akin to godliness.

But to New Englanders, industriousness was a necessary, but not sufficient, cause for salvation. The state of one's soul was, in the end, an individual matter, and despite their industrious application to mundane affairs, these colonists were repeatedly forced back upon their own consciences in search of the righteousness of their acts. The ministry, whose sermons on hell-fire and damnation were scarcely calculated to lend peace of mind to their congregations, did not relieve their uncertainty.

The Southern colonists, it should be noted, fared somewhat better. Their theology did not keep them mentally poised on the brink of a flaming abyss in which sinners were cast to death by the hands of an angry God. But to the New Englander, the search for consolation in the contemplation of the "Great Beyond" was indeed a difficult one, and it is for this reason that the Puritans were forced into the realm of philosophical speculation and the examination of philosophical ideas.

By the turn of the 18th century, urbanization and its concomitant secularization, as well as the rapid expansion of industry and trade, had begun to weaken the theocratic organization of the New England Colonies. Theological and philosophical speculation gave way, to some extent, to the pursuit of worldly goods as an end in and of themselves.

Nevertheless, until the outbreak of the Revolution, common law, industriousness and an uncertain, fearful relation to the Almighty formed the major elements of the Puritan character. And it is against this ideological backdrop that the figures of funeral practice, and their specific death customs, take on comprehension and become more than items of incidental interest.

Burial Practices: Early New England recognized death as a natural, inevitable, commonplace reality. "The grave was as familiar as the cradle, and the New Englander never saw any reason to ignore or disguise it."[7]

Old New England graveyards were familiar places to the living, as well as resting places for the dead. Gravestones did not merely identify bodily remains, but, through inscriptions in the form of epitaphs, also served as a medium of popular literary expression. As Wallis points out, "The manner of expression may be ribald and ridiculous, pompous and lugubrious, eloquent, or serenely simple."[8]

Yet, the fact remains that the dead were not alienated from the living in Colonial times; rather, the unlettered inscriptions spun a thin thread of remembrance to the unique personalities of those who had passed on. Andrews says:

> Sickness, death, and the frailties of human life were perennial subjects of conversation and correspondence, and few family letters of those days are free from allusion to them. From infancy to old age death took ample toll — so great was the colonial disregard for laws of sanitation, so little the attention paid to drainage and disinfection. The human system was dosed and physicked until it could hold no more.[9]

Death was never denied. In fact, the most persistent symbol of early New England days was probably the skull and crossbones. Shepard's view is that, as the Colonial period advanced, the slow change from the gravestone death-skull to the winged cherub indicates the expulsion of the basic doubts of the early Puritan as to immortality and the development of hope for an ascent into paradise.[10]

The diary of Samuel Sewall, a ranking judge in the Massachusetts Bay Colony, kept a diary covering the late-17th and early 18th centuries. This record is regarded by American historians as one of the most revealing documents of the time, performing for the American scene much the same function that *Pepys' Diary* performs for the English. With almost punctilious morbidity, Sewall notes the daily deaths in Massachusetts, and, with gruesome regularity, he parades Indian raids and accidents, killings, hangings and natural deaths.

But it was not these but sickness that was most feared in the small settlements. Epidemics of smallpox struck repeatedly. Of Sewall's prodigious family of 15 children, more than half died in infancy or childhood. It was not unusual for a colonist to lose a wife or two or three, and remarriages were the order of the day.[11]

Alice M. Earle, patient chronicler of New England social customs, sums up her studies of Colonial burial thus:

> One cannot keep from being impressed, when studying almanacs, diaries and letters of the time, with the strange exaltation of spirit with which the New England Puritan regarded death. To him the thoughts of mortality were indeed cordial to the soul. Death was the event, the condition... of which he constantly spoke, dreamed and thought; and he rejoiced mightily in that close approach, in that sense of touch with the spiritual world. With unaffected cheerfulness he yielded himself to his own fate, with unforced resignation he bore the loss of dearly loved ones, and with eagerness and almost affection he regarded all the gloomy attributes and surroundings of death.[12]

The earliest New England burials were models of simplicity and quiet dignity. Not wishing to commit what they considered the "popish error" of saying prayers over the dead, the mourners merely followed the coffin and stood silently as the grave was filled. Lechford, describing a 17th-century funeral, remarks:

> At burials nothing is read nor any funeral sermon made, but all the neighborhood or a goodly company of them come together by tolling the bell, and carry the dead solemnly to his grave and then stand by him while he is buried. The ministers are most commonly present.[13]

Although funeral sermons might have been preached in church *after* the burial, by the end of the 17th century, the English practice of having a funeral sermon said over the body in the meeting house or in the church was again observed. Sewall notes critically the choice of text and emphasis of numerous funeral sermons, remarking that, at the burial of one Goodman Pilsbury: "Mr. Richardson Preached from I Cor. 3:21, 22 going something out of 's Order by reason of the occasion, and singling out those Words *Or Death*."[14]

Following the English fashion, early New Englanders wrote laudatory verses, which they attached to the bier or the hearse. The latter consisted of a framework that supported the coffin and upon which candles were placed; it had little resemblance to the modern vehicle in which the casket is transported.

The early Colonial press found fruitful occupation in the printing of broadside sheets and pamphlets. Black-bordered and dismal, these were often crudely and gruesomely decorated with the macabre symbols of death: skull and crossbones, scythes, coffins, hourglasses, all-seeing eyes, skeletons, and winding sheets. (***See Plate 20***.)

Edification found rich meat in funerals. Funeral sermons for leading men of the Colonies were often printed, as were the exemplary confessions made by criminals prior to their execution. It can be truthfully said that the whole social complex surrounding death and burial of the New Englanders was richly portrayed in popular verse, with imagery as grim in many ways as that of the death-dance period of the Middle Ages. Executions of criminals were public, and ministers worked feverishly with the doomed, exhorting them to confess at the gallows. The first stammered words of repentance were greeted with cheers by the assembled citizenry.

Mourning took on an extensive social character. Rings, scarves, gloves, books, verses and products of needlecraft all were used by the colonist in the process of paying tribute to the dead. The custom of making gifts to the living to announce funerals was brought to the Colonies from England, where it had been part of the feudal funeral. In its new home, it flourished in the late-17th century and survived through most of the 18th. Earle remarks: "in the case of a funeral of any person prominent in State, Church or Society, vast numbers of gloves were given away."[15]

The quality of those distributed at the same funeral varied with the social status or the degree of blood relationship or friendship that the recipient had with the bereaved. The excesses that developed in this funerary gift-making became evident in the fact that, at the funeral of Governor Belcher's wife in 1736, more than 1,000 pairs of gloves were given away.[16]

As towns expanded through peaceful trade and growing industry, funerals took on what seemed to many a wanton lavishness. Judge Sewall, who appreciated keenly the pleasures of funeral ceremonies and recorded carefully his gifts of rings, scarves and gloves in his diary, was led to remark on the extravagance of the early 18th-century ceremonies. Moreover, in 1721, 1724 and 1742, the General Court of Massachusetts passed laws prohibiting "Extraordinary Expense at Funerals."[17]

A letter to the *Boston Evening Post*, June 20, 1737 (***see Figure 2***), points to sumptuary legislation passed by the General Assembly of the Province of Massachusetts as early as 1651.

Figure 2. Early Colonial Letter to Editor Protesting Extravagances, Especially at Funerals.

PLATE 20

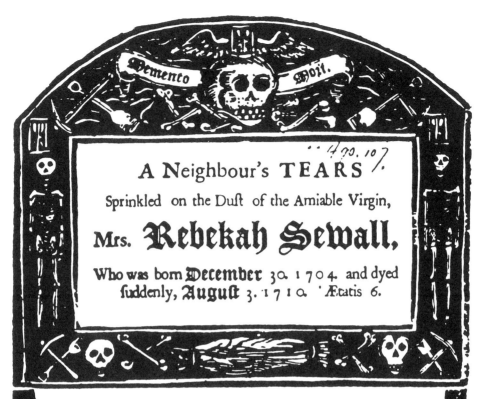

A Neighbour's TEARS

Sprinkled on the Dust of the Amiable Virgin,

Mrs. **Rebekah Sewall,**

Who was born December 30. 1704. and dyed suddenly, August 3. 1710. Ætatis 6.

Heav'ns only, in dark hours, can Succour send ;
And shew a Fountain, where the cisterns end.
I saw this little One but t'other day
  With a small flock of Doves, just in my way :
What New-made Creature's this so bright ? thought I
Ah ! Pity 'tis such Prettiness should die.
Madam, behold the Lamb of GOD ; for there's
Your Pretty Lamb, while you dissolve in Tears ;
She lies infolded in her Shepherd's Arms,
Whose Bosom's always full of gracious Charms.
Great JESUS claim'd his own ; never begrutch
Your Jewels rare into the Hands of Such.
He, with His Righteousness, has better dress'd
Your Babe, than e're you did, when at your breast.
'Tis not your case alone ! for thousands have
Follow'd their sweetest Comforts to the Grave.
Seeking the Plat of Immortality,
I saw no Place Secure ; but all must dy.
Death, that stern Officer, takes no denial ;
I'm griev'd he found your door, to make a trial.
Thus, be it on the Land, or Swelling Seas,
His Sov'raignty doth what His Wisdom please.
Must then the Rulers of this World's affairs,

20. Portion of Colonial Broadside.

For persons of importance, their funeral-glove collection grew to considerable size. When Andrew Eliot, minister of the North Church in Boston, tallied his take for 32 years, he found that he had received 2,940 pairs of funeral gloves. These were in addition to funeral rings and scarves. In fewer than 50 years, Sewall received 57 mourning rings. Earle gives other instances showing the drain that this gift expense made upon families:

> We can well believe the story of Doctor Samuel Buxton, of Salem, who died in 1758, aged eighty-one years, that he left to his heirs a quart tankard full of mourning rings which he had received at funerals; and that Rev. Andrew Eliot had a mugful. At one Boston funeral in 1738, over two hundred rings were given away. At Waitstill Winthrop's funeral sixty rings, worth over a pound apiece were given to friends. The entire expense of the latter-named funeral — scutcheons, hatchments, scarves, gloves, rings, bell tolling, tailor's bills, etc., was over six hundred pounds. This amounted to one-fifth of the entire estate of the deceased gentleman.[18]

So strongly ingrained was this peculiar fashion that even pauper funerals demanded the distribution of a minimum number of pairs of gloves.

Despite the growing concern about burial expense and the legislative attempts to curb the practice of spending a sizable portion of the estate for gifts at funerals, the colonists persisted in making the disposal of the dead an occasion for celebration. Perhaps the epitome of extravagance was reached at the funeral of Andrew Faneuil in 1738, when 3,000 pairs of gloves were given away and more than 1,100 persons accompanied the funeral cortege.[19]

In a typical New England town, a funeral in the middle of the 18th century would reveal the following basic pattern.[20] Upon death, neighbors, or possibly a nurse if the family was well-to-do, would wash and lay out the body.

The local carpenter or cabinet-maker would build the coffin, choosing a quality of wood to fit the social position of the deceased. In special cases, "coffin furniture," i.e., metal decorations imported from England, would be added to the coffin.

Relatives and friends within a few days' travel would be notified immediately, for it was not customary to let the body lie in state. If the weather was warm, the body, as Sewall put it, would be "embowelled and put in a Cere-Cloth" (alum, pitch, or wax-soaked sheet), and, of course, rings, scarves or gloves would be distributed to all those invited to the funeral.

Funeral services would begin in the church, with prayers and a sermon said over the pall-covered bier. Ministers looked upon funerals as an occasion to deliver some of their most inspired remarks, and it was not uncommon for their funeral sermons to be printed and circulated among the public, featuring a conventional black-border and skull and crossbones on the cover. (***See Plate 21***.)

The procession to the grave was on foot, with under-bearers actually carrying the coffin on the bier, while pallbearers, men of dignity and consanguinity (related somehow to the deceased), held the corners of the pall. If the distance was far, fresh under-bearers were used, and, in any case, the procession went slowly and was marked by numerous rest stops.

In many towns, there were no gravediggers so neighbors consequently supplied the necessary

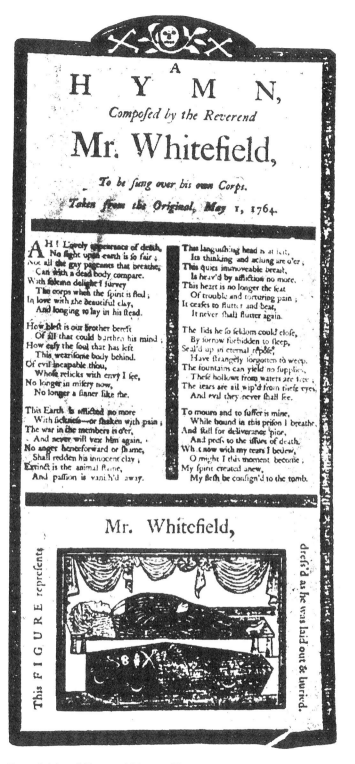

21. Broadside of Funeral Hymn Showing Burial Dress and Coffin.

labor. Usually, the sexton would have dug the grave and tolled the bell to announce the funeral. Unlike his English cousin, however, the Colonial sexton exacted a fee for both services. In some towns, such as Salem, these fees were regulated by municipal ordinance.

The funeral service at the grave was simple: a brief prayer followed by the ritual commitment of the body to the earth. The filling of the grave marked the formal end of the funeral ceremonies.

Samuel Sewall gives us a description of an upper-class funeral:

> Friday, Feb. 10, 1678/8. Between 4. and 5. I went to the funeral of Lady Andros, having been invited by the Clark of the South Company. Between 7. and 8. Lychus (Lynchs), [i.e., links or torches] illuminating the cloudy air. The Corps was carried into the Herse drawn by Six Horses. The Souldiers making a Guard from the Governour's House down the Prison Lane to South-meetinghouse, there taken out and carried in at the western dore, and set in the Alley before the pulpit, with Six Mourning Women by it. Was a great noise and clamor to keep people out of the House, that might not rush in too soon. I went home, where about nine a'clock I heard the Bells toll again for the Funeral. It seems Mr. Ratcliffs Text was, Cry, all flesh is Grass. The Ministers turn'd into Mr. Willards. The Meeting-House full among whom Mr. Dudley Stoughton, Gedney, Bradstreet, &. 'Twas warm thawing wether, and the wayes extream dirty. No volley at placing the Body in the Tomb. On Satterday, Feb. 11. the mourning cloth of the Pulpit is taken off and given to Mr. Willard. My Brother Stephen was at the Funeral and lodged here.[21]

But there was more to the Colonial funeral than the ritualized disposal of the dead. Relatives and friends, having traveled various distances, needed to be fed and housed. In addition, the neighborhood was always involved, and, in keeping with the general mood of exhilaration (undercut with latent apprehension), festivity, even frolic, was mixed with the gloom of the funeral ceremonies.

The serving of liquors was as universal as it was generous. Funeral bills were often top-heavy with the expense of strong beverages. A typical example is a bill for the mortuary expenses of David Porter, of Hartford, who drowned in 1678:[22]

By a pint of liquor for those who dived for him 1s
By a quart of liquor for those who brot him home 2s
By two quarts of wine and one gallon of cyder to jury of inquest 5s
By 8 gallons and 3 quarts wine for funeral L1-15s
By barrel cyder for funeral 16s
1 coffin 12s
Windeing sheet 18s

In addition to drink, food in vast quantities was supplied. At the funeral feast of Calie Dawes in Boston, 1797,[23] rum, wine, beer, gin and brandy were served along with a dinner that featured beef, ham, bacon and fowls for the funeral's baked meats, supplemented by fish, oysters, 150 eggs, peas, onions and potatoes, followed by cheese, fruit and sweetmeats. The total funeral cost was $844 — a small fortune for the time, and equivalent to between $5,000 and $10,000 in modern purchasing power.[24]

PLATE 22

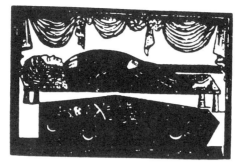

An ELEGIAC
POEM,

On the DEATH of that celebrated Divine, and eminent Servant of JESUS CHRIST, the late Reverend, and pious

GEORGE WHITEFIELD,

Chaplain to the Right Honourable the Countess of HUNTINGDON, &c. &c.

Who made his Exit from this transitory State, to dwell in the celestial Realms of Bliss, on LORD's-Day, 30th of September, 1770, when he was seiz'd with a Fit of the Asthma, at NEWBURY-PORT, near BOSTON, in NEW-ENGLAND. In which is a Condolatory Address to His truly noble Benefactress the worthy and pious Lady HUNTINGDON,—and the Orphan-Children in GEORGIA; who, with many Thousands, are left, by the Death of this great Man, to lament the Loss of a Father, Friend, and Benefactor.

By PHILLIS, a Servant Girl of 17 Years of Age, belonging to Mr. J. WHEATLEY, of BOSTON :—And has been but 9 Years in this Country from Africa.

HAIL happy Saint on thy immortal throne !
To thee complaints of grievance are unknown ;
We hear no more the music of thy tongue,
Thy wonted auditories cease to throng.
Thy lessons in unequal'd accents flow'd !
While emulation in each bosom glow'd ;
Thou didst, in strains of eloquence refin'd,
Inflame the soul, and captivate the mind.
Unhappy we, the setting Sun deplore !
Which once was splendid, but it shines no more ;
He leaves this earth for Heaven's unmeasur'd height :
And worlds unknown, receive him from our sight ;
There WHITEFIELD wings, with rapid course his way,
And sails to Zion, through vast seas of day.

When his AMERICANS were burden'd sore,
When streets were crimson'd with their guiltless gore !
Unrival'd friendship in his breast now strove :
The fruit thereof was charity and love
Towards America———couldst thou do more
Than leave thy native home, the British shore,
To cross the great Atlantic's wat'ry road,
To see America's distress'd abode ?
Thy prayers, great Saint, and thy incessant cries,
Have pierc'd the bosom of thy native skies !
Thou moon hast seen, and ye bright stars of light
Have witness been of his requests by night !
He pray'd that grace in every heart might dwell :
He long'd to see America excell ;

A greater gift not GOD himself can give ;
He urg'd the need of him to every one ;
It was no less than GOD's co-equal SON !
Take him ye wretched for your only good ;
Take him ye starving souls to be your food.
Ye thirsty, come to this life giving stream,
Ye Preachers, take him for your joyful theme ;
Take him, "my dear AMERICANS," he said,
Be your complaints in his kind bosom laid :
Take him ye Africans, he longs for you ;
Impartial SAVIOUR, is his title due ;
If you will chuse to walk in grace's road,
You shall be sons, and kings, and priests to GOD.

Great COUNTESS ! we Americans revere
Thy name, and thus condole thy grief sincere :
We mourn with thee, that TOMB obscurely plac'd,
In which thy Chaplain undisturb'd doth rest.
New-England sure, doth feel the ORPHAN's smart ;
Reveals the true sensations of his heart :
Since this fair Sun, withdraws his golden rays,
No more to brighten these distressful days !
His lonely Tabernacle, sees no more
A WHITEFIELD landing on the British shore :
Then let us view him in yon azure skies :
Let every mind with this lov'd object rise.
No more can he exert his lab'ring breath,
Seiz'd by the cruel messenger of death.
What can his dear AMERICA return ?

22. Facsimile Portion of Broadside Elegy, Written by a Slave Girl.

The cost of wine at one funeral in Virginia came to more than 4,000 pounds of tobacco. In light of such expenditures, it is not surprising that more than one Colonial assembly passed laws designed to keep the friends of the deceased from eating and drinking the widow and orphans out of house and home.[25]

In discussing this period, Hawthorne notes the expressive release that these funeral feasts gave:

> They were the only class of scenes so far as my investigation has taught me, in which our ancestors were wont to steep their tough old hearts in wine and strong drink and indulge in an outbreak of grisly jollity. Look back through all the social customs of New England in the first century of her existence and read all her traits of character, and find one occasion other than a funeral feast where jollity was sanctioned by universal practice. Well, old friends! Pass on with your burden of mortality and lay it in the tomb with jolly hearts. People should be permitted to enjoy themselves in their own fashion; every man to his taste — but New England must have been a dismal abode for the man of pleasure when the only boon-companion was Death.[26]

Andrews makes the astute observation that a funeral was both a social function and a public event, and therefore drew crowds of people, children among them, who frequently acted as pallbearers. The Puritan conscience could not allow an opportunity to teach to remain unexploited. It was hoped that the little ones "might be impressed with the significance of death as the inevitable end of a life of trial and probation."[27]

In New York and Virginia, the pattern of funerals differed somewhat. Dutch funerals took place three or four days after death and were accompanied by extensive and important ceremony. The best parlor was used for funerals, prayers were said, and the pall-covered coffin and bier were carried to the churchyard by 12 pallbearers. After interment, the procession returned to the house, where food, tobacco and drink were distributed while festivities became the occasion.

A "Monkey spoon" — so-called because of an irreverent jest; possibly because the crudely executed apostle intended for the handle resembled more the animal than the saint — was often given to each pallbearer. (***See Plate 23***.) Ceremonies were under the direction of the licensed official called "aanspreecker," and, in the main, funerals were attended only by the adult males.[28]

Early Virginia funerals, like horse races and weddings, were important occasions. Bruce has pointed out the lively nature of the eating and drinking that went along with the funeral ceremonies.[29] Often, a "furious fusillade" preceded the festivities, although, at different times, the law did not permit such waste of powder and shot.

As was the case with the New Englanders, the consumption of liquor was often enormous and likely to impoverish the decedent's estate. "The expenses incurred in burying John Griggs, of York County," notes Bruce, "were estimated at sixteen hundred pounds of tobacco. The provision of food and drink for the persons present on this occasion included turkeys, geese, and other domestic poultry, a pig, several bushels of flour, twenty pounds of butter, sugar and spice, and also twelve gallons of different kinds of spirits."[30]

PLATE 23

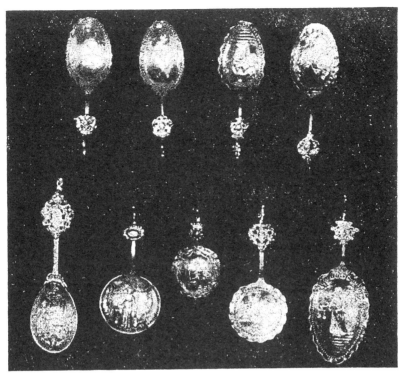

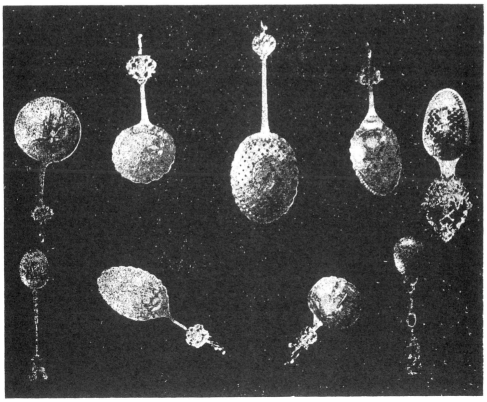

23. "Monkey Spoons" Used by Early Dutch Colonists.

Many deplored the excesses in eating, drinking and the firing of guns. Some made provision in their wills for more decorous behavior at their funerals, including Colonel Richard Cole, who provided mourning clothes for all those present at his funeral, but nothing in the line of food, drink and fusillades.

Even in so solemn a matter as a funeral, informal controls served the Colonial fathers no better than they served their ancestors, who used the medieval waking of the dead as an excuse for carousing. Drinking at funerals exceeded the minimum bounds of propriety traditionally associated with Christian burial, and also violated the ceremonial dignity that quickly marked funerals as soon as the Colonies became stable and prosperous.

In order to prevent the waste of gunpowder at drinking frolics, and to forestall false alarms, the Virginia Assembly in 1655 — 48 years after the settlement of the colony — ordained that no persons should "shoot guns at drinking, marriages and funerals only excepted."[31]

Social Change in Late Colonial America: During the 18th century, Colonial society was subjected to serious upheavals resulting from two revolutions, one political and the other basically economic. The culmination of the political revolution was the war of liberation from England; yet, the roots of this conflict were in the less-obvious commercial and industrial revolution that gave America its urbanism, industrial manufacturing centers, and the outlines of a social-class system. Both revolutions, however, had distinct consequences for Colonial modes of mortuary behavior.

Bridenbaugh makes clear the relationship between the breakdown of traditional Puritan controls and the changing standards of living that came about with increasing urbanization:

> As the towns approached maturity, urban moral standards began to diverge widely from those of the countryside. Within the towns, also, wealthy aristocrats, as in other societies, increasingly pursued a manner of living radically different from that of middle and lower classes. The center of morality was shifting, and wealth and urban conditions brought about new and more elastic codes of conduct...
>
> In every town the profits of peaceful trade led to great display, which seemed to many to be mere wanton extravagance. Aged Samuel Sewall observed with alarm the "Affection and the use of Gayety, Costly Buildings, Stilled and other Strong Liquors, Palatable, though expensive Diet, Rageth with great Impetuosity, and... (lead) to Sensuality, Effeminateness, Unrighteousness, and Confusion." Elaborate and costly funerals were said to be ruining those who could ill afford the luxury of "gloves, scarfs, and scutcheons."... Similar complaints against display and declining moral standards emanated from New York and Charles Town.[32]

As commercial relations with England became strained by the Embargo Acts, there was a consequent reduction of trade between the colonists and the homeland. Taking a hitch in their economy, the colonists, among other things, began to limit themselves to what mourning paraphernalia they had on hand. Once this wore out, there was a noticeable diminution in the use of clothes, scarfs, gloves and other items of mourning that might have been imported. Weeden observes:

The economy enforced to avoid importations from Great Britain brought in sensible changes in the management of funerals and their attendant ceremonies. The full suits worn by all the connections were dispensed with, bands of crepe for the gentlemen and black ribbons for the ladies being substituted. The gloves, formerly being distributed generally, were now only presented to the "pall-holders."[33]

Although earlier sumptuary laws had been ineffective in curtailing extravagant display and gift-giving at funerals, these and more-recent legislative measures had, in light of the seriousness of the situation, a greater urgency to them. In 1788, there appeared in the *Massachusetts Sentinel* a reminder by "The Inspectors of the Police" that a law, established before the Revolution, specifically referred to the display of mourning, and, to refresh the minds of the public of Boston, the law was hereby reprinted as follows:

TO PREVENT EXCESS AND VAIN EXPENSE IN MOURNING, ETC. It is hereby ordered, that in future no scarfs, gloves or rings shall be given at any funerals in this town, nor shall any wine, rum or other spirituous liquor be allowed or given at, or immediately before or after any funeral in this town, under pain that the person or persons giving, allowing or ordering the same shall respectively forfeit and pay the sum of *twenty shillings* for each offense.

And it is further ordered, that whatever male person shall appear or walk in the procession of any funeral in this town with any new mourning or new black or other new mourning coat or waistcoat or with any other new black apparel, save and except a black crepe around one arm, or shall afterwards, on account of the decease of any relation, or other person or persons, put on and wear any other mourning than such piece of black crepe around one arm, shall forfeit and shall pay the sum of *twenty shillings* for every day he shall put on and wear or appear in the same.

And no female, of whatsoever degree shall put on, or wear or appear at any funeral in this town, in any other mourning or new black clothes whatsoever other than a black hat or bonnet, black gloves, black ribbons and a black fan, on pain of forfeit and pay the sum of *twenty shillings*; and also forfeit and pay a like sum of *twenty shillings* for every day she shall at any time, or after such funeral, put on or wear or appear in such new black clothes as or for mourning, other than black hat, or bonnet, black gloves, black ribbons, and a fan as aforesaid.[34]

In 1790, the town of Salem published some regulations about funerals in the papers, among which were specific items referring to sextons and undertakers:

For each Tolling of the Bell 8 d.

The Sextons are desired to toll the bells only four strokes in a minute.

The undertakers service in borrowing Chairs, waiting upon the Pallholders and warning the Relations, etc. to attend 8.

B. Doland and B. Brown are appointed by the selectmen to see that Free Passages in the Streets are kept open.

The appearance of these and similar regulations and restrictions on matters pertaining to mourning and the conduct of funerals indicates, for one thing, a gradual weakening of the theocratic tradition of government, as well as the early performance of specific funeral tasks in the context of secular, or non-religious, activities. Concurrent with the Revolutionary War, it appears, came the shift to simpler mourning customs, the inclusion of funeral practices more specifically under legislative scrutiny, and the proliferation of funeral tasks as specialists in other occupations. (The latter development is the subject matter of the next chapter.)

Meanwhile, a word must be said further about the general socioeconomic trend of the 18th century and its bearing on Colonial mortuary behavior. With the growth and prosperity of commerce and trade, the seaport towns developed into flourishing trade centers, comparable to the port cities of England. "Within these towns," Bridenbaugh notes, "merchant grandees accumulated riches so rapidly as to raise their position above that of other townsmen."[35]

The upshot of this process was the formation of social classes, based not upon lineage, but upon established commercial success, occupations and social function. Symbols of class position were sought and found in the style and size of mansion, the mode of attire, form of transportation (carriage transportation was a la mode), etiquette, manners, customs and world outlook. The beautifully appointed townhouse, the exquisite furniture, furs, jewels and silks, coaches, slaves, governesses, riding horses, and the like — all were combined to ensure social stratification in town life of the 18th-century colonists.

As the years of peaceful prosperity deepened, so did the class barriers. Yet, mobility from one class to another was never categorically blocked, as would be the case in a caste system. Laborers, seafarers, servants and even slaves could aspire to, and often gain, higher socio-economic class position. Likewise, the *nouveau riche*, by affecting the symbols and the demeanor of the established "upper" class, might find social acceptance at a higher level, although the consolidation of such position might take several generations.

The relevance of such socio-economic development in Colonial America to the history of funeral service becomes clear when we try to make intelligible the difference between the festivities and spontaneous expression of human impulse of the early Colonial funeral with the status of the dead — as *reflected* by the degree of display and the level of expense, and the later town-burials where the funerals *affected* a class position that was seldom anchored in traditional acceptance. This element of class pretension marks the significant difference between the religion-permeated, but socially uproarious, funeral of 17th-century Colonial America and the status-conscious, but religious-tinctured, funeral of the following century.

It is evident that the early American Colonies differed regarding the role of the established Church of England. The Massachusetts Bay Colony rejected it and set up an independent theocracy, headed by its own framework of social and political organization. Singularly enough, ecclesiastical law was generally rejected in the Colonies in favor of a more flexible common law, tempered by common sense, but some canon law was brought into usage in the realm of the burial of the dead. Nevertheless, as indicated earlier, there was no consistent body of law and precedent to inform and direct Colonial funeral behavior, as was the case in England.

English industriousness, with its roots in the Protestant ethic of making a calling out of one's work, served to energize the colonists and keep them alert to the possibilities of bettering their social and economic lot — bounded, of course, by Puritan middle-class morality and religious humility. Although burial practices varied in different settlements, Colonial funerals generally combined three functions: sociability, religiosity, and the reaffirmation of the established social status of the deceased. While the crisis of the Revolution led to specific changes in mourning customs, the more fundamental and persisting change was toward the use of funerals as an instrument to express status aspirations and pretensions by the socially class-conscious members of an expanding urban society.

Even though it is possible that undertakers operated in the American Colonies in the 17th century, Habenstein uncovered very little evidence in the operations at that time of such specialists who "made their living as funeral directors, called themselves by that name, and were popularly recognized as such, as was the case in England from about 1685 on."[36]

A fragment of evidence seeming to support their claim to existence in the early 18th century may be found in Earle, who, speaking generally of the Colonial period, remarks that "the undertakers could charge but eight shillings for borrowing chairs, waiting on pallbearers and notifying relatives to attend."[37] More likely, however, she is referring to the funeral regulations of Salem, made public in 1790.

In an effort to discover the earliest appearance of the "undertaker" in America as a member of a specific, recognized occupation, Habenstein examined copies of all the extant American city directories from the 18th century, and most of those for major cities from the first half of the 19th.[38] The earliest directory printed in America was for the city of New York in 1786.[39] Although each citizen was identified as to occupation, no one was listed in this directory as an "undertaker"; several sextons are designated.

In a section of the same volume, captioned "Annals of New York City For the Year 1786," the funeral of the Honorable Abner Nash is described. The procession included the clerk of the church from which he was buried, 60 charity boys, clergy from other churches, his physician, pallbearers, relatives, and the sexton, but no undertaker.

Evidence that funeral undertaking was emerging as a distinct occupational specialty becomes apparent in the first quarter of the 19th century, when public announcements by undertakers first became common. Prior to this, the few newspaper advertisements telling of both male and female tradespeople are scattered and infrequent. The richest data to indicate the emergence of the new occupational group were derived from the early registries and directories of New England and Atlantic Coast towns and cities.

Chapter 6 examines how these various factors combined to give rise to the American funeral undertaker of the 19th century — an occupational specialist — organizing within the scope of operations the major tasks necessary to the care and disposal of the dead.

CITATIONS AND REFERENCES IN CHAPTER 5

1. Massachusetts Historical Society, *Proceedings*, Vol. 17, pp. 168-169.

2. *Ibid.*, p. 169.

3. Gerald W.C.F. Johnson, *Our English Heritage* (Philadelphia and New York: J.B. Lippincott Co., 1949), p.156 *seq*.

4. Percival E. Jackson, *The Law of Cadavers*, 2nd ed. (New York: Prentice Hall, 1950), p. 22. This is not to exclude the presence of a Spanish Church and a French Church in early America.

5. *Ibid.*, p. 27. Only secular law regarding burial prevails in America today.

6. The reciprocal relation of religion and commercial pursuits has been brilliantly analyzed by the German economic historian Max Weber in *The Protestant Ethic and the Spirit of Capitalism*, trans. Talcott Parsons (London: George Unwin, 1930).

7. Zephine Humphrey, *A Book of New England* (n.p. Howell Sosken, 1947), p. 211.

8. Charles L. Wallis, *Stories on Stone; A Book of American Epitaphs* (New York: Oxford University Press, 1954), p. xi.

9. Charles M. Andrews, *Colonial Folkways*, Vol. VIII of The Chronicle of America Series, ed. Allen Johnson, 50 Vols. (New Haven: Yale University Press, 1918), p. 92.

10. Presented by Humphrey, *op. cit.*

11. Samuel Sewall, *Sewall's Diary*, ed. by Mark Van Doren (New York: Macy-Masius, 1927).

12. Alice M. Earle, *Customs and Fashions in Old New England* (New York: Charles Scribner's Sons, 1894), p. 386.

13. Quoted by Earle, *ibid.*, p. 364.

14. Sewall, *op. cit.*, p. 39.

15. Earle, *op. cit.*, p. 374.

16. William B. Weeden, *Economic and Social History of New England 1620-1789*, 2 vols. (Boston and New York: Houghton Mifflin Company, 1890), Vol II, p. 538.

17. See Carl Bridenbaugh, *Cities in the Wilderness*, a volume of the Ronald Series in History, ed. by Robert C. Binkley and Ralph H. Gabriel (New York: The Ronald Press, 1938, and Alfred A. Knopf, 1955), pp. 387, 412, *passim*.

18. Earle, *op. cit.*, p. 376.

19. *Ibid.*, p. 374.

20. *Ibid.*, Chapter XV. See also Andrews, *op. cit.*, pp. 92-95.

21. Sewall, *op. cit.*, pp. 54-55.

22. Earle, *op. cit.*, p. 370.

23. Somewhat fancifully reconstructed in Fairfax Downey's *Our Lusty Forefathers* (New York: Charles Scribner's Sons, 1947), pp. 209-219, based on an account given in the *Proceedings of the Massachusetts Historical Society*, vol. 54.

24. *Ibid.*

25. Habenstein, "The American Funeral Director," *op. cit.*, p. 86.

26. Andrews, *op. cit.*

27. *Op. cit.*, pp. 94-95.

28. An interesting and more complete account of early Dutch funerals is found in Mrs. John King Van Rensselaer's *The Goede Vrouw of Manan-ha-ta* (New York: Charles Scribner's Sons, 1898), pp. 54 ff.

29. Philip Alexander Bruce, *Social Life of Virginia in the Seventeenth Century* (Richmond, Va.: Whittet and Shepperson, 1907), pp. 218-222.

30. *Ibid.*, 220-221, quoted from *York County Records*, Vol. 1675-84, p. 87, Va., St. Libr.

31. Edward Eggleston, "Social Life in the Colonies," *The Century*, XXX (July 1885), p. 393.

32. Bridenbaugh, *op. cit.*, p. 393.

33. Weeden, Vol. II, *op. cit.*, p. 740.

34. Henry M. Brooks, *The Days of the Spinning Wheel in New England* (Boston: Tickner and Company, 1886), pp. 95-96.

35. Bridenbaugh, *op. cit.*, p. 411.

36. Habenstein, "The American Funeral Director," *op. cit.*, p. 95.

37. Earle, *op. cit.*, p. 380.

38. This research was undertaken at the Library of Congress, repository of the best collection of city directories and registries.

39. "The New York Directory for 1786, with Description of New York in 1786" by Noah Webster (New York: Trow City Directory Co., 1786).

Chapter 6

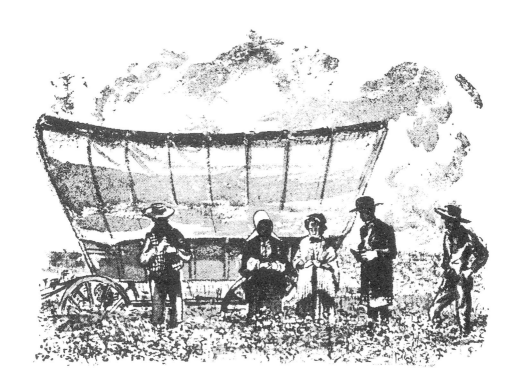

Early American Funeral Undertaking

If we limit the meaning of "funeral directing" to an occupation that provides a set of tasks for the care and disposal of the dead, takes the form of a personal service, and operates as a business enterprise, then it is clear that in this limited, modern sense, funeral directing as an occupation was born in America during the 19th century. As with most emerging vocations, however, funeral directing did not spring forth full-grown, but in its earlier stages evolved by slowly adding specific funeral tasks previously carried out generally, and largely by other occupations.

In dealing with the early funeral undertaker in America, this chapter will present the various classes of tradesmen who were in some way involved in the disposal of the dead at that period when "funeral undertaking," the predecessor of modern funeral directing, was emerging as a newcomer among the occupations of the early 19th century.

Tradesmen Undertakers: From England, where undertaking had been an occupation involving the furnishing of mourning paraphernalia in the style of an earlier feudal society since 1685 (if not before), America received very few persons dedicated solely to such trade. On the frontier, one man was as good as another, and hereditary titles, privileges and social classes did not make much sense. The fact that such social-class distinctions were less likely to be introduced into the Colonies worked against transplanting the English "Dismal Trader" into America.

The only place where such persons might find root would be in the Colonial towns, but historical records do not show "undertakers," except as underwriters of commercial ventures, in the Colonies until the second half of the 18th century. One of the first was Blanch White, who announced in *The New York Journal of General Advertisers* of January 7, 1768:

> Blanch White, Upholsterer and Undertaker, from London, on the New-Dock, next Door but one to Alderman Livingston's; Makes all kind of Upholstery-Work, in the newest Fashions and on the most reasonable Terms; Likewise all kinds of Field Equipage, Drums, Etc. Funerals furnish'd with all things necessary and proper Attendance as in England.
>
> Mrs. White begs leave to acquaint the Ladies and Gentlemen that she washes all sorts of Gauze Laces, caps, on the Wires; Silk Stockings, etc. in the neatest Manner, she having a proper frame and a Stove for bleaching. Flounces and Trimmings for Ladies Robes, neatly pinck'd; also Shrouds and Sheets.[1]

Further evidence of the English influence in early funeral undertaking in the New World comes not from the Colonies, but from Montreal, Canada, where, in the 1820 directory of "Merchants, Traders, and Housekeepers," one finds another woman who combined the role of upholsterer and undertaker:

> Mrs. Benjamin Birch, Funeral Undertaker,
>
> 20 Campeau Str. Forster & Fry
>
> Upholsterers & Undertakers, Cabinet
>
> Makers, Furniture Show Rooms

Interestingly enough, the husband of Mrs. Birch is listed at the same address as "Shoemaker."

In the Colonial period, cabinet-making was often found with upholstering, and to this combination undertaking occasionally was added. Such was the case of William B. Purves, who advertised himself in a Charleston, South Carolina, city directory in 1835 as "Cabinet Maker, Upholsterer & Undertaker."

Yet, it was more frequently the case that cabinet-makers, chair-makers and the like first supplied coffins only; and then, over a period of time, extended the range of their functions from producer of a necessary material article, i.e., the coffin, to that of provider of non-material personal services. These craftsmen were not likely to have been English and trained in the undertaker's trade; possibly only a few knew the skills of being "in attendance" and had mastered the art of furnishing all manner of funeral paraphernalia. But the rapid expansion of America, and the absence of clear and uniform Church regulations over funerals, provided an opportunity for craftsmen to develop these skills as added specialties to their current occupations. Moreover, such actions were squarely in keeping with the spirit of industry and enterprise characteristic of Colonial society.

As early as 1799, coffin-making, as part of a cabinet-making business, was combined by Michael Jenkins in Baltimore, Maryland, with funeral undertaking. Jenkins, already a well-known furniture maker, set up a partnership with Thomas Combs and advertised in the *Federal Gazette and Baltimore Daily Advertiser*, May 10, 1799:

Cabinet and Chair Manufactory
Combs and Jenkins
No. 17 Water Street between
Calvert and South Streets

At about the same time, Jenkins was appointed coroner for the city of Baltimore and, shortly after, he extended his activities to include undertaking.[2]

Records of the business indicate that in 1799, coffins were made and sold, with one charged to the account of Wm. Jenkins, a brother of Michael: "Aug. 10, for a Mahogany Coffin...L7, S10, D0"

Although the partnership was dissolved in 1802, Michael Jenkins continued cabinet- and furniture-making with the undertaking business until his death on September 8, 1832.[3]

The record of Jacob Knorr's establishment is a remarkable one. In 1761, Knorr, a German Quaker, set up a two-story joiner's shop in Germantown, Pennsylvania, and, in addition to his cabinet-maker's business and lumberyard, made coffins upon demand. (*See Plate 24*.)

He continued to operate in these various capacities until his death in 1804, at which time his two sons, George and Jacob Jr., the executors under his will,[4] sold the property, as it was unlawful for executors to purchase property in which they were interested financially. In 1807, it was transferred back to Jacob Jr., and, in a series of transactions, the property eventually came into the hands of Samuel Nice, the nephew of George Knorr.

Until this time, the owners had continued the functions that Jacob Knorr started before the outbreak of the Revolutionary War. Company bills dated prior to 1800 indicate the production of coffins as the major "undertaking" in providing goods and services to the bereaved.

Samuel Nice continued to operate the concern until 1865, when he sold the property to B. Frank Kirk, his son-in-law, and William Johnson Nice. They, in turn, tore the original buildings down and set up a new undertaking establishment dedicated solely to the business of caring for the dead.

Although these buildings have again been torn down and newer, more-spacious ones built, the buildings are on the same site. Likewise, though the original family name connected with the business (Knorr) has disappeared, there has been a line of kinship relation running through the operation of the coffin-shop-turned-undertaking-turned-funeral-directing establishment for more than 250 years! When the undertaking aspect of the establishment actually involved more than the making of a coffin cannot be determined. Nevertheless, as an example of the early combination of cabinet- and coffin-making enterprise, there is likely no similar business with such a long pedigree. (*See Plate 24*.)

The combination of cabinet-making with various undertaking functions appears with some frequency during the first half of the 19th century, with these composite businesses springing up during the western expansion following the War of 1812. (*See Plates 25 & 26*.) For example, a furniture- and cabinet-making business was established in Vincennes, Indiana, by Andrew Gardner in 1816, the same year that Indiana was admitted to statehood. Fourteen years later, the cabinetmaking firm of H.B. Deusterberg and Sons was founded in the same town. As time progressed, both of these firms shifted to funeral undertaking as their major occupational function.

These firms, along with the W.D. Diuguid firm (established 1817) in Lynchburg, Virginia; J.J. Shepherd and Son (established 1827) in Pembroke, Massachusetts; and the Boston firm of J.S. Waterman, cabinet-maker (founded 1832), make up a partial list of early cabinet-makers who added undertaking to their trade. Although the firms named do not exhaust the list of early cabinet-making and furniture-business firms that began undertaking early in the 19th century, they have been included specifically to illustrate the fact of persistence of operation, as nearly all of them are still in business under the name of the founder.

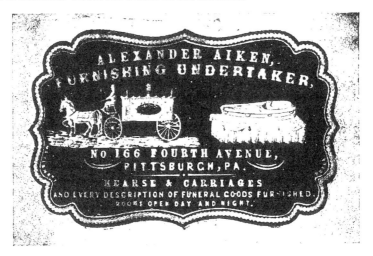

Figure 3. Trade Card of Furnishing-Undertaker, Post-Civil War Period.

Other cabinet-making undertakers added further services. Thomas Chartres let it be known in the 1829 Baltimore city directory that, besides selling cabinet furniture and making cabinets, "Funerals attended on the shortest notice, and Hacks and Hearse provided, if required."

Obligingly, Andrew Oakes, cabinet-maker, undertaker and coroner of Kings County, informed the public in the Brooklyn city directory of 1843 not only of the practice of these various crafts and functions, but also that lost children might safely be left with him until the parents could be found.

The occupational advances made by Sherman Blair, and revealed by the New Haven, Connecticut, city directories, are instructive:

1840......... Sherman Blair, Cabinet Maker

1841......... Sherman Blair, Cabinet manufacturer

1846......... Sherman and R. Blair, Cabinet manufacturer and undertakers

1853......... Blair's Cabinet Furniture, Upholsterers and undertakers

Another tradesman-undertaker variation appears somewhat later as the "furnishing-undertaker" — an undertaker who not only offered services on occasion at funerals, but who also furnished other undertakers with necessary supplies and paraphernalia. The appearance of the furnishing-undertaker took place concurrently with the emergence of the small "combination operator" — the cabinet-maker, carpenter, sexton, or liveryman who performed funerals as a sideline and who would not likely have the necessary supplies and paraphernalia at hand. (*See Plate 27.*)

PLATE 24

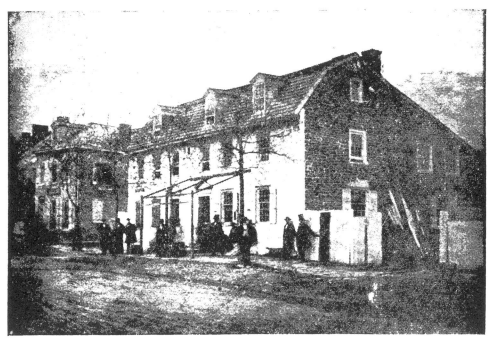

24A. Knorr Undertaking Establishment, Germantown, Pennsylvania, Mid-19th Century.

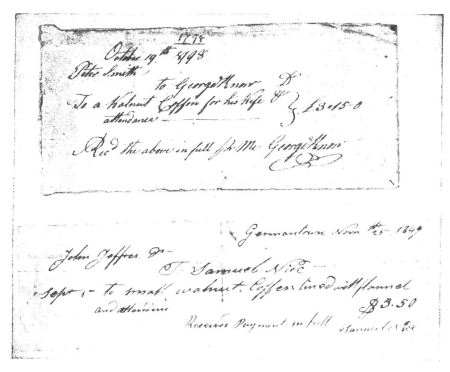

24B. Late-18th- and Mid-19th-century Bills for Coffins and "Attendance."

At the same time, once established, the furnishing-undertaker served to encourage more people to enter the field of undertaking, as newcomers need no longer feel concerned about the initial outlay for the merchandise and equipment required to start in business. Henceforth, it became possible for even more individuals with limited facilities and modest business expectations to open a new establishment. The fact that all of the funeral essentials could now be "furnished" made irrelevant the particular craft, skill or business of the person who wanted to become an undertaker.

It seems to have been the historical function of the furnishing-undertaker, then, by supplying all of the funeral-undertaker's material needs, to have introduced a dynamic force for change in the nature of funeral service practice. Not only was the field opened wider to new practitioners, but *personal service, unhampered by obligations to craft or trade, could also become a central preoccupation of the undertaker*.

Before this was to happen, however, other classes of persons were already involved in the performance of mortuary tasks. One of these was the keeper of hacks and carriages. As cities grew and the material resources of the townsfolk increased, livery stable keepers were faced with an expanding demand for carriages for funerals. Foot processions and carrying coffins by hand were not only losing their appeal, but because of the increasing distances, were also becoming burdensome and onerous, and the rental of carriages, buggies and other vehicles for funerals became more general.

Well before 1750, those in Boston who had social-class pretensions could rent coaches and black horses for funerals from Samuel Bleigh and Alexander Thorpe.[5] But by the first quarter of the 19th century, the use of carriages and horse-drawn hearses began to spread more generally throughout the population. In the 1824 city directory for Baltimore, we find the proprietor of a livery stable adding funeral-undertaking functions to his vocation.

Soon, others followed and, in the following several decades, certain phrases in the advertisements became standardized, especially "will attend personally and take proper measure that a decent order be preserved." (***See Figure 28, Chapter 9***.)

When a business changed hands, the new proprietor would often continue the identical advertisement of his predecessor, substituting only his own name.

It was not unknown for a man of enterprising spirit to attempt to provide the full round of funeral services, each as a part, however, of one of the several trades he would ply. The advertisement in the Providence directory of 1856 is instructive:

GARDNER T. SWARTZ

Livery Stable Keeper, Undertaker

Tomb Proprietor and Dealer in ready-made

coffins, of all kinds and at all

prices, near the corner of

Pine and Dorrance — Street

Providence

PLATE 25

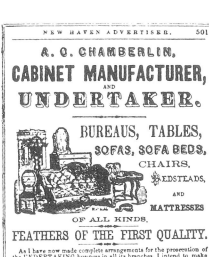
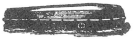
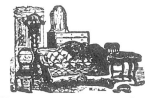

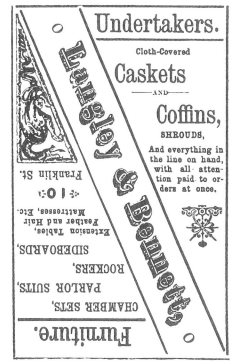

25. Advertisements of Mid-19th-century Tradesmen & Undertakers and Their Combination Establishments.

If Swartz had also "tolled the bell and dug the grave," his "undertaking" would have run the gamut of all necessary functions, short of religious services, for proper mid-19th-century care of the dead.

The period was not without its occupational oddities. John Dobbin rented hearses and hacks in Baltimore. (*See Plate 28.*) The town messengers of Charleston, Massachusetts, in 1838, and Cambridge, Massachusetts, in 1848, were also funeral undertakers. Moreover, if Andrew Oakes could take care of lost children as well as dead bodies, then Z. Cotton, "undertaker," could also pull teeth and frame pictures. (*See Figure 4.*)

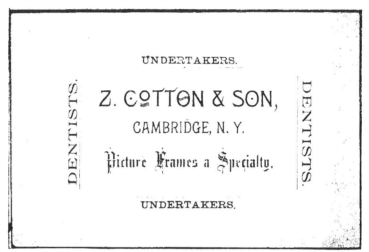

Figure 4. "Professional" Card, Mid-19th Century.

Performers of Personal Service: Well before funeral-undertaking in America evinced any positive signs of developing into a distinct occupation, the care of the dead in early America had been in the hands of those who rendered such attention as a personal service. Friends and neighbors were the first to come to the aid of the bereaved, and, as has usually been the case in small-community life, certain members, quite often adult females, would develop a rough skill in laying out the dead, or, over a period of years, would have given assistance often enough to feel an informal responsibility to offer their services in cases of community or neighborhood deaths.

The first advance toward connecting such informal personal services with a recognized occupation was seen in the tendency for the family nurse or nurse-governess to assume a slightly more formal responsibility for the preparation of the dead for burial. Judge Sewall writes in 1685:

> Having read to my Wife and Nurse out of John; the fourteenth Chapter fell now in course, which I read and went to Prayer: By that time had done, could hear little Breathing, and so about Sunrise, or little after, he fell asleep, I hope in Jesus, and that a Mansion was ready for him in the Father's House. Died in Nurse Hill's Lap. *Nurse Hill washes and layes him out...* Thursday, Decr. 24th 1685. We follow Little Henry to his Grave: Governour and Magistrates of the County here, 8 in all, beside my Self, Eight Ministers, and Several Persons of note... I led Sam., then Cous. Savage led Mother, and Cousin Dumer led Cous. Quinsey's wife, he not

PLATE 26

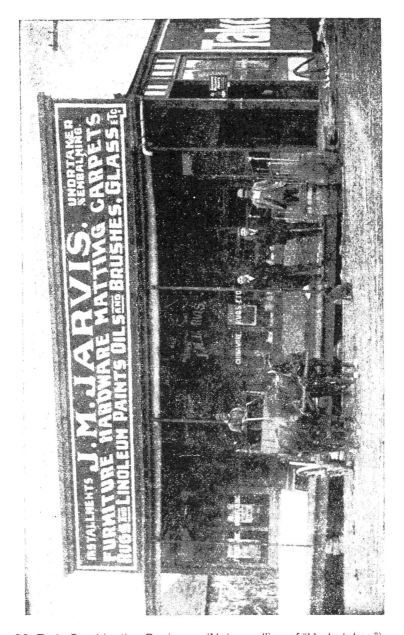

26. Early Combination Business. (Note spelling of "Undertaker.")

well. *Midwife Weeden and Nurse Hill carried the Corps by turns*, and so by Men in its Chestnut Coffin 'twas set into a Grave (The Tomb full of water) between 4 and 5. At Lecture the 21. Psalm was Sung from 8th to the end.[6] (*Italics the authors'*.)

Nurses also practiced healing arts outside of particular families and cared for the sick in small communities, and again, in the case of a death, they extended their personal services to include laying out the dead. Sewall notes, for example, that "This day one of my Shirts goes to lay out a Man dead at Nurse Hurds of this (small pox) distemper, being a Stranger."[7]

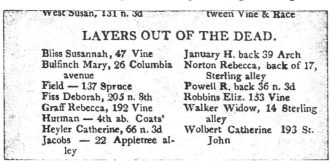

Figure 5. Females Who Performed Undertaking Tasks, Philadelphia city directory, 1810.

Although the midwife often shared with the nurse many of the tasks involved in burials, yet by the end of the 18th century, laying out the dead in larger cities had become a specialty in its own right. The Philadelphia city directory for 1810 added to the section listing occupational specialists, such as "Doctors," "Midwives" and "Bleeders with Leeches," the category of "Layers Out of the Dead."

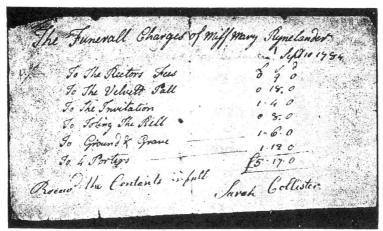

Figure 6. Late-18th-century Funeral Bill,
Showing Participation by Female in Arranging for Services.

In 1810, three persons were listed under such heading. All were likewise listed, however, in the general registry as "nurses."

Looking back through the general registry sections of directories, one finds Rebecca Powell listed in 1801 as "Widow, layer-out-of-the-dead." An earlier case of a female undertaker (although this evidence is less satisfactory since there is no heading attached) finds Sarah Collister

PLATE 27

CHAS. W. COMPTON,
Funeral Furnishing Rooms,
No. 148 MARKET STREET,
Opposite Insurance Buildings,

Where a large assortment of

Ready-made Coffins of various Styles and Prices
can be furnished at the shortest notice.

COFFIN PLATES NEATLY ENGRAVED.
ALSO,
BURIAL DRESSES, CAPS, &c.,
OF NEAT AND SUITABLE PATTERNS.

Having enlarged my former Stock to 16 Coaches, some of the most expensive in this City, also new and elegant Hearses suitable for all ages, enables me to have the most extensive facilities in conducting the Undertaking business in a reasonable and satisfactory manner.

ALSO, MY SUPERIOR
IMPROVED PATENT CORPSE PRESERVER,
ARRANGED SO THAT BODIES CAN BE SEEN AT ALL TIMES WHILE UNDER PRESERVATION.
UNDERTAKERS SUPPLIED AT WHOLESALE.

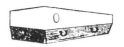

W. V. W. VREELAND.
(Successor to TOLLES & VREELAND,)

WHOLESALE COFFIN WAREROOMS,
AND GENERAL FURNISHING
UNDERTAKER'S ESTABLISHMENT,
125 Market Street, (up stairs.)

COFFINS OF ALL KINDS,
ALSO,
SHROUDS AND DRESSES,
AND ALL THINGS PERTAINING TO THE BUSINESS CONSTANTLY ON HAND, WHICH WILL BE SOLD AT REDUCED RATES. ALSO,

FIRST CLASS HEARSES AND COACHES
FURNISHED.

326 BURIAL CASKETS.

W. W. ROBERTS,
UNDERTAKER,
12 and 14 Pratt St.
Hartford, Conn.

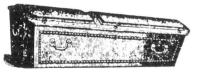

Manufacturer and Dealer at Wholesale and Retail in
Burial Caskets,
INVENTOR and PATENTEE of the
New Round Top Rosewood Caskets,
and of several new designs in Rosewood and Walnut.
ALL KINDS OF
Caskets, Coffins, Shrouds, Caps,
and everything in my line of business furnished at low prices.
HEARSES furnished for Funerals.
All orders promptly attended to by night or day.

SAMUEL PECK,
FURNISHING
UNDERTAKER,
L. B. NEWTON, Practical Assistant.
56, 58 AND 60 HIGH ST., NEAR CHAPEL.

Burial Caskets

Always on hand, of my own make, and of the most desirable patterns suited to all classes.

The Stein Patent
Cloth and Velvet Covered Caskets

GLOBE DRAPED AND PLAIN PATENT CASKET,

Robes, Shrouds, Habits, Linings, Etc.,

We are now prepared at all hours, by day or by night, to furnish everything pertaining to the laying out and burial of deceased persons, giving special attention to preserving and retaining the natural appearance, with or without the use of ice. My assistant, having had long experience, cannot fail to give satisfaction to the friends of deceased persons, relieving the family as much as possible from care and anxiety.
Please call and examine in new style Caskets, especially the "Elm City," (patent applied for) just completed, note prices and see the improvements being made, then, if called upon to select for friends, you can act understandingly.

NIGHT BELL, WITH PERSON ALWAYS IN ATTENDANCE,
A share of the public patronage solicited.

MANUFACTURER AND DEALER IN
Undertakers' Goods.
THE TRADE SUPPLIED ON LIBERAL TERMS.
Telegraph dispatches promptly attended to.

27. Furnishing-Undertaker Advertisements, 1860 and 1870.
(The term "coffin" changes to "casket" in many such ads during this period.)

submitting a bill for different funeral tasks performed in conjunction with the burial of Miss Mary Rynelander, Sept. 10, 1784. (*See Figure 6*.)

Despite their early appearance in the emerging occupation of undertaking, women became less conspicuous in such endeavors as the 19th century got well underway. As the number of services expanded and funerals involved a wider range of tasks to be performed, and as undertaking began increasingly to reflect the spirit of business enterprise, other categories of tradesmen, craftsmen and functionaries came to dominate the occupation.

Religious Functionaries: Until the 19th century, churchyard and church cemetery burial, though not universal, continued as the major mode of sepulture in America, as well as in England. Likewise, the church caretaker, or sexton, has always been associated with churchyard burial and the care of the cemetery.

The sexton in America, however, faced with incompletely defined laws of sepulture, the growing magnitude of cemeterial care as burial grounds expanded, and the inducements of business enterprise, found opportunities to extend his mortuary functions far beyond those of his British counterpart.

Consequently, at the beginning of the 19th century, to the conventional "tolling of the bell" and "digging of the grave," such new undertaking tasks as laying out the body, being "in attendance," directing the procession, and, later, furnishing undertakers with the merchandise and paraphernalia of funerals, were taken over by the sextons.

Apparently by 1800, there was an expanding market for sextons, full- or part-time, in New England, and it might well have been those who went into sexton's work from some other trade who incorporated undertaking functions into the bundle of tasks they were already performing. The evidence of the Boston city directories points in this direction, for by tracing back through the general registers of earlier years — from 1818 when sextons were listed separately as town officers, and forward to 1834 when "undertakers" were first listed as town officers — we can build occupational histories that follow the pattern of craftsmen to sexton, to undertaker. Thus, Thomas Murray in 1807 was a tobacconist; in 1818, sexton; and in 1834, an undertaker. John Law was a cordwainer in 1796; in 1807, a sexton; and in 1817, still a sexton. Records run out at that point on him.

But nearly 50 years of occupational history are reflected in the record of Samuel Winslow, who is listed first in 1796 as housewright; in 1807 as housewright and sexton; in 1818 as sexton; in 1834 as undertaker; and in 1843 still as undertaker, although the general registry indicates he had not given up sexton's work altogether. William Cooley, sexton of Brattle Square Church, took up undertaker's work in the 1840s and continued both functions, but by 1849, he had established a coffin warehouse (*see Plate 28*) and, within a decade, had given up sexton's work to function as undertaker and proprietor of the coffin warehouse.

One of the most notable of the earlier sexton-undertakers was the Reverend Stephen Merritt, who began his undertaking business in 1846, with the first entry on his books dated August 1,

PLATE 28

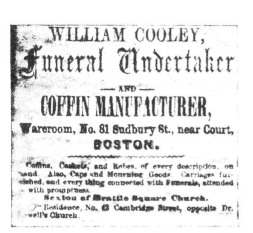

28A. Undertaker, Manufacturer and Sexton, 1849.
(Note early use of term "casket.")

28B. Undertaking as Part-time Work.

28C. Early Advertisement Indicating Use of English-style Trade Sign by American Undertaker.

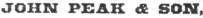
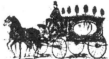

28D. (Left) Livery Stable Keeper and Undertaker, Baltimore, 1847.
28E. Advertisement Showing Use of Term "Funeral Undertakers," Boston, 1873.

1846. In addition to the undertaking tasks, he was cartman, assistant captain of the watch, and a lighter of the oil lamps. He was also an assistant foreman of the Mazeppa Engine Company No. 48; an assessor; and spent his evenings at the Eighteenth Street Episcopal Methodist Church, where he was the sexton. Again, we have an example of undertaking as a sideline or specialty — in this case along with a profusion of "specialties."[8]

Other cases involving the combination of sexton-undertaking became numerous as the 19th century gets well underway. Brooklyn in 1840 had W.B. Disbrow, sexton-undertaker; Joseph Miller, of the same city, three years later advertised himself in the city directory as sexton and undertaker, and gave the address of his "warehouse."

Before the century was half over, all the major cities of America, with the possible exception of Baltimore, had sexton-undertakers. By that time, many had become large-scale furnishing-undertakers, such as Isaac Brown, who advertised in the city directory of New York, 1852-53:

> BROWN, ISAAC H., Sexton of Grace Church and general furnishing undertaker — coffins of all kinds and everything requisite for funerals always on hand. Interments procured in all the public cemeteries in or out of the city... Orders left at his residence... at any hour of the day or night will be promptly attended to.

A final point on sexton-undertakers refers to the prerogative they held over burial in the churchyards under their care. Until William Ensign, one of the first "independent undertakers" of Paterson, New Jersey, took his case to the law courts shortly after 1850, sextons controlled the permits to bury in churchyards and church cemeteries. Such monopoly on sepulture obviously had its advantages for sexton-undertakers and might have provided another reason for their rapid expansion in numbers during the first half of the 19th century.

Municipal Officers: There is some indication that municipal concern with the burial of the dead occurred at a very early point in Colonial history. Landauer notes that one specialty connected with funerals was the "Inviter to Funerals," who actually might have called personally upon those expected to attend. In New York City in 1684, John van Gelder was "approved by the court of mayor and alderman" as "Inviter to funerals." For all who shall employ him, he is to "comport himself Civally."[9]

The same authority, in discussing two of these public officials, notes that they were licensed, were to receive equal profits, and were obliged to attend the burial of the poor without charge. By 1715, the Common Council had a specified set of charges running from "eight to eighteen shillings according to the age of the deceased."

That this public monopoly of the function of inviting to funerals was not a disregarded statute is evidenced by the fact that, in 1755, a suggested reform made much of the fact that violation of the ordinance was punishable by a fine of forty shillings.[10]

Early American funeral-undertakers sometimes found themselves members of town officialdom, charged with duties pertaining to public health and sanitation. By the nature of their work, the undertaker traditionally has been expected to have the technical skills and knowledge qualifying him for the role of coroner — and this specialty, in fact, has remained in close affinity to the undertaker's work for more than a century. Several of the earliest funeral-undertakers, such as Michael Jenkins of Baltimore, Maryland, and Andrew Oakes of Brooklyn, New York, were coroners.

Yet, there were funeral-undertakers in New England who, as municipal officers, functioned, among other things, as the *town* undertaker. An advertisement in the 1838 city directory of Charlestown, Massachusetts, for example, lists:

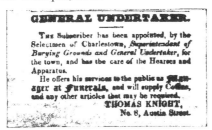

Figure 7. Charlestown, Massachusetts, Town Undertaker, 1838, Advertisement in City Directory.

Often, the undertakers would be town health-officials appointed by the mayor, as in Boston in the 1830s. In different towns, their status varied, however, from superintendent of all mortuary necessities, or city registrar of deaths, down to city messenger. Hollis Chaffin of Providence, Rhode Island, for example, was one of the town's official undertakers in 1856, but also ran an "old peoples' asylum" and kept the city pound!

In many New England towns and cities, it was the practice to bring funeral-undertaking under the supervision of the city registrar, whether or not he would be the town undertaker. All bills for services and merchandise would be itemized on a form provided by the city and approved by him. (***See Plate 29***.)

In summary, the *occupation* of undertaker, specifically named as such and accepted in popular usage, appeared in America in the first half of the 19th century. Although in the latter part of the 18th century, a few people who had formerly been engaged in the undertaking field in England might have been practicing in the Colonies, it is doubtful if the newly developing Colonial society offered substantial footing for what was, in England, an established trade. Rather, out of the circumstances of the reformed nature of early Colonial religious values, the rudeness of the early settlements, and the rise of norms that stressed community controls and the values of mutual aid, the functions of undertaking were first spread out in various ways among neighbors, relatives, clergy, craftsmen, and nurses or family attendants.

The distinctive character of American undertaking, as we know it today, is a consequence of a conjunction of circumstances peculiar to Colonial life, not the least important of which was the assumption of undertaking functions by other established occupations and offices. Thus, the woodworker who, in the earliest Colonial times, made a coffin upon demand, as society and economic opportunity expanded about him, found that it made economic sense to turn a part of his shop into a wareroom or coffin warehouse. The sexton, too, found that, in addition to tolling the bell and digging the grave, or supervising such, he could direct the funeral arrangements and provide materials and equipment that were increasing in general demand.

Similarly, the proprietor of hacks and coaches found that funerals often involved rather extended journeys and that the *order* of the funeral procession could not simply be left to chance or individual discretion. Thus, it was a short step from furnishing a hearse or coach for funeral use to the furnishing of other funeral paraphernalia and to assuming a processional directing function.

On the other hand, one of the earliest functionaries to whom one of the most sacred tasks, laying out the body, was first delegated, i.e., the nurse, could find small justification in a male-dominated society for extending her function to include placing the body in a coffin, conducting the funeral ceremonies, organizing the procession and leading the last rites. Among Colonial customs, there was only small precedent for female services or trade functions, although female undertakers were no novelty in England.

Moreover, the "occupational jump" required to extend one's tasks from laying out the body to the functions listed above seems far greater than was necessary to be made by sexton, cabinet-maker and liveryman.

E.L. Devore enriches this basic summary with a few vivid details:

> The burial of the dead as a distinct and separate business is of comparatively recent origin or necessity. Many of you can remember when a ready-made coffin was an unheard of thing. At that time when a death occurred, the family of the deceased called in their most intimate friend, to whom they left the arrangements for the funeral. He would go to a cabinet-maker or carpenter and together they would work all night by candlelight preparing a coffin. The ordinary one was made of pine and covered with alpaca. When something better was wanted it was made of walnut or cherry, rubbed with beeswax and polished with a hot smoothing iron.
>
> When the coffin was brought to the house, if the deceased was a female the ladies took charge of the preparation of such, as dressing, placing in the coffin, etc.; and if a man, the men performed the same offices. The farm wagon answered for a hearse. I have heard it said that in one part of this state that the coffin containing the remains of a child was generally carried by this friend on horse-back, on a pillow placed on the front of the saddle. In one of the adjacent counties the first hearse ever seen had only two wheels. The body was about the shape of a "Boyd grave vault" and was drawn by one horse, it being led by some one riding alongside. As the country became more thickly settled the cabinet makers began to make coffins "to order" and take charge of funerals, and step by step they advanced until they became known as "undertakers" as well as furniture dealers. In the cities these men gradually limited their business to undertaking.[11]

In America before 1859, then, we find that undertaking had taken on the characteristics of a service occupation with a set of tasks and functions organized into a pattern of behavior toward the dead that basically included the laying out, the coffining, and the transporting of the body

PLATE 29

COFFIN WAREHOUSE,
19 BLOSSOM STREET.
Residence, 48 Poplar Street.

COFFINS AND TRIMMINGS CONSTANTLY FOR SALE.
GRAVE CLOTHES,
OF VARIOUS QUALITIES.
Bodies preserved in Ice, in the best manner possible.
Coffin Plates Engraved.

Boston Jan. 26th 1872

Miss E. A. Doe,

To **N. P. WHITNEY, Undertaker, Dr.**

For burial of Emma B. Doe aged 68 years.
At Woodlawn Mass,

For services at the House, ————————————— $
" placing corpse in the Coffin,   1.50
" carrying corpse and depositing the same in the Tomb or Grave,
     including assistance and 2 horse 5 miles,   10.00
" carrying corpse into Church,
" opening and closing Tomb,
" lighting Cemetery,
" use of Pall,   .25
" digging Grave   feet deep,
" extra charge for frost,
" disinterring and removing bodies, &c.
                              $11.75

Approved for $ ————

City Registrar.

To one coffin with handles & plate 24.20
To one black tibet robe — 12.00
Cash for Receiveing Tomb — 15.00

$62.95

Rec'd Paym't

N. P. Whitney
By
W. H. W.

29. Boston Funeral Bill, Itemized on Form Supplied by City Registrar.

to the grave. Around these central functions, certain auxiliary services, such as the furnishing of paraphernalia of mourning, i.e., clothing, emblems, remembrances, etc., were to some degree included. The role of the clergy was important since the clergyman supplied the funeral's sacred ritual and gave spiritual comfort to the bereaved.

The first half of the 19th century is therefore crucially important in the evolution of the modern funeral director because this period witnessed the gathering and organization of all of the basic undertaking functions under a conventionally recognized name, the "funeral-undertaker" or, more simply and commonly, the "undertaker."

CITATIONS AND REFERENCES IN CHAPTER 6

1. *The Arts and Crafts in New York 1726-1776* (New York: Printed for the New York Historical Society, 1938), pp. 141-142.

2. C.R. Francis, "Funeral Directors Since 1799" *The Embalmers Monthly*, July 1935 reprint, collection of NFDA, Milwaukee, Wis.

3. *Ibid*.

4. Photostatic copy of this will is in the collection of NFDA, Milwaukee, Wis. Other evidence was made available by Kirk & Nice, Undertakers, Germantown, Pa.

5. Bridenbaugh, *op. cit.*, p. 412.

6. Sewall, *op. cit.*, pp. 28-29.

7. Sewall, *op. cit.*, p. 96.

8. "Stephen Merritt Burial Company Memorial," pamphlet found in the Bella C. Landauer Collection of the New York Historical Society. The firm is currently in operation.

9. Bella Landauer, "Some American Funeral Ephemera," *The New York Historical Society Quarterly*, Vol. 36, April 1952, pp. 222-224.

10. *Ibid.*, pp. 223-223.

11. Speech by E.L. Devore. Archives of NFDA, Milwaukee, Wis., n.p., n.d.

Chapter 7

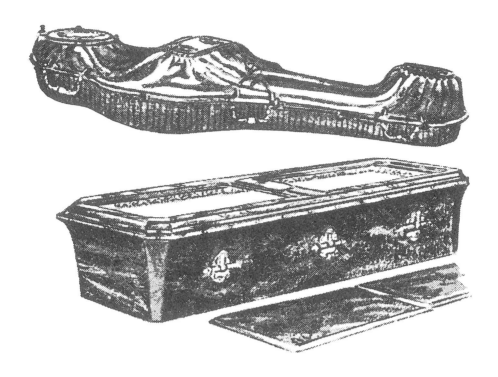

Coffins, Burial Cases and Caskets

How much time, energy, emotion and materials a group of people, whether family, community or nation, will expend on the funerals and disposition of their dead varies by geographical area, historical period and, to a much lesser extent, by level of material wealth. Five thousand years before Christ, the early Egyptians buried their dead in simple graves at the east end of their villages. A few thousand years later, a high proportion of this same civilization's energies were taken up in the care, preservation and disposal of the dead. Today, however, Egyptians have relatively simple burials in comparison with those of three and four thousand years earlier.

The mere passage of time guarantees nothing about the burial customs of peoples, nor does geographic location. Americans spend more money on funerals than do their Latin American neighbors, although the latter spend far more time observing mourning ceremonies.

Moreover, the money Americans spend on funerals does not follow any simple rule, such as "the poorest spend the least and the wealthiest spend the most." Proportionate to their income, the situation is often reversed, and U.S. courts invariably allow a greater percentage of a smaller estate to be spent legitimately on funeral charges. Most funeral directors are aware of cases where those who could afford the most spent the least, and vice versa. One must approach the subject of expenditure of wealth and energy in the burial of the dead with caution for few general statements can safely be offered.

While we have already seen something of the history of coffined burial in cultures that contributed to today's American culture, this chapter focuses on the growth and transformation of interest in burial in coffins and in the multiplication of shapes and designs in the United States. It also explores the changing meaning and functions of the burial receptacle — from the crude wooden coffin of early times to today's more elaborately constructed, aesthetically pleasing caskets.

17th- & 18th-century Coffined Burial in America: The great 17th-century exodus from England to the American Colonies contained a large proportion of skilled craftsmen who brought with them, as part of their cultural baggage, the English medieval craft tradition. A craft was a trade or occupation, the "Art and Mistery" of which was acquired only after a long period of training under a master craftsman.

The household of the master craftsman sheltered one or more journeymen or apprentices. The master not only trained these, but was businessman, as well, dealing with the consumer and producing goods, either upon order or believing he could find a customer for them. Limited only by the willingness of the customer to purchase the goods produced, this craft system afforded adequate opportunity for the development of fine craftsmanship and individuality of product.

Craft organization was not corporate — although the Europeans of the 17th century knew something of the division of labor to make quantity-production possible.

Although Bridenbaugh, an authority on the Colonial craftsman, does not specifically mention coffin-making as one of the crafts represented among the tradesmen immigrants of the 16th century, it is more than likely that the cabinet-makers and carpenters knew coffin-making as a sideline. It is also possible that coffin-makers were among those not encompassed within his study.[1]

The early colonists in America, beset by sickness, starvation and the urgent demands made by a strange, hostile and vigorous country, undoubtedly first buried their dead in the bare earth. With the growth and increasing prosperity of the settlements, however, the custom of burying in a coffin soon made its appearance. Dutch, as well as New England and Virginia colonists, wrapped the dead body in a shroud — a cerecloth might be used to preserve the body for short periods — and placed it in a coffin before burial.

Earle speaks of the coffin as the usual adjunct to the early Colonial burial, and, in one instance cited earlier, presents a funeral bill for David Porter in 1678[2] that includes a "coffin" (12 shillings) and a "windeing sheet" (18 shillings).

Judge Sewall recounts a visit to the family tomb in 1698 where:

> 'Twas wholly dry, and I went at noon to see in what order things were set; and there I was entertain'd with a view of, and converse with, the Coffins of my dear Father Hull, Mother Hull, Cousin Quinsey, and my Six Children... 'Twas an awfull yet pleasing Treat...[3]

From his earlier entry of 1685, we also know that the coffin of one of Sewall's daughters was made of chestnut. The fact that his parents had been buried in coffins seems to indicate that the practice was, at least among the upper classes of a middle-class society, fairly common in the second half of the 17th century.

Students of funeral history have found in the 1683 burial of Roger Williams an early instance of the practice, although by this time, the custom might already have become fairly well established. That the Dutch colonists of the 17th century used coffins in their burials is amply attested by such social historians as Mrs. John King Van Rensselaer, who, in one of her tales of the early Dutch colonists, describes the funeral of a young girl who was buried in a white coffin.[4]

The growing use of coffins is indicated in the fact that, as early as the mid-18th century, slaves occasionally were given coffined burial. It is recorded that Job Townsend Jr. of Newport, Rhode Island, who had learned joinery under his father and set up a shop for himself in which he fashioned furniture of every sort, on one occasion sold to J.R. Rivera a coffin for a Negro slave and "two rolling pins."[5]

By 1750, the development of occupations in the cities of the American Colonies exhibited a subdivision of the crafts. Increasing opportunities for specialization were made possible by growing markets and a steady labor supply. Bridenbaugh points out that:

> Woodworking provides an example of this breaking down or specialization within a trade, for in the city it was divided and subdivided into rough carpentry, joinery, wood turning, carving, coffin making, cabinetmaking, looking-glass making, picture framing, wagon making, coach making, and a variety of other categories to meet the constantly widening demands of the colonial population.[6]

Occasionally, a craftsman in one of these restricted areas, forced by competition or tempted by a chance of increased profit, reversed the trend and supplied any article requested by a buyer. For instance, even though cabinet-making in Philadelphia had become a fairly large and flourishing business by the latter part of the 18th century, permitting a genuine division of labor, a bill rendered by William Savery in 1774 to Joseph Pemberton included charges for mending a knife case, globe, and hobby-horse; nailing a carpet on the stairs; putting a bottom on a rocking chair; and making a mahogany staircase and a walnut coffin with silver handles.[7]

It is highly doubtful that coffins were ever imported during the Colonial period. The ocean voyage was costly and slow, and an individual funeral, particularly in a culture that did not practice embalming, could not wait until an order had been filled from abroad. Moreover, the colonists did not stockpile coffins. Importing and stockpiling would not have made sense when there were cabinet- and coffin-makers available locally who, on demand, could and did turn out very respectable coffins. "Coffin furniture" (trimmings and fittings) were imported during the 18th century; the manufacture of such goods began in this country only after 1800.

Although there was plenty of iron-making in the Colonies during the 18th century — by 1775, they were producing one-seventh of the world supply — early American coffins were made of wood. Different varieties of wood revealed the economic status of the person buried. Hardwoods, polished or stained, went into the more expensive coffins and served the well-to-do while, for the most part, the lowly pine, painted with a mixture of lamp black and glue water, sufficed for the less-fortunate. The shape was nearly always octagonal, a conventional Old World form, with all the sides flat.

Although the coffin traditionally symbolized the trade of English undertakers, who as far back as 1680 displayed trade signs, such as "The Four Coffins" and "Naked Boy and Coffin"[8] to indicate their craft, early American undertakers generally did not follow suit. An exception, found in the 1847 Baltimore city directory, reads: "R. Frederick, Undertaker of Funerals and Chair Maker, opposite the Engine House, Sign of the Gold Coffin." (**See Plate 28, Chapter 6**.) A more common sketch accompanying the advertisements of the early 19th century shows a hearse in the midst of a procession of several carriages.

Coffin-making as a specialty in woodworking appears with the growth of an urban population in early America.[9] As noted in the previous chapter, cabinet-makers and carpenters alike lent their efforts to making coffins when the demand was present, and nearly all earlier "undertakers" made the care of the dead only a sideline to their regular trade.

Others, however, turned to coffin-making as a full-time occupation, while some of the more enterprising began to furnish coffins and funeral paraphernalia to those who possessed the rudiments of service skills but did not have the materials to furnish to the families of the deceased. Thus, there emerged the "coffin shop," followed by "coffin warehouses" and "furnishing-undertakers."

As early as the mid-18th century, coffin-makers in America could buy "coffin furniture," i.e., decorations, plates, handles, etc., for their trade. In the *Boston Gazette*, May 29, 1758, there appears an advertisement:[10]

> COFFIN FURNITURE to be sold by Arthur Savage Tomorrow Evening at his Vendue Room, about 50 sett of Neat Polished Coffin Furniture, consisting of Breast-plates, Angels, Flowers, etc.

Similar advertisements are found in the *Pennsylvania Pocket*, as in 1799 when John Norman is found selling:[11]

> Coffin Furniture Made and Sold by the subscribers in Front Street between Market and Arch Streets, Philadelphia. Persons wanting large quantities are requested to give timely notice as materials are very scarce. The best prices are given by them for block tin, pewter and lead. Pocket and sheet Almanacks for the year 1780 are likewise sold at the subscribers, elegantly engraved on copper, having a curious likeness of His Excellency General Washington; also, a great variety of children's books, Paper hangings, etc.
>
> Thomas Nevell, Thomas Bedwell, John Norman.

Early Coffin Shops and Coffin Warehouses: The period of Westward expansion following the War of 1812 was marked by the rapid growth and spread of coffin shops focused exclusively on the production of burial receptacles, and by the beginning of coffin warehouses. The firm of John L. Dillon, Coffin and Shroud Warehouse, of New York, founded at this time, was one of the first of its kind in America. With the appearance of such small but vigorously productive enterprises, the emphasis in funerals began to shift in the direction of the *coffin*, especially regarding price, quality and diversity of purpose.

The reproduction of the funeral bill presented by John L. Dillon to Baldwin and Spooner in 1825 (*see Figure 8*) offers more than a simple illustration of funeral service provided by an undertaker who bought coffins from a manufacturer. The fact that the item "Mahogany Coffin,

Coffins, Burial Cases and Caskets

Lined, Trimmed, Hinged, and Mounted... $24.00," is listed first is especially noteworthy when comparing this bill to David Porter's (mentioned earlier in this chapter and in Chapter 5), which was rendered about a century and a half earlier. In the Dillon bill below, the charge for the coffin constitutes nearly two-thirds of the entire bill, while in the earlier specimen, the twelve-shilling price of the coffin is almost inconsequential — less than one-fourth the cost of liquors alone!

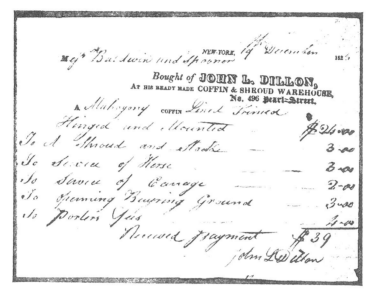

Figure 8. Early 19th-century Funeral Bill.

The evidence gathered from city directories, funeral bills, newspaper and journal advertisements, and records of early funeral establishments indicates that possibly one of the most significant developments in early 19th-century funeral business was this growth of coffin shops and coffin warehouses, paralleled by an increased popular attention given to the burial receptacle as a major item in burials.

Although the pattern was not immediately established, from this period on it becomes increasingly clear that American burial, although modified by backward glances toward the late English feudal period, is beginning to build a solid pattern of its own upon its simple Judeo-Christian-English foundation. This pattern was in keeping with a democratic New World social system in which no well-defined social classes separated by insurmountable barriers existed.

Variation in Early Function and Type: Although Americans had earlier turned their increasing attention to burial in coffins in funeralizing their dead, only about 1800 did they begin to make a determined effort to improve the function, style and composition of these receptacles. Throughout the 19th century in America, by means of experimentation carried out by a considerable number of people, the old-fashioned coffin slowly transformed into the modern casket.

Coffin- and casket-makers sensed goals that, at one time or other, they tried to reach, especially concerning improvements: their product should have increased utility; it should better indicate the importance of the dead person and his or her family; it should provide more protection against graverobbers and the forces of dissolution; and, finally, it should be more artistic and more beautiful to better harmonize with the aesthetic movement in burials.

The order in which these goals are listed roughly indicates the sequence in which each received major emphasis from American 19th-century coffin- and casket-makers, although some of them — such as the use of the coffin to display the wealth or importance of the dead — obviously were present throughout most of the history of Western civilization. Other themes, as will be seen in the discussion of particular types of coffins, have waxed and waned in popularity and usage.

The practice, if not the basic idea, of coffined burial is part of the American inheritance from later British folkways. We have seen that by the time the American Colonies were being heavily settled, many, if not the majority, of Englishmen were being buried in coffins. One function served was purely utilitarian — a simple, unadorned wooden receptacle was used to encase the dead body before burial. For those of higher station, the coffin, by its quality of materials, workmanship and adornment, served to indicate the social-class differences that separated their group from other groups.

In addition, well-to-do merchants and professional people, the aristocracy and the nobility would, after death, lie in state for an extended length of time. For these, in conjunction with generally crude preservation methods to render the decomposing body less offensive, a lead inner-coffin was employed. Thus, in Paris on July 20, 1792, the American naval hero of the Revolutionary War, John Paul Jones, was buried in a lead coffin, his limbs wrapped in tinfoil. The efficacy of the method was demonstrated when, in 1905, after a six-year search, his still-recognizable body was located.

With the growth of medical science in England and the increased need for cadavers for use in anatomical studies, the practice of graverobbing and body snatching became common enough to rouse the populace to a state of alarm concerning the safety of their dead. British trade undertakers of the late-18th century were aware of this concern and advertised coffins of iron and other ghoul-proof innovations in burial receptacles. The trade card of one read:

> IMPROVED COFFINS — The fastenings of these improved receptacles being on such a principle as to render it impracticable for the grave robbers to open them. This security must afford great consolation at an aera when it is a well-authenticated fact that nearly one thousand bodies are annually appropriated for the purpose of dissection.[12]

The importance placed on iron coffins is also shown in an 1822 advertisement:

> The only safe coffin is Bridgman's Patent Wrought Iron one, charged the same price as a wooden one, and is a superior substitute for lead.[13]

In America, during the first half of the 19th century when medical schools were few and far between, the theme of protecting the dead from ghouls appears to have had considerably less force in shaping the design of burial receptacles. It did play a more important part later in the century, however, when grave vaults were introduced into the burial complex.

In strong competition with the desire to render the dead safe from human harm was the need to preserve the dead — not for eternity, but rather for a period sufficient to permit family members and relatives separated by considerable distances to make the journey and attend the funeral. Conversely, the preservation of the body for a short span of time could also permit its transportation back to the family burial ground from the more-remote parts of the country.

Yet, even before 1850, there was apparent an emerging impulse to encase the body in a receptacle whose primary claim to public acceptability lay in the fact that it was beautiful, and thus suitable for use in funerals. Already underway was a gradual drift in mood from gloom to beauty. That this drift had an increasing and lasting vitality should be clear to anyone seeking to learn the origin of the use of the casket in modern funeral practice. (A corresponding development is found in the emphasis on restorative art as one of the most valued aspects of the embalming process.)

The key, then, to understanding the historical development of coffin styling and composition is to be found in the dynamic interplay of five major themes in defining and fulfilling the proper function of the burial receptacle. These themes were utility, status indication, preservation of the body, protection, and aesthetic representation. In the illustrations of some of the more outstanding receptacle types that follow, the presence or absence, emphasis or de-emphasis of these various themes will be evident.

Stone and Metal Coffins: Coffins of material other than wood make their appearance in the first half of the 19th century, though it is possible that, in rare instances, iron coffins might have been used in an earlier period of American history. Although James A. Gray of Richmond, Virginia, received the first American patent on a metallic coffin in 1836, a year earlier, patents had been granted to John White and Associates of Salina, New York, for coffins made of "stone or marble" and of "hydraulic cement." These patents were allowed to expire in 1849, either because the coffins were hard to manufacture, were too heavy to be handled, or had little aesthetic appeal or popular acceptance.

Nevertheless, the granting of these patents signaled a deluge of ideas in the design and composition of burial receptacles. By 1860, patents had been sought for coffins not only of iron, cement, marble and artificial stone, but also of potter's clay; cement and wood; iron and wood; and zinc, iron and glass combined. Before the turn of the century, the list was enlarged to include burial receptacles made of elastic materials, including vulcanized rubber; fabricated metals of various kinds and combinations; papier-mâché; aluminum; cloth and wood; wood and glass; and coffins with inner-coffins.

In one arresting case, an 1876 patent was granted for "coffins or caskets and their ornaments of celluloid, which, in a dissolved or plastic state, is cast in forms or molds, by which process the coffin or casket bodies as well as their lids are manufactured."

The Fisk Metallic Coffin: Perhaps the most remarkable coffin ever patented and put into widespread use in America was the Fisk, "An Air-tight Coffin of Cast or Raised Metal," patented in 1848. Although it was specified only as an "improvement in coffins" (metallic coffins having been patented earlier), it contained innovations in design that recalled at once the ancient Egyptian sarcophagus, the iron torpedo, and the strong box.

In the original letters-patent sketch (*see Figure 9*), the side view shows the top half of the two shells, which form the coffin, cast to fit the form of a person flat on his or her back with arms folded. A glass plate kept the face visible, similar to a diving helmet. The formfitting character reduced weight (an important drawback of earlier metallic coffins) and, at the same time, reduced the air space.

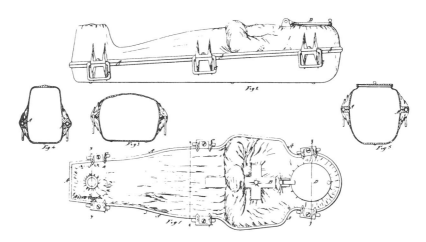

Figure 9. Patent Sketch of Fisk Metallic Burial Case, 1848.

Its inventor, Almond D. Fisk, claimed to have created "a new and useful manner of constructing an Air-tight Coffin of Cast or Raised Metal... with the least possible quantity of metal, by means of which lightness is obtained... (from which)... the air may be exhausted so completely as entirely to prevent the decay of the contained body on principles well understood; or if preferred, the coffin may be filled with any gas or fluid having the property of preventing putrefaction."

The Fisk Metallic Burial Case patent, issued for 14 years, expired in 1862. During this period, Fisk apparently licensed or franchised a number of manufacturers to use his patent, while continuing to produce the Fisk burial case himself under the partnership name of Fisk and Raymond. Located at Newtown, Long Island, New York, the firm had an office and salesroom in New York City, where they sold their cast-iron cases for $7.00-$40.00.[14]

During the Civil War, advertisements for Fisk coffins for sale by W.M. Raymond Co., Long Island, suggest that Fisk, by the time his patent expired or shortly thereafter, was already dead. In any event, in 1865, the U.S. Congress approved a measure "for the relief of the heirs of Almon (*sic*) D. Fisk," permitting them to apply for a seven-year extension, as though the patent had not expired.[15]

The Raymond Co. apparently continued to make the Fisk coffin, but other companies also manufactured the product, among them A.C. Barstow Co. of Providence, Rhode Island, and W.C. Davis & Co., stove founders of Cincinnati, Ohio.

There is not much to suggest large-scale production in the early years after the patent had been granted in 1848. The cost, for one thing, was considerably above that of wooden coffins, and its use, in most cases, was undoubtedly restricted to the well-to-do. That this was the case in at least one significant instance is shown in the testimonial appearing in the *New York Tribune* in April 1850:

FISK'S METALLIC BURIAL CASES

The entombment of John C. Calhoun in one of these cases has elicited the following letter, signed by many Hon. U.S. Senators — "Gentlemen: We witnessed the utility of your ornamental Patent Metallic Burial Case used to convey the remains of the late Hon. John C. Calhoun to the

Congressional Cemetery. It impressed us with the belief that it is the best article known to us for transporting the dead to their final resting place."

The signatures on this letter were Jefferson Davis, Henry Dodge, Henry Clay, Dan'l Webster, and Lewis Cass.[16]

A year before, when former President James K. Polk died, his body was interred in the city cemetery of Nashville, Tennessee, wrapped with a silk winding sheet and buried in an old-fashioned, raise-lid-style coffin, which was covered with black broadcloth, lined with copper and tightly sealed.

The Large-scale Manufacture of Metallic Burial Cases: The widespread use and commercial success of the Fisk Metallic Burial Case is, to a considerable extent, to be associated with the founding of a manufacturing concern capable of standardizing production on a mass basis and distributing the product in the Eastern and Midwestern United States in large-scale quantity lots.

The development of metallic burial-case manufacture on a significant scale begins with the acquisition of manufacturing rights from Fisk by M.H. Crane and J.R. Barnes of Cincinnati, Ohio. This firm was organized August 15, 1853, under the name of Crane, Barnes and Co. Five months later, it was succeeded by Crane, Breed & Co., consisting of M.H. Crane, A.D. Breed, and John Mills. In 1860, W.J. Breed purchased the shares of John Mills and the firm continued under that ownership and title until 1882, when it was incorporated as the Crane and Breed Mfg. Co.

It should be noted that, with the introduction of metallic burial cases into the funeral business of America at mid-century, the basis of manufacture and production of burial receptacles underwent a very significant change. Although the cabinet and carpenter shops might still produce wood coffins in substantial numbers, the day of small coffin shops dominating the scene began to wane. Put another way, the small coffin shop, devoting most of its production to a craftsman's product, emerged at the end of the Colonial period and continued to flourish during the first half of the 19th century, but with the appearance of metallic burial cases, a new mode of coffin construction based on *mass-production* methods emerged and became the leading method of manufacture in the second half of the century.

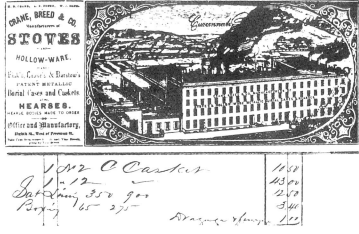

Figure 10. Mid-1860s Illustration of Crane, Breed & Co. Factory:
"Stoves, Hollow-ware, Fisk's, Crane's & Barstow's Patent Metallic Burial Cases and Caskets"

The mid-1860s illustration of the Crane, Breed & Co.'s factory in Cincinnati indicates the significance of the departure from the small coffin shop with its craftsmanship orientation. (*See Figure 10.*) Stove manufacturers, instead of woodworkers, were now in the business of burial case production — and a big business it was to become.

The success of the metallic burial case began with the demonstrable proposition that it preserved the body. "We assert," a 1858 Crane, Breed & Co. brochure declared, "and refer to our numerous testimonials for the proof, that the bodies of the dead have been preserved in Metallic Burial Cases for months and not unfrequently for years, without any perceptible changes." This allowed distant relatives to journey to the deceased's home and "behold again the features of their departed friends."

Other claims calculated to commend the cast-metal case to the public were advanced: protection of the body against water seepage and vermin; safeguarding against infection and contagious diseases (not a small consideration in a century noted for its plagues and epidemics); and, finally, the facilitation of removal of the body for reburial.

The latter point was not incidental. Many of the dead did not reach their final resting place at burial. Quite often, in towns and cities, the dead were deposited in public vaults "for the winter."

Moreover, the rapid growth of towns had already made the removal of graveyards to more-remote or suburban areas imperative. In older cities, scarcely one of the pauper burying grounds, or "potter's fields," of the large cities was located on its original site by mid-century. And most of the cemeteries that had been already moved were to be moved again, and perhaps even once more, by 1900. Although regular burial grounds were less likely to be moved, there was no guarantee that one would ever "sleep for eternity" in an urban cemetery.

It is worth repeating that the large-scale shipment of bodies back to family homesteads or family vaults no doubt received its greatest impetus with the mass return of the Civil War dead to their homes, and with the growth of steamboat and rail transportation. The metallic burial case thus provided an improved device for returning bodies from a distance for burial with ancestors and other relatives.

From Pragmatic to Aesthetic: When patented, the Fisk mummy case was far removed from the realm of artwork. (*See Figure 11*.) As produced in 1853 by Crane, Barnes and Co., the form had been retained much like the original, with some simplification of line and design.

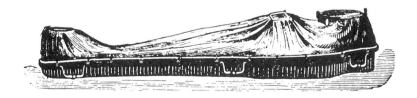

Figure 11. Fisk Mummy Case, Style of 1853.

Increased public acceptance led the company to announce, in a circular dated 1854, increased facilities, stepped up production and "new patterns, combining many important improvements in style and finish." The most important pattern changes included the new "Bronzed Case" line, i.e., cast-iron with bronze finish, bedecked with highly wrought ornaments, representing drapery, flowers, emblems of mortality, etc.

"Much that has hitherto contributed to shock the feelings of the sensitive and delicate," the brochure goes on to say, "is now dispensed with altogether. We are, therefore, warranted in saying that in all the essentials of an appropriate and befitting depository for the dead, the cases we now offer to the public surpass any that have hithertofore been in use."

Two styles, the "Ornamental" and the "Cloth Covered," were offered in this line. The latter had its lower half covered with "fine French cloth, trimmed with silk fringe." (*See Figure 12*.)

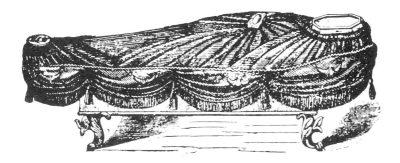

Figure 12. Cloth Covered, "Bronzed Case," 1854.

Simultaneous with the issuing of the "Bronzed Case" line, there appeared in 1854 the "Plain, or Octagon" pattern, finished in imitation rosewood (the finish glued to the metal surface somewhat resembling "decalcomania," in which designs were transferred from paper to porcelain or glass) and polished equal to the finest furniture. (*See Figure 13*.)

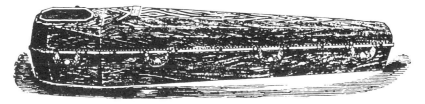

Figure 13. "Plain or Octagon" Metallic Burial Case.

A variety in sizes and depth was offered. Plain lining consisted of cambric and cotton wadding, priced separately. Those with lining cost slightly extra in the "Ornamental" line, but the refinements of the "Cloth Covered" included a substantial increase in price. In 1854, the wholesale price of a six-foot "Ornamental Bronzed Case" was $20.50, with plain lining $2.00 extra. For the "Plain, or Octagon" type of case, the price was $1.75 extra. The cost of a "Cloth Covered Case," including lining with white satin and silver-plated mountings, was an additional $21.00.

Until the appearance of the casket, a coffin covered or draped with fine fabric in the current European style constituted the luxury level of burial receptacles. Yet, in the words of an 1862 Crane, Breed & Co. catalog, the "Bronzed Case" line, despite Crane's refinement of the original

Fisk "mummy case" pattern: "Repelled the sensitive and failed, in a measure, of meeting the wants of the refined."

The "Covered Case" marked the ultimate in the attempts of the company to enhance the aesthetic appeal of the original pattern, and although it fell out of favor, the idea of *beauty in burial cases* led to a new and rather distinctly American form of burial receptacle, the *casket*. The "Plain, or Octagon" burial case, with its enlarged glass, improved sealing flange (composition sealing was all-important in metallic cases), and high degree of transportability, nevertheless continued in favor through the 1850s.

The Metallic Burial Casket: In a "Specification of Letters Patent" dated April 19, 1859, A.C. Barstow of Providence, Rhode Island, remarked on the changing sensitivities of American burial-case taste:

> The burial cases formerly used were adapted in shape nearly to the form of the human body, that is they tapered from the shoulders to the head, and from the shoulders to the feet. Recently, in order to obviate in some degree the disagreeable sensation produced by a coffin on many minds, the casket, or square form has been adopted; and of this kind, the metallic burial cases have for many reasons been preferred.

Barstow then goes on to note that the waste space in many of the metallic cases, and the increased weight, constituted serious objections to their use. His innovation was designed to improve burial cases of the square variety, i.e., caskets, by reducing the excess space through "ogee" design. (***See Plate 30***.) The system of overlapping ribs has its counterpart in some form of metallic caskets currently in use.

But the origin of the American casket is difficult, if not impossible, to place. Claims for the earliest straight-sided burial case have been made running back to 1830. In the popular mind, the term "casket" suggests a "jewel box" or container for something valuable. When we read of "Iron Casketts" on the import lists of dutiable articles in the Colonies, the reference is to an iron box or container and not a burial receptacle.

The Boston city directory of 1849 offers the first recorded indication of the introduction of "casket" into American burial usage. "William Cooley, Funeral Undertaker and Coffin Manufacturer," advertised "Coffins, caskets and robes of every description..." (***See Plate 28, Chapter 6***.)

It is quite likely that the idea of a straight-side receptacle might well have been independently conceived by several coffin manufacturers at approximately the same time. In the course of the next 50 years of experimentation in burial receptacle styles and materials, such simultaneous invention was to happen many times, as duplicating claims for something new in the way of stone, cement, glass, terra cotta and the like were to pour into the U.S. Patent Office.

Three firms specializing in the manufacture of coffin furniture — the McGraw and Taylor Co., and a firm headed by Joseph Applegate, both of New York, and the William M. Smith & Co. of Meriden, Connecticut — might well have been involved in the earliest ventures in straight-sided coffins, or "caskets" as they were later to be called. In default, however, of compelling evidence to support the claims that any of these concerns was the earliest to produce such an item, the records sustain William Cooley of Boston, Massachusetts, as the first to offer caskets to the American public.

PLATE 30

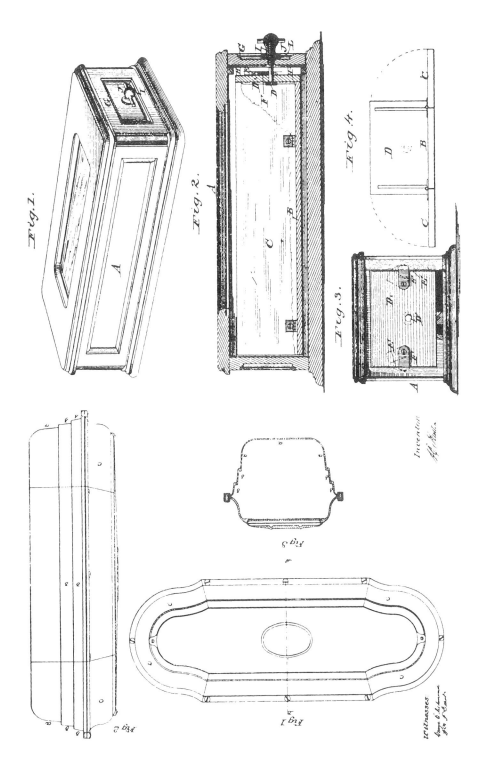

30B. End Seal Airtight Burial Casket, Patent Sketch, 1877.

30A. Early Metallic Burial Case, "Ogee" Design to Reduce Excess Space.

More significantly, the change in burial-receptacle pattern from the various earlier burial cases manufactured by Crane, Breed & Co., to the Crane's Patent Casket, occurring between 1858 and 1862, undoubtedly marks the introduction of the new style on a mass-production basis, and gives it its *popular* birthright. (It might be observed that the changeover was preceded by a short-lived, in-between model, the zinc "shoulder casket" in 1857. (***See Figure 14.***)

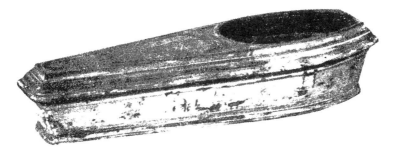

Figure 14. Zinc "Shoulder Casket" Burial Case, 1857.

It can be seen that the "sarcophagus principle" of shaping the casket top to the human form had already given way, and, for the modern form of casket to appear, only a "rectangularizing" of the receptacle was necessary. (***See Figure 15.***)

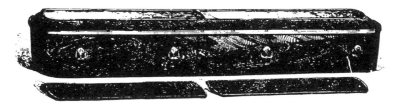

Figure 15. Casket, Modern Rectangular Form, About 1860.

In presenting the new style of burial receptacle, the 1862 manufacturer's brochure pointed out that it possessed such advantages as being simple; "chaste," i.e., pure and simple in design, not ornate; and airtight. The last characteristic, it was claimed, would check the spread of contagion and, for a time, would arrest the process of decomposition. Like the "Plain Case," it was described as "invaluable as a means of transporting the body of a deceased friend to a distant part of the land, or even to a foreign land, for sepulture."

Perhaps the most radical change in the construction of this casket, versus the burial case, was in its top, which consisted of two large sections of plate glass, between which the nameplate was located. Each of the glass sections had an ornamented cap that could be screwed on before or after the funeral ceremonies.

Thus, the *encasing* of the body, the primary idea expressed in earlier burial receptacles, is now modified toward the *presentation* of the dead in a burial receptacle designed to provide an aesthetically pleasing setting for its visually prominent and dramatically centered object of attention.

From 1862 on through the remainder of the century, improvements were made in the metallic casket, and also in the wooden case. (***See Plate 31***.) The weight of the cast-metal receptacles continued to offset other advantages, and the appearance of the lighter metal and cloth-covered wooden burial cases and caskets caused casket manufacturers for the rest of the century to be acutely conscious of the competing principles of durability, preservation and aesthetic quality of the metallic burial cases and caskets, as opposed to the lightness and pleasing exterior of the wooden and the cloth-wooden types.

In the early 1870s, Crane, Breed & Co. supplied the first true sheet-metal casket to the trade. While it retained the top of the new casket, the body was of sheet metal made over iron flanges at bottom and top. Designated the "Oriental," this casket and the earlier "New Casket," an improved version of the earlier Crane's Patent Casket, were the leading metallic receptacles on the market.

In the process of shedding weight, the lighter sheet-metal caskets gradually came to replace the heavier caskets of cast-iron. Summarizing this development, a brochure by the Crane and Breed Casket Company states:

> Increasing adaptability of steel and the ease with which it could be formed into more ornamental shapes, added to the lightness of the material, and finally displaced the heavier caskets;... (but) the difficulty of adopting the more durable metal zinc to these modern forms forced the abandonment of that metal for a time.[17]

The term "casket" did not immediately replace "burial case" — a term sometimes used generically to designate all burial receptacles, sometimes to indicate a coffin built along Egyptian mummy-case principles, or some modification or refinement thereof — or "coffin," the traditional term taken over from earlier English usage. Instead, a period of confused burial-receptacle terms existed from the 1850s through the Civil War. Patent applications throughout this period and later show the highest usage for the term "coffin" — primarily because this was the first category of burial receptacles used by the U.S. Patent Office.

Although terms such as "burial case" and "burial casket" were to gain increasing use after 1870, it is not until the 1890s that the term "casket" came to dominate the language of burial receptacles in patent literature. In popular language, the term "burial case" enjoyed a mild vogue just before and after the Civil War, but gave way to "coffin" and "casket," both of which are interchangeable in America for the conventional straight-lined rectangular receptacle. The wedge-shaped octagonal "coffin" no longer exists in America, but the American "casket" has yet to be popularly accepted in England and Europe. The American funeral director's "coffin" signifies the Continental form of receptacle.

These statements must be made with the reservation that, although "casket" is the term generally accepted in America today, a few firms still cling to the older names, probably because these have been long identified with their businesses. Thus, "Coffin Companies" and "Burial Case Companies" were still represented in the roster of firms at the 1955 Massachusetts Conference of Casket Manufacturers.

Cloth Burial Cases: The success of the metallic burial case was based on the demonstrable claim of body preservation, in addition to the unique design of the earliest Fisk "mummy case" innovation. Its continued acceptance derived to a great extent from successful large-scale manufacture and distribution of the product, and also from the willingness of its manufacturers to vary the style and materials to produce a burial receptacle that continued to please the eye.

While the "metallic" never compromised its preservation function, its form, as noted earlier, slowly moved from the sarcophagus mummy-case to the rectangular casket. A somewhat different development in the manufacture of burial receptacles, however, is found in the story of the introduction of the mass-produced, wood-constructed, metal-reinforced, cloth-covered burial case.

Although the use of cloth to cover the more luxurious of burial receptacles had been practiced by English and Continental undertakers from the beginning of the 19th century, if not earlier, its incorporation into American burial usage, as noted before, dates closer to 1850. The development of a *line* of cloth-covered burial cases as the main item of manufacture began in 1871 with Samuel Stein and his Stein Patent Burial Casket.

Stein reflected all the genius of the innovator, and it is credit to his persistent belief in the idea of a light, strong and aesthetically pleasing cloth-covered casket that the changing pattern of American burial rapidly moved from the more ponderous type of burial receptacles. Stein, originally trained as a cabinet-maker in Austria after a wandering career in Europe and America, settled down shortly after 1850 in Rochester, New York, as a builder of showcases.

Around 1870, the idea of a casket built along showcase lines with glass sides occurred to him. After experimenting for some time, he actually produced a model of such a casket and secured a patent on it. It proved "too innovational" for the times, however, and he soon modified it by replacing the glass sides with wood, and then covering these panels with cloth.

Although the patent for this casket was granted late in 1872, Stein had already begun a small shop a year earlier to manufacture a cloth-covered casket. His first triumph was securing an order for a casket to be used for the funeral of James Gordon Bennett, proprietor and editor of the *New York Herald*, who died June 1, 1872. Its appearance aroused a host of comment, and leading New York papers described its radical features in mixed tones of awe and astonishment. Said the *New York Sun*:

> The casket in which the remains of Mr. Bennett are enclosed is remarkable for its elegance. It is nearly square, and made of a species of wood said to be more durable than any metal. The side of the panels are covered with the most costly Lyons velvet. The handles, of which there are eight, are of solid silver. They represent two hands grasping a rod about eight inches long. The lid is in two parts, or panels, and made of French crystal plate glass. Two panels of Lyons velvet are made so as to cover the glass when required. The lid is hung on heavy silver hinges, and is secured by two heavy locks. The entire casket is surrounded by a massive moulding of silver, forming a framework which will survive the lapse of ages. The inside is upholstered with white satin, silk and Venetian lace, heavy silken tassels dropping from each corner.

PLATE 31

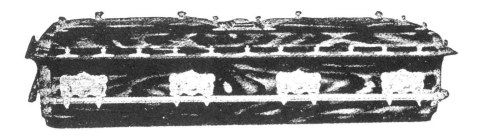
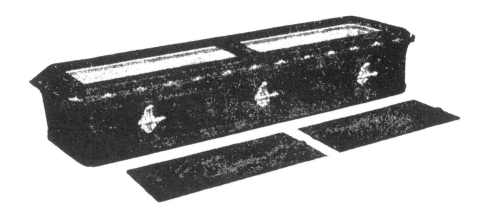
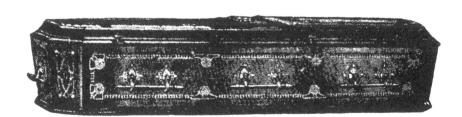
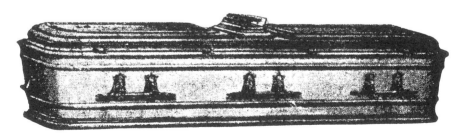

31. Examples of the Casket-maker's Art, Late-19th Century.
(The top two are metallic; the bottom two are wood.)

Quite modest in its origin, the Stein Manufacturing Company had begun with a handful of workmen and a room of about 1,000 feet of floor space. (*See Figure 16*.) As it prospered, it expanded its establishment and, in 1890 when it merged with the National Casket Co., it occupied nearly 100,000 square feet of space and was producing 600 cloth-covered caskets weekly.

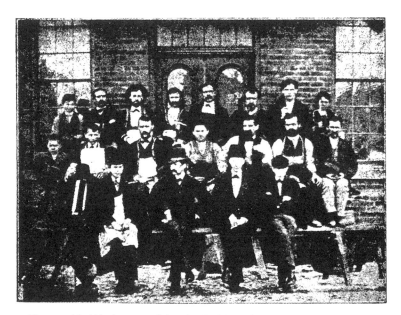

Figure 16. Workmen of the Stein Manufacturing Co. in 1873.

In the early years of the concern, however, all was not easy sailing. On the competitive side, the metallic cases offered a durability that could scarcely be matched by the cloth-covered receptacle, although, as early as 1874, a brochure claimed for the Stein cases that, "in regard to decay they will outlast any metal casket ever placed in the ground." In addition, the traditional wooden coffin, handmade with highly polished sides, still had the favor of many undertakers who preferred to make their own.

But if the specially made casket for James Gordon Bennett introduced the cloth-covered casket to the country, it was the Stein casket display at the Philadelphia Centennial of 1876 that impressed the public mind with the advantages of this new form of burial receptacle. Stein decided, in what was a bold move, to make a display of modern burial receptacles, as manufactured by his company, available to the public. To this end, he engaged space in one of the main exhibition halls.

Because of the objections of other neighboring exhibitors, however, permission to display the Stein caskets was revoked. Stein's response was to secure the necessary permission to exhibit in a separate building *of his own construction*, which was completed only a few hours before the exposition opened.

The success of this exhibit resulted not only in putting the Stein Manufacturing Co. on the map, but it also reinforced the fashion of placing coffins and caskets on display in coffin shops and in undertaking establishments, where such receptacles were made.

In the early history of this company, a third milestone occurred in 1885 with a casket order for the funeral of former President Ulysses S. Grant. The "Style E State Casket," made with the finest black broadcloth, heavy silver metal mountings, and a flat top with full French plate glass, was chosen. (***See Figure 17 & Plate 32***.) Its inner metallic case was especially finished on the interior and set off by a pillow on which the general's initials were embroidered. The result, claimed a company brochure, was a "real triumph," adding, "another real influence on the general acceptance of the cloth covered casket was exerted."

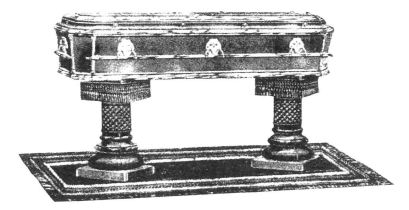

Figure 17. Stein "Style F State Casket," Similar to President U.S. Grant's Casket.

"Also-rans" in 19th-century Burial Receptacles: During the 19th century in America, three types of burial receptacles were commonly used: the traditional wooden coffin, the metallic "mummy case," and the cloth-covered, metal-reinforced burial case. In the course of time, all three were gradually modified in an effort to improve their appearance.

While these three were more or less in general use, many other receptacles were dreamed of, or even produced, during the same time but failed to gain popular acceptance. These were the "also-rans" of the coffin-casket industry.

Two influences were at cross-purposes in this experimentation. The first was a potential market for a more artistic or more serviceable funeral receptacle; the second consisted of the "hard facts" of actual production and distribution. As a result of the latter, many innovators and inventors never managed to get their proposals beyond the "idea stage." Some could not secure capital to begin production; others found themselves owning patents but without means of manufacturing; and still others found that while they could get limited quantities of the patented funeral receptacles produced, they could find no ready market to support further operations. By the operation of economic factors, a number of poorly conceived or impractically designed caskets were thus kept *off* of the market.

Outstanding examples of such "also-rans" are found in early U.S. patent files. It is interesting to note that all three patents issued in 1835 — the first in America — for coffins of cement and artificial stone were not produced, and these patents expired 17 years later without the public even having the opportunity to accept or reject the innovation.

Dogged by the problem of weight, those who saw a future in coffins of some form of earth-composition continued to seek a shape or combination that would permit the production of a burial receptacle that might at least be lifted, if not carried, by pallbearers. One variation arose in 1855 when David Sholl received a letters-patent for a coffin composed of terra cotta, or pottery ware. (*See Figure 18*.) Records do not show the fate of this innovation, although its lighter weight put it one step beyond the earlier cement types.

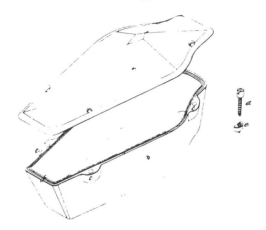

Figure 18. Terra Cotta Coffin, 1855, Patent Sketch

Some 16 years earlier, Moses Leonard of Syracuse, New York, had sought to perfect, and had even patented, a coffin made from a combination of wood and cement. The "cement" in this case was a mixture of rosin, beeswax and pulverized stone. Whether the major obstacle to the production of this type of coffin developed in the mixing of the ingredients to produce suitable cement, or because of the weight once made, historical records do not show. In any event, it failed to reach the market and wooden coffins remained the only choice available.

An intermediate step between the cement coffin and its eventual form as a burial vault was the invention patented on May 1, 1880, by William H. Bachtel of Canton, Ohio, of the "coffin, burial-casket, or vault of clay or other plastic materials."

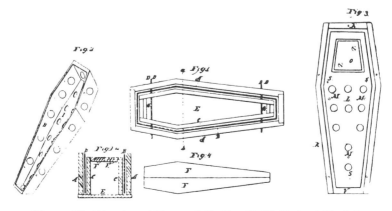

Figure 19. Wood and Cement Coffin, 1839, Patent Sketch

PLATE 32

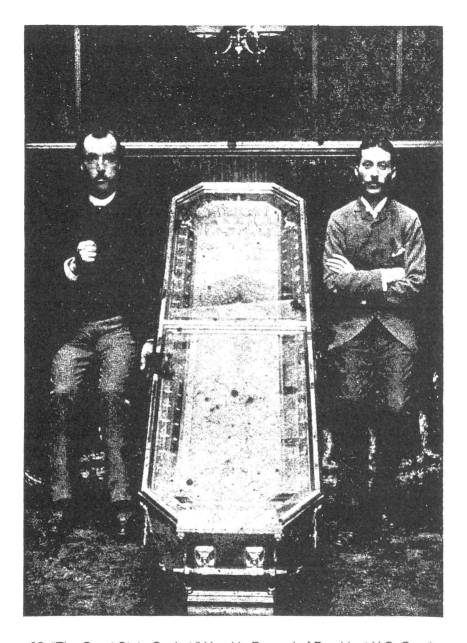

32. "The Grant State Casket," Used in Funeral of President U.S. Grant.

Most arresting, perhaps, in a review of burial receptacle forms and compositions that failed for one reason or another to gain popular acceptance in 19th-century burials is the story of glass coffins and caskets. This type first makes its appearance in the patent files in 1859, when John R. Cannon of New Albany, Indiana, received a letters-patent for "...certain new and useful improvements in the Construction of Coffins" consisting in "coffins of glass." (*See Figure 20*.)

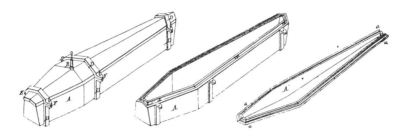

Figure 20. Coffin of Glass Plates and Iron Bands, 1859, Patent Sketch.

The coffin envisioned by Cannon was long, narrow and hexagonal, with all sides made in sections of glass. Cement was used to keep the receptacle airtight, and iron bands, as used in a strong box, held the lid secure. A small air pump atop the coffin was used to remove a portion of the air, "so that there being less pressure of air on the outside than there is on the inside of the body, it will be caused by the air within to fill out and assume a more life like appearance — besides this by removing a portion of the air there will be less liability of the body's decaying."

Other advantages claimed for this glass coffin were its non-conductive properties, durability, cheapness, ease of manufacture and transparency. Its inventor claimed: "...when the body within it is made to assume a more life-like appearance by removing a portion of the air, the said body may be at any time seen and observed by the friends and relatives of the deceased."

Despite the many advantages claimed by its inventor, this glass coffin did not make serious inroads into the market versus other more-conventional burial receptacles.

Less than a year later, however, George W. Scollay of St. Louis, Missouri, secured a patent for an improved glass coffin, built more along the rectangular casket lines, yet essentially acting as a specimen-container in that the receptacle was not to be filled with "poisonous liquour, to destroy the animalcula," but was to constitute an airtight container "from which the air can be abstracted (*sic*), and into which can be introduced any one or more of that class of gases, which in the absence of air or oxygen, will destroy animal life, and consequently the animalcula, that develop in the body after death." The coffin was to be molded, and had a special rib-flange construction better designed to make it airtight. (*See Figure 21*.) The emphasis, however, was more upon preservation than display.

Following these innovations, John Weaver of Baltimore, Maryland, and Isaac Shuler of Amsterdam, New York, both received letters-patent for coffins with glass panels, each emphasizing the display function. Likewise, between 1870 and 1890, the profusion of patents granted for coffins and caskets incorporating glass into their structure indicated a growing concern with the transparency feature of glass versus other physical properties.

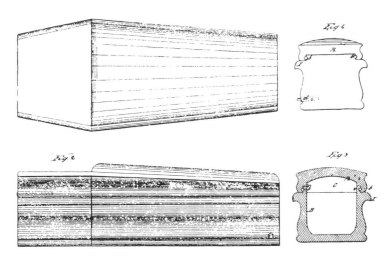

Figure 21. Glass Coffin, Airtight, with Rib-Flange Construction, 1880, Patent Sketch.

Nevertheless, the casket made wholly of glass was not destined to be retained as part of the fashion of modern burial, although two offshoots, the glass panel and the glass liner, remain in use today. The experience of Samuel Stein and his early (about 1870) "Showcase casket" (mentioned earlier) is indicative of an imminent desire on the part of the late-19th-century burying public not only to display a body in its physical entirety, but also to place it in a handsome setting, part of which is comprised by the casket. Thus, although some of the glass cases were undoubtedly fine pieces of casket construction, their artistry and workmanship on the whole went unrewarded by the public.

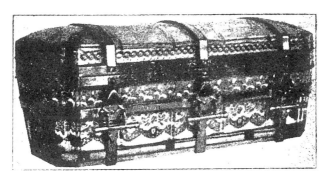

Figure 22. Glass Casket, Late-19th Century.

Glass caskets might be one of the great failures in 19th-century burial receptacles, but it is evident that the use of some glass in modern caskets persists. Likewise, cement and stone, while never feasible as the major substances for burial receptacles, eventually found use in the construction of burial vaults.

Many other new ideas and substances had a less-fortunate life history. Such, for example, was the case with celluloid, offered to the American public in 1876 by Aaron Pitman of Matawan, New Jersey; with papier-mâché, patented as "a substance which is positively imperishable," by Jefferson Evarts of Madison, Connecticut, in 1868; and with "caoutchouc" (unvulcanized natural rubber), "air-tight and very light," patented a year later by Cornelius Hurlburt of Springfield, Massachusetts.

Additionally among the "also-rans" were innovations such as the willow coffin, made of basketry or wickerwork, suggested by protagonists of burial reform but never patented, and, as far as can be determined by historical record, never produced for actual use.

Another remarkable form of casket that did not survive the 19th century was the cruciform, or cross-shaped, burial case (*see Figure 23*) manufactured specifically by the Oswego Cruciform Casket Co. of Oswego, New York, whose popularity ran a relatively short course in the late-19th century.

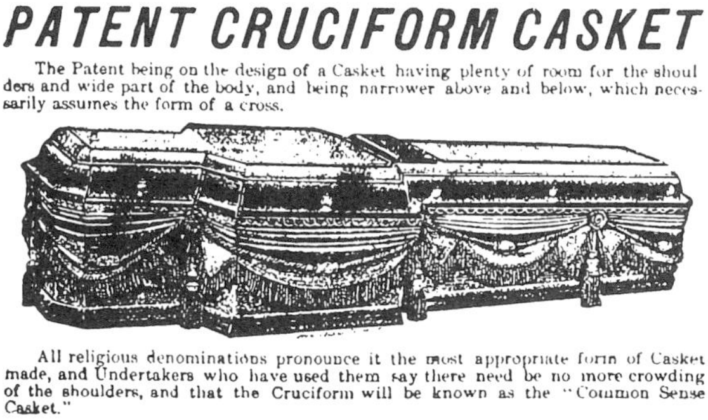

PATENT CRUCIFORM CASKET

The Patent being on the design of a Casket having plenty of room for the shoulders and wide part of the body, and being narrower above and below, which necessarily assumes the form of a cross.

All religious denominations pronounce it the most appropriate form of Casket made, and Undertakers who have used them say there need be no more crowding of the shoulders, and that the Cruciform will be known as the "Common Sense Casket."

Figure 23. Cross-shaped Casket, 1877.

Another failure for what might logically seem to have been a sure winner was the burial casket of John Homrighous of Royalton, Ohio, patented in 1878. This receptacle had what the inventor claimed was the answer to the undertaker's most pressing need — an adjustable casket, suitable for the largest and smallest cases. Again, no records exist to show if this model ever got into production.

Life Signals: An interesting, somewhat bizarre, but nevertheless important image in the minds of many people during the 19th century was the horrifying prospect of being buried alive. The foundation for such morbid preoccupation stems from an earlier period of the great plagues and epidemics, when, in the frenzied haste of disposing of the dead, the stricken might well be mistaken for dead.

Even in classical antiquity, there were customary acts performed by the bereaved that functioned as crude tests of death, such as the Roman *conclamatio*, the Greek washing of the body with warm water, and the Hebrew wake, or watch, in the sepulcher. In America, this concern might be expressed in prose and poetry, but with the focus of popular attention on the burial receptacle during this period, there was a corresponding increase in inventions designed to indicate to the living whether life still existed in the grave.

The earliest of these "life signals" to be patented came from the drawing board of Christian Eisenbrandt of Baltimore, Maryland, who, in a specification of letters-patent dated November 15, 1843, claimed a "new and useful improvement in coffins" that he termed "a life-preserving coffin in case of doubtful death." His invention (*see Plate 33*) featured an arrangement of wires and pins, and a spring lid, that enabled the occupant to cause the coffin lid to spring open by the slightest movement of hand or head.

PLATE 33

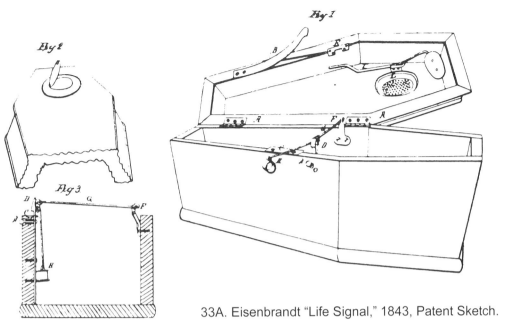

33A. Eisenbrandt "Life Signal," 1843, Patent Sketch.

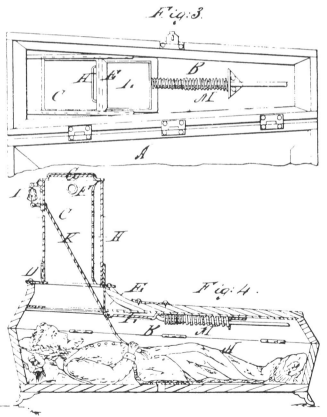

33B. Life Signal to be Used with Electrical Alarm, Patent Sketch.

While Eisenbrandt's life-preserving coffin obviously had utility only before the coffin was buried in the earth, the next four similar devices to appear in the patent files were designed to operate even after the body was interred. The first of these, invented in 1868 by Franz Vester of Newark, New Jersey, consisted of a square tube containing a ladder and a cord, one end of which was to be placed in the hand of the person laid in the coffin, while the other extended up to a bell on the top of the tube, which was attached to the head of the coffin. (***See Plate 33***.)

A very similar idea is expressed in the invention of Theodore Schroeder and Hermann Wuest of Hoboken, New Jersey, whose "Improvement in Life-Detectors for Coffins," patented in 1871, consisted of a narrow round tube, similar to a speaking tube, attached to the head-end of the coffin in such manner that the rope within it might be pulled by the buried person, releasing an air opening in the mouth of the tube and simultaneously setting off an electrical alarm. (***See Plate 34***.)

If the name of the inventor could be considered a recommendation, the invention of Albert Fearnaught of Indianapolis, Indiana, should have had instantaneous public acceptance. His "Grave-Signal," patented in 1882 (*see Plate 35*), consisted of a rather elaborate device to release a flag, if its occupant were to move a hand, through the end of a tube that projected up from the foot of the grave.

A final example of a life signal is offered in the invention of John Krichbaum of Youngstown, Ohio, whose "Device for Indicating Life in Buried Persons," also patented in 1882, consisted of a rather formidable arrangement of pipes, bars, tubes and cross-pins (*see Plate 36*), that would, upon a movement of the hands of "persons being buried in a trance," open an air vent and, at the same time, give indication that there was life in the coffin below.

As far as the authors' research has been able to ascertain, these inventions did not provoke more than a ripple of attention from the world of undertaking and funeral service, and it is doubtful if any were marketed. Yet, the mere fact that this number, and possibly more, were brought to a patentable stage suggests how widespread the fear of being buried alive was at the time.

Stories of people buried alive are legendary and, true or not, always attract much attention. Newspapers of today seldom fail to publicize the occasional reports of persons who "come alive" after being thought dead. One of the effects of embalming by chemical injection, however, has been to dispel fears of live burial.

Another creation of the inventive mind, the "coffin torpedo," applied to the problem of protecting the grave from prowlers, "resurrectionists," ghouls or graverobbers. (A "resurrectionist" was someone who stole bodies from graves to sell to anatomists, i.e., a "body snatcher.") This device, made of iron and about an inch in diameter and six inches long, contained an explosive charge and a mechanism set to go off with the tampering of any coffin that had properly been prepared. One such type of coffin torpedo was actually put on the market by the Clover Coffin Torpedo Manufacturing Company of Columbus, Ohio, and described fully in an 1878 issue of *The Casket*.

PLATE 34

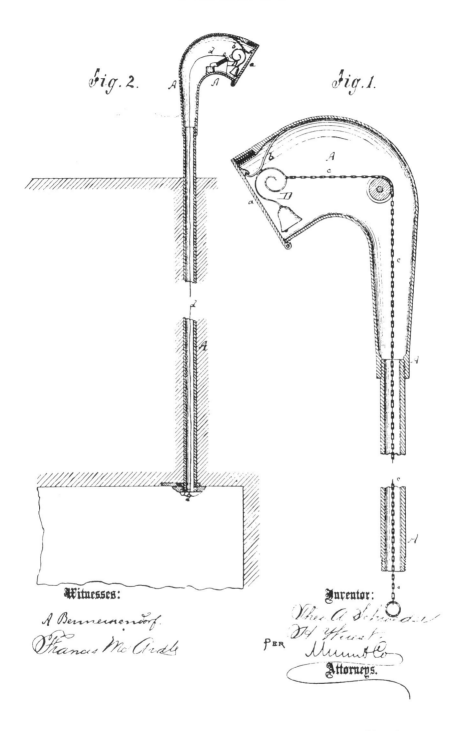

34. Life Detector, Mechanical Principle, 1871, Patent Sketch.

PLATE 35

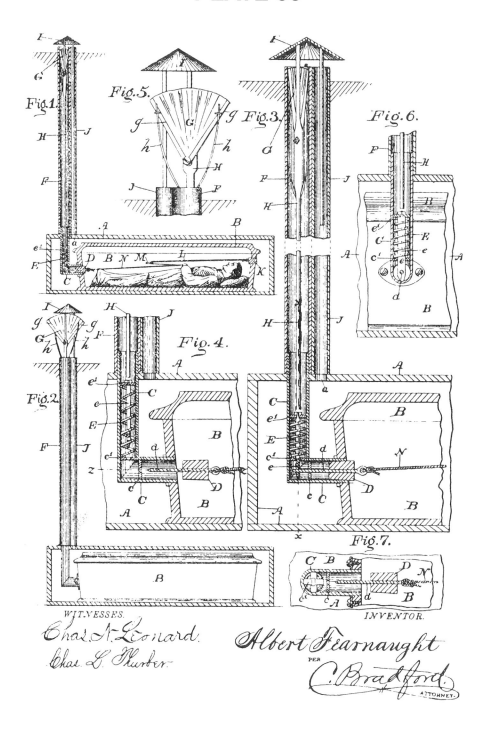

35. Grave-Signal by Albert Fearnaught, 1882, Patent Sketch.

PLATE 36

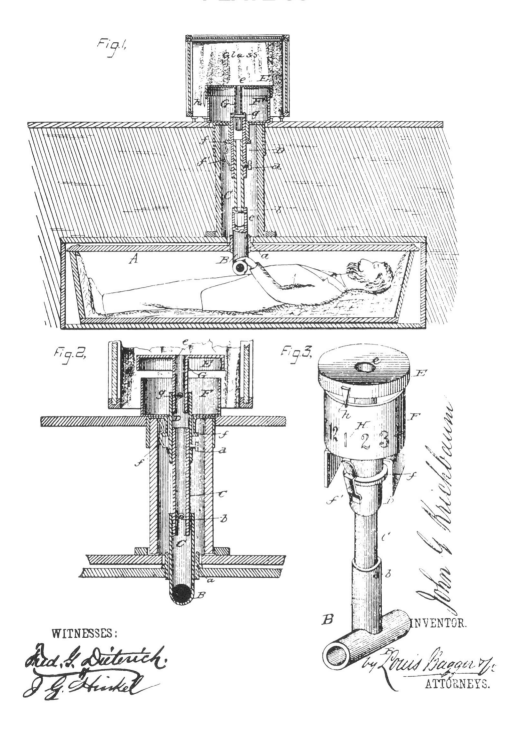

36. "All Weather" Device for Indicating Life in Buried Persons, 1882, Patent Sketch.

Burial Vaults and Outside Boxes: Although the use of the burial vault has not been solely an American burial practice, the growth and development of the vault as an item of manufacture, and the thinking behind its popular usage, cannot be divorced from the general picture of changing American taste in funeral service and interment.

It is, of course, true that the basic idea of permanently protecting the body from ghouls and the elements persisted in various cultures and civilizations extending back before antiquity. The Egyptians customarily enclosed their mummies in a case that, at times, might best be described as a coffin, decorated and inscribed with its renowned "coffin texts." During other periods, the crudeness of the outside case and its obviously utilitarian purposes makes the term "vault" seem more appropriate. The stone coffins of the Greeks and Romans were more likely to be simply stone slabs laid together to form a crude protective box or vault. Also, English barrows often have been noted to contain a similar type of slab vault, especially where chalk, a favored material for use in such cases, might be found.

Throughout the 19th century, occasional attempts were made to line the grave with rock, stone or brick, cut or laid in such fashion that the body was, to some extent, separated from the earth about it. Later, concrete slabs were used, and, before the century had ended, one form of lining consisted of "sectionals," i.e., concrete slabs sealed together with a sand-cement mortar.[18]

As early as 1872, however, Jacob Weidenmann of Hartford, Connecticut, commenting that "various costly expedients have been resorted to (to preserve the dead) such as building brick-graves, covering coffins with a large body of cement, and the like," in his specification forming part of a letters-patent, offered a "cheap, effective, and durable impermeable covering for coffins and caskets." His improvement in burial cases, he claimed, was a common coffin-box of wood, used ordinarily to encase a coffin, but so designed as to permit cement to be poured into it and around the coffin to form a vault. The term "vault" was not specifically used, however, nor does it seem to have come into popular usage until later in the same decade.

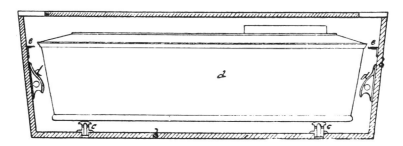

Figure 24. Cement Mold Type of Burial Case, 1872, Patent Sketch.

The "burial safe," an example of which is represented by the invention of Andrew Van Bibber of Cincinnati, Ohio, in 1878 (*see Plate 37*), was specifically designed to protect the body from ghouls and marauders. The theme of protection of body and casket from the earth and the elements in the design of such "mort-safes" is virtually ignored.

PLATE 37

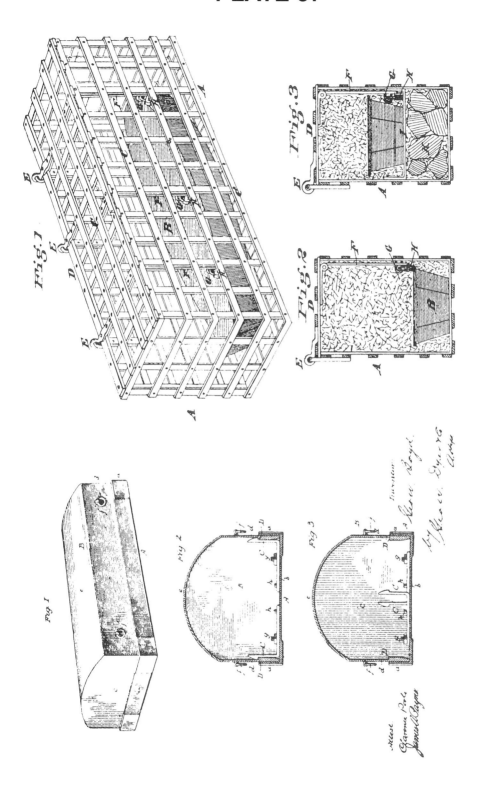

37B. Burial Safe, to be Lowered Into the Grave, 1878, Patent Sketch

37A. Boyd Metal Grave Vault, 1879, Patent Sketch.

Another form of earth material, slate, was brought into use for grave lining somewhat later in the century, and grooved-and-bolted slate vaults were marketed before the more-easily manufactured concrete vaults appeared and eventually dominated the stone and stone-composition portion of the burial vault industry.

Yet, despite the early appearance of cement mixtures in burial receptacles and coffins, the concrete vault, as it is known today, did not come into prominence until shortly after 1900. Many firms, particularly in the Great Lakes area, had their beginnings at this time. Some of these had been making other concrete products, and many of them had been engaged in concrete construction work.[19]

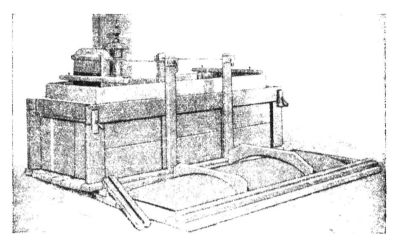

Figure 25. Metal-clad Wood Mold for Concrete Vaults.

The number of patents granted in connection with concrete burial vaults is greatest during the period 1900-1920. This development, it has been noted, brought about an active trade in molds and territories for vaults of uniform design to be sold under a trade name. Where gravel, sand and cement are available, concrete vault-making can and usually does occur. Even though the size of a business might not be great, the competitive advantage of lower shipping costs can permit profitable operations. Thus, the weight and bulk of vaults has militated against the concentration of their manufacture into a few large companies.

On the other hand, the metal vault shows a more clear-cut continuity in its development. Metallic coffins of the mummy-case type, the prototype of which is to be seen in the Fisk Metallic Burial Case, in the course of several decades of use and improvement, established the fact that metal sheets of one sort or another could be sealed together in such fashion as to provide relatively permanent protection of the body from the earth and elements. As this burial receptacle was changed to improve its appearance, there arose a popular repugnance against placing an object of such beauty directly in the ground.

Since Colonial times, *some* box or container to enclose and protect both body and casket seems to have been demanded by those burying their dead. Consequently, as the term "casket"

PLATE 38

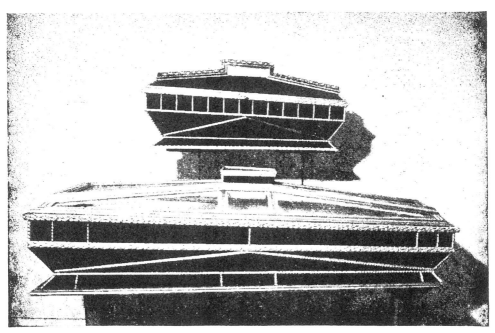

38A. Handmade Glass Caskets, Built About 1900, Found in Bozeman, Montana.

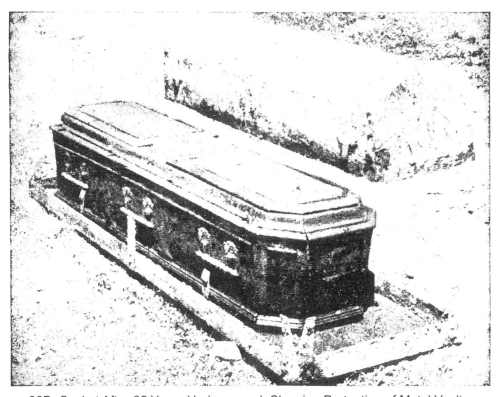

38B. Casket After 65 Years Underground, Showing Protection of Metal Vault.

and the kind of receptacle it implied came into popular use, the "burial case," originally thought of as a form of coffin, was now extended in terminology and as a physical object to mean a type of protecting container for the coffin or casket.

In rough fashion, then, the terminological sequence starting in the late 1840s ran "mummy-case," "burial-case," "coffin-case," "casket-case" or "casket-burial case" and, finally, some time in the late 1870s, "grave vault."

Still, as pointed out earlier, there was considerable overlap, both in terminology and conceived function, of the case used to protect the receptacle that held the body. William H. Bachtel of Canton, Ohio, in offering "Coffins of Clay or Other Plastic Material," patented 1881, claimed by the improvements over his 1880 model "to produce a coffin, burial casket, or vault that will be much lighter, more easily handled than those composed simply of baked or burned clay." His would have a vitreous surface.

Jacob Coover of Chambersburg, Pennsylvania, on the other hand, offered in 1883 a grave vault that, upon examination, turned out to be a mode of reinforcing wooden outside-boxes in such a way that they could sustain a cover of iron, which, if desired, could in turn be covered with cement — an early application of the idea of iron-reinforced concrete that was to prove fruitful in the 20th-century construction of large buildings.

The final stage for setting the type of metal grave vault, which today remains substantially in the same form and function, begins with the famous "burial-case" (*see Plate 37*) patented in 1879 by George W. Boyd of Springfield, Ohio. This outer receptacle consisted of the conventional two parts, cover and bottom, made of "wrought-metal plates riveted together like boiler-plates" that could, if desired, be "nickel-plated, bronzed, or otherwise ornamented." The cover actually comprised most of the vault, and the bottom consisted of a narrow iron frame into which the former was locked.

The crux of the invention was to be found in the "manner of securing the ring-catches which lock the two parts of the vault together, enabling them to be transported in one piece without locking..."

Summing up the purpose, Boyd stated further in his specification that his object was:

> ...to prevent the resurrection of human bodies, by providing a case or vault for containing the burial-casket, coffin, or other case in which the body may be put, which will be burglar-proof, so that it cannot be opened after being once closed, and will be made of such strong material that it cannot be broken into at any point, and at the same time will be portable and easily conveyed from place to place, and will be cheap to manufacture when compared with other devices for the same purpose.

Paul Pence, an officer in The Champion Company for many years, relates the story of the Boyd Vault in this manner:

> In 1879, a man by the name of Boyd was running a machine shop in Springfield. Mr. Boyd was impressed by the number of grave robberies which were going on at that time. He conceived the

PLATE 39

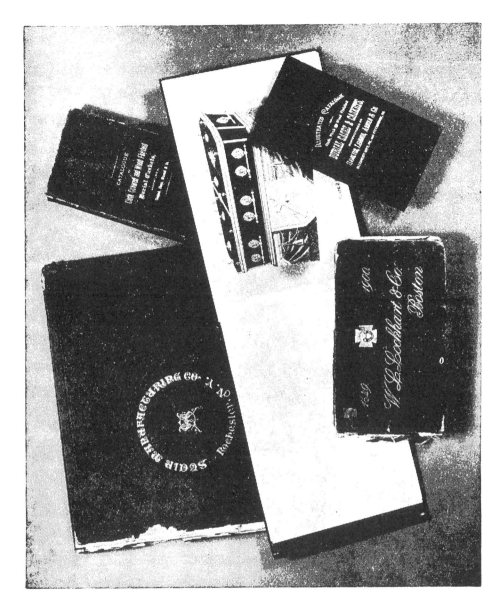

39. Catalogs of Coffin and Casket Manufacturers, Late-19th Century.

idea of a burglar-proof vault which would be a defense against grave robbing. The result was the Boyd Vault which was originally aimed at protection against grave robbing. However, the principle of the Boyd Vault, unknowingly to Mr. Boyd, was the air seal type. Thus, the Boyd Vault was originally made to sell for protection against grave robbing, but developed into the present air sealed burial vault.

After Mr. Boyd had developed the burglar-proof metal burial vault, he found that he had a good idea, but no way to exploit it. He contacted Mr. Scipio Baker, who was then developing a sales organization to distribute embalming fluid for The Champion Company and sold Mr. Baker the original Boyd patent. Mr. Baker had a sales organization but no manufacturing facilities, so he made arrangements with the Springfield Metallic Casket Company to make this vault for him and the Champion Company salesmen sold the vaults. Later the Champion Company provided manufacturing facilities and started to produce the Boyd Metal Burial Vault which they have done to this time.

In the 1890s, shortly after The Champion Company began manufacturing its own vaults, the Springfield Metallic Casket Company began producing vaults patterned somewhat after the Boyd, which they called The New Baker Patent Burglar-Proof Grave Vault, also made of cold rolled steel. It is interesting to note that the air-seal principle, operating on the principle of the diving bell, was not recognized for its function in keeping interiors of vaults airtight until many decades later, and that Baker's "improvements" included putting the cover for the vault near the top, thereby losing the air-seal advantage.

The Champion Company also put out the Baker-type vault through the first decade of the 20th century. These two companies dominated the production and distribution of grave vaults through the rest of the century, and, along with other concrete and metal-vault producers established somewhat later, shared and continue to share in the production and distribution of the burial vault as an important item in the American funeral bill of goods.

Another variant of the burglarproof vault, known as the "end sealer," was made like a safe-deposit box with a hinged door. The casket was placed inside this vault, necessarily either alongside the grave, or on planks or a lowering device that was set up over the grave, and then it was all lowered as one unit after the vault had been sealed. These vaults were known as "burglar-proof" and were made specifically for that purpose. It was felt that their construction and the difficulty of raising the entire vault would prevent ghouls from robbing the graves.[20]

Despite these developments, the sale of vaults based on the need to protect the body from ghouls and burglars was slow. By 1915, five to ten percent of all funerals included vaults, nearly all of metal. As the fear of graverobbing gradually diminished, the basic function of the vault became that of protection of the casket and its contents. Eventually, the aesthetic principle that had been so efficacious in changing the form of burial receptacles made itself felt in regard to vaults, so that, today, these receptacles are designed for eye appeal, as well as for their basic protective purpose.

PLATE 40

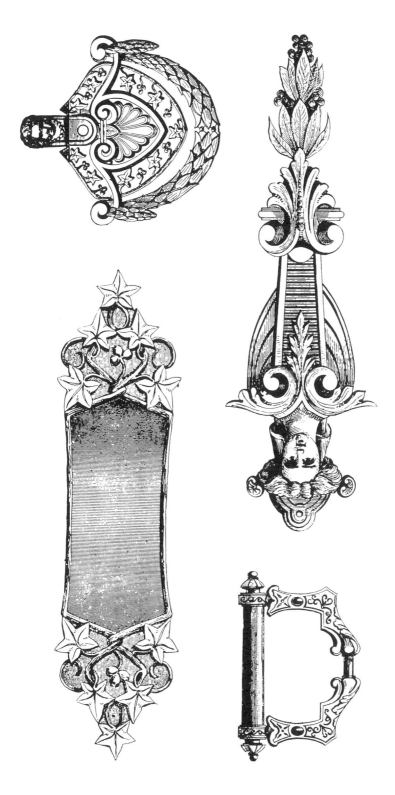

40. Ornamental Casket Trim and Hardware, From a Manufacturers Catalog, Late-19th Century.

A final mention of the wooden "outside," or "rough," box is needed. From the time that the coffin became more than a utilitarian receptacle for the corpse, some sort of outside container or protective arrangement has been put into use as a part of the burial procedure. That this container should often be of wood is not surprising, especially during times when wood was cheap and plentiful. In fact, up until about 1875, the ordinary unfinished outside, or rough, box was buried simply to get rid of it.

The growing and insistent demand for protection from man, beast or elements, however, quite generally outmoded the wooden outside box, although never completely so since a receptacle is nearly always used to encase the modern casket, and such a container need not necessarily be concrete, metal, or a combination of both. Probably the peak use of wooden boxes came after the introduction of the metallic vault, but before the rise of the concrete burial-vault industry early in the 20th century. As early as the late 1870s or early 1880s, the Stein Manufacturing Company was producing fine cedar, chestnut, oak and mahogany outside boxes. Prices ranged from $25 to $30 for adult sizes, depending upon the quality of the wood, metal hardware and workmanship.

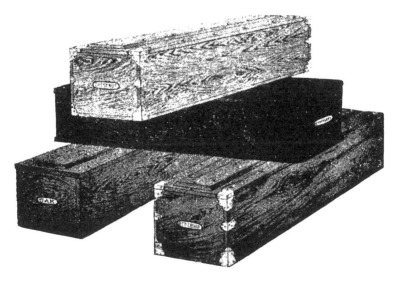

Figure 26. Finished Outside Boxes, Used in Late-19th Century.

Even in outside boxes, woodworkers displayed much ingenuity in their product. In the *Western Undertaker* of December 1889, J. Wittig of Marinette, Wisconsin, advertised a skillfully contrived burial box that displayed the craftsmanship of a cabinet-maker. He described his creation as the "Undertaker's Friend."

In spite of a well-made product, however, the wooden container for the coffin or casket could not, apparently, continue to fulfill the demand of the American public for an outer container or vault that would provide substantial and enduring protection for a sacred body encased in an inner, aesthetically pleasing receptacle.

Coffins, Burial Cases and Caskets 217

An equally important factor was the resistance of cemetery managers and authorities to the wooden box, due to problems of grave upkeep, especially in perpetual-care cemeteries. Most cemeteries today demand the use of either a metal or concrete vault in burials.

Balance Sheet on Wood, Cloth and Metal: It would be erroneous to assume that metal, and wooden, cloth-covered caskets, made a clean sweep of the market for burial receptacles during the second half of the 19th century. The number of large-sized manufacturers producing these items during this period was never great. In 1886, *The Casket Directory of Manufacturers and Jobbers of Funeral Supplies* listed 13 concerns dealing with cloth caskets and covered work, six dealing with metallic cases and caskets, and four with composition caskets.

At the same time, an association of makers of wood coffins claimed some 20 large manufacturers as members. Again, there were more shops producing casket hardware and trimmings than those manufacturing the three kinds of coffins listed in this directory.

Yet, the field of manufacturing and wholesaling burial goods was much larger than any directory would indicate. In point of fact, there were 769 establishments engaged in such ventures in 1879. When the U.S. Census Bureau redefined factories to exclude "hand and neighborhood shops" in 1889, the figure dropped that year to 194.[21]

It seems clear that since most hand shops produced coffins as their main items of funeral goods manufacture — usually in the context of furniture manufacture and cabinet-making or carpentry; and since the hand shops outnumbered the factories by a tremendous margin; and, finally, since cloth-covered and metallic cases were produced in only a handful of factories, probably less than two dozen — a majority of the coffins and caskets made and used must have been of wood. The balance, moreover, has favored wood, up until the current period.

In the last analysis, the acceptance of metallic, and wooden, cloth-covered cases and caskets, reflects the tendency of Americans to express themselves through the material objects they use. The basic appeal of the new types and patterns has been to the sense of beauty, and the varieties of materials used singly or combined attest to the willingness of Americans to bring the area of mourning behavior under canons of taste set not by ancient and venerable traditions, but by popular fashion, and by seeking objects not only different but also improved.

CITATIONS AND REFERENCES IN CHAPTER 7

1. See Carl Bridenbaugh, *The Colonial Craftsman* (New York: New York University Press, 1950), p. 3 *seq.*

2. Earle, *op. cit.*, p. 370.

3. Sewall, *op. cit.*, p. 138.

4. Van Rensselaer, *op. cit.*, pp. 63-66.

5. Bridenbaugh, *The Colonial Craftsman*, *op. cit.*, p. 82.

6. *Ibid.*, p. 75.

7. *Ibid.*, pp. 80-81.

8. Sir Ambrose Heal, *The Signboards of Old London Shops* (London: B.T. Batsford Ltd., 1947).

9. Bridenbaugh, *The Colonial Craftsman, op. cit.*, pp. 65-96.

10. Quoted in George F. Dow, *Everyday Life in Massachusetts Bay Colony* (Boston: The Society for the Preservation of New England Antiquities, 1935), p. 128.

11. From the Collection of the Massachusetts Historical Society.

12. Sir Ambrose Heal, *London Tradesmen's Cards of the XVIII Century* (London: B.T. Batsford Ltd., 1925), p. 22.

13. James M. Ball, "Resurrection Days" in *Lectures of the History of Medicine* (Philadelphia: W.B. Saunders Co., 1933), p. 114. Iron coffins were first patented in England in 1796.

14. Pamphlet: "Fisk's Metallic Burial Cases" (1850). Collection of Edward C. and Gail R. Johnson.

15. Thirty-eighth Congress, Session II, Chapters 36-40-44-51.

16. *Reader's Digest*, Jan. 1953.

17. *The Evolution of the Modern Casket*, brochure, ms. photostat, Collection of NFDA, Milwaukee, Wis., n.p.

18. Cf *The First Fifty Years Were the Hardest: A Brief History of the Concrete Burial Vault Business* (Columbus, Ohio: National Concrete Burial Vault Association, 1953), p. 3 ff.

19. *Ibid.*, p. 3.

20. Personal communication to Howard C. Raether from Harry J. Gilligan.

21. Gebhart, *op. cit.*, pp. 223-224.

Chapter 8

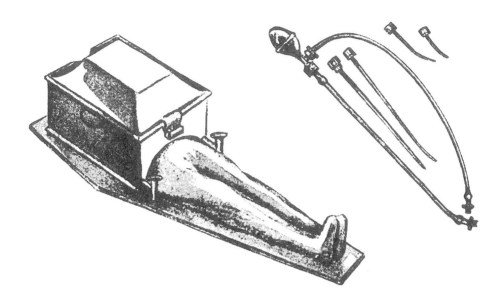

Preservation: The Ice Age Into Embalming

In its treatment of the body after death, mankind has run a gamut of procedures that might startle the imagination of the uninformed. The data of the ethnographer and anthropologist are rich with variations in death customs the world around. One of the major decisions a society must make about its dead is whether the corpse should be preserved. The answer to this, and to other questions related to major crises in the lives of human beings, tends to be phrased by custom and tradition.

When attention is turned, however, to the role of preservation of the dead in an emerging 19th-century American society, the outstanding phenomenon appears to be the rapid rise, spread and acceptance of the need for body preservation as a necessary preliminary to its proper interment. Another interesting aspect of this development is the attention, ingenuity and effort directed to the preservation of the dead by many persons who acted independently of, and often unknown to, one another.

In puzzling out an interpretation of the facts of changing embalming practices in America, however, the historian must first look backward to tradition and custom for clues, and, lacking an adequate explanation there, look to the "situational" or immediate circumstances of the change.

Customary Aspects of Preserving the Dead: The growth of methods, and the limitations on the practices, of embalming the dead on the European continent before American Colonial times have been presented in earlier chapters. Briefly, in looking for an explanation underlying these early developments, note that the practice of letting the nobility and persons of substantial rank and status lie in state for a period of about a week reaches back into classical antiquity. Also, if this custom did not at first find acceptance and support in Christian belief and practice, it nevertheless reappeared in the Christian care of the dead through the Middle Ages.

It was also reinforced indirectly by the practice, at the close of this period, of the preservation and distribution of portions of the bodies of religious leaders to churches, shrines and other places to be hallowed by the presence of such relics.

Likewise, as the pretentious medieval funeral of an earlier feudal period became an object of imitation and emulation by the socially mobile merchant and commercial classes in Renaissance times, the preservation of the dead — as crudely performed by physicians, surgeons and barber-surgeons for nobility and important clergy — was arrogated to themselves by various classes of tradesmen and artisans. These "undertook" the organization of funeral obsequies and provided the paraphernalia for funerals for those to whom elaborate mourning behavior in the fashion of the nobility, a class to which they did not belong, was primarily an affectation.

Body-preservation techniques, in light of this development, tended to deteriorate by the turn of the 18th century to the "sawdust and tar" level, and were lost as a prerogative reserved for branches of the healing arts.

The growth of cities and the organization of funeral service in 18th- and 19th-century England within the context of the tradesman's service also gave rise to a need to preserve the dead along lines totally different from those reflected in the desire to have the body, as a mark of social status, lie "in state." This "need" appeared as a consequence of the inability of the poorest urban classes to pay funeral expenses. Thus, the corpse necessarily remained unburied and without the benefit of funeral ceremonies until the requisite amount of money could be raised.

The impulse to give the dead a "decent Christian burial" has always been strong in Western society. These factors underlay the early appearance of burial associations and burial societies, which remain today as a social element in the structure of modern institutionalized insurance.

In sketching out the background for the rise of embalming in America as an integral part of the funeral service, it is probably fair to state that the influence exerted by cultural extension from Europe and the tradition of the Western world were both instructive, in that the practice of letting bodies of important personages lie in state, as well as the custom, dictated by need rather than tradition, of the poorer classes to delay burial, provided cues for the funeral behavior of the early colonists.

There is little, however, to suggest that these usages were of a compelling nature. Rather, the search for a more complete and satisfying explanation for the rapid spread of embalming in America needs to be extended to the particular circumstances of a new way of living in a new world, and as an important aspect of the emergence of new social forms emphasizing *taste* and *style* in American funeral behavior.

Chapter 5 discusses Colonial funeral customs and offers several clues to the genesis of embalming as a widespread practice in America. On the one hand, the small settlements fostered a community spirit that, among many ways, was expressed in either church or family graveyards. Thus, the family plot has always been a common element of cemetery organization in America.

From the middle of the 17th century on, the well-to-do were likely to have family tombs in which various generations were buried. Much importance was attached to being gathered not only *to* but also *with* the fathers. Whether relatives gravitated toward urban centers, edged toward the frontier, or merely took up residence in other parts of the Colonies, the traditional impulse to gather beside the bier of the departed relative was apparently no whit diminished by the distance separating one from the other. Upon the death of a dear friend or relative, colonists would set out on what might be several days' journey to participate in the funeral, comfort the immediately bereaved, and share in the social gatherings that automatically followed the get-together of scattered relatives and friends who seldom met except on occasions such as these.

In order for such gatherings to take place, it became necessary, in many instances, to use whatever preservative methods were available at the time to restrain the putrefaction of the corpse while the funeral was delayed, since a funeral lost much of its significance without a corpse as the central figure. The early colonists used several crude methods, such as disemboweling, filling its cavity with charcoal, immersing the body in alcohol, or wrapping the body in a cloth soaked in alum (a "sere sheet").

In 1773, in a letter to Barber Dubourg, Benjamin Franklin anticipated cryonics by nearly two centuries as he speculated on the possibility of embalming in wine. "I wish it were possible from this instance to invent a method of embalming drowned persons, in such a manner that they may be recalled to life, however distant."[1]

A felt need for preservation produced a number of ingenious efforts to find a satisfactory preservative. The stories that tell of embalming persons in beverage alcohol are many. Lord Nelson, according to some of his biographers, was returned to England from Trafalgar in a barrel of rum.[2] When a young woman, Nancy Martin, died at sea in 1857 at the age of 27, her father did not wish her buried at sea, so he had her body thrust into a cask of alcohol and returned to this country. The cask and its contents were buried in Oakdale Cemetery, Wilmington, North Carolina.[3]

Even in less-dramatic circumstances, upon occasion, when the body was sent elsewhere for burial, it was encased in a metal container, usually of lead, soldered airtight, and again encased in an outside coffin of wood.

In the decades marking the expansion of America following the War of 1812, Americans found themselves increasingly separated from one another, both as members of kinship groups and of communities. The village life of the Colonial period to some extent was founded upon mutual aid and protection. The towns in Colonial America were likely to be patterned after the European model, in which people did not live on their farms but went out from towns to work in their fields. The pattern of defense was to live together rather than to attempt to fortify each dwelling.

But the first half of the 19th century found pioneers giving over small settlements in which houses huddled together in favor of scattered, often isolated, homesteads. The compact village did not appear as commonly west of the Appalachians as it did in New England.[4] After the danger of American Indian raids passed, it was safe for rural people to live scattered over a farming community.

Thus, in many cases, expediency dictated the place and, to a certain extent, the mode of burial. Yet, the impulse to be buried in the same earth as one's ancestors persisted, as did the tradition of the family burial plot. The need for more adequate and reliable methods of body preservation was generated in intensity just to that extent that the desire to be buried "home" called for transportation of the body for increased distances.

In a period marked by the rise of individualism and the spirit of enterprise, American ingenuity met this demand in a host of different fashions, and usually without reference to the state of technological advance in other geographic regions or, for that matter, in other countries. Thus, while in England and France the utility of chemical embalming had long since been demonstrated, though without any appreciable popular acceptance, American methods of preserving the dead well into the Civil War period were based on the simple rudiments of refrigeration.

After this period, with considerable overlap, was the attempt to preserve bodies by using airtight burial cases, as described in Chapter 7. Not until shortly before the Civil War was the principle of chemical embalming by injection brought into the American funeral complex.

Corpse Coolers and Cooling Boards: In 1843, a patent for the first "corpse preserver" based on the principle of ice refrigeration was granted to John Good of Philadelphia. It did not find its way into the commercial market, however, and the patent was allowed to lapse in 1850.

In May 1846, two years before the appearance of the Fisk Metallic Burial Case, two Baltimore undertakers, Robert Frederick and G.A. Trump, received a patent for a "Refrigerator for Corpses." In their specification, Frederick and Trump indicated that their invention was an innovation that rested upon a conventional principle:

> Various devices have from time to time been essayed for preserving bodies after death by the application of ice; but where applied directly to the body it was troublesome and ineffectual, wetting it and thereby rendering it more subject to decomposition. Another process has been to place the body in a coffin shaped case, said case being surrounded with ice, but this method was objectionable on account of the space that must intervene between the ice and those parts of the body more desirable to congeal. Experience has proved that it is now only necessary to freeze the trunk or abdomen and the chest; but no apparatus has heretofore been made that would with any degree of certainty effect this object on all sized persons without an immense expenditure of ice... By our invention we effect this, and with a very small quantity of ice we freeze the corpse as much as is necessary, while at the same time, our apparatus is portable and convenient.

Their "corpse cooler" consisted of a common cooling board, on which the body was laid out, and a concave, metal, ice-filled box that fit the torso and was equipped with lid, spigot and handles. (*See Plates 41 & 42.*)

PLATE 41

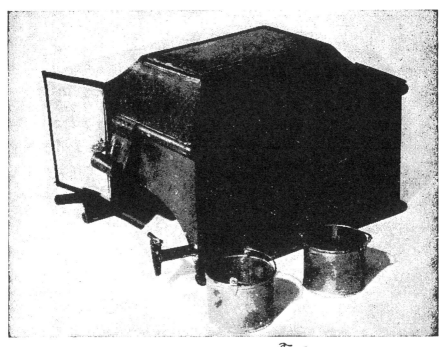

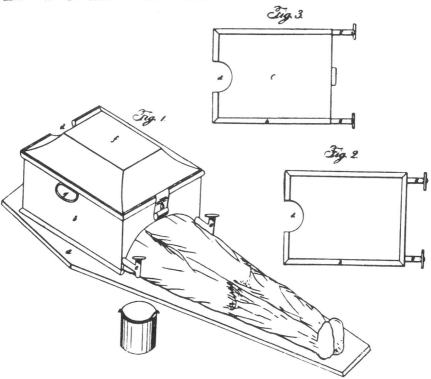

41. Corpse Cooler of Frederick and Trump, 1846, Patent Sketch.
(Top, an actual cooler; Bottom, the patent sketch.)

The Frederick and Trump corpse cooler not only was patented, but also successfully marketed to a substantial number of undertakers who were happy to find a cooling device that was portable and economical. Moreover, it could be used *after* the body was dressed, so that, shortly before the funeral, the body could be lifted, fully dressed from the corpse cooler and placed in the coffin.

Such was its obvious utility that no other type of cooler could seriously challenge its dominance for the next two decades. The predecessor for the cooler of the type likely to be found in early city morgues was patented in 1868 by Charles Kimball, of Quincy, Massachusetts. This consisted of a large refrigerator with two compartments, one for the body and the other for ice. This Kimball cooler had an early competitor in the corpse preserver of Howard V. Griffith of Altoona, Pennsylvania, patented in 1870. (*See Plate 42*.)

In the same year, R.C. Andrus of Poughkeepsie, New York, patented a corpse preserver (*see Figure 27*) that consisted of a set of ice-cases, all built along the Frederick-Trump principle — one to encase the head and another for the chest. A case for the limbs was optional. The cases were to be made of zinc or wood.

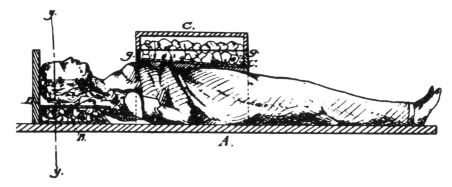

Figure 27. Corpse Cooler Consisting of Several Ice Cases, 1870, Patent Sketch.

Corpse coolers continued to be patented until roughly 1875, and, for many undertakers, ice cooling became so much a part of their services that they persisted in using coolers and cooling boards until the dawn of the 20th century. By then, however, the "cooling board" had taken on the function of an embalming table, and for some time after the cooling operation had ceased to be a part of it, the embalming table was still called a "cooling board."

The "Airtight" Receptacle: Early, metallic burial cases, described in some detail in the previous chapter, were presumed to have both preservative and protective properties. In the cycle of their development from crude "mummy cases" to aesthetically pleasing metal caskets, the preservative function came to play a role of somewhat lesser importance.

Nevertheless, there were some 19th-century receptacles that had as their basic virtue bodily preservation by keeping it enclosed in an "airtight" manner. Others operated on the principles of introducing, or creating within, a gas that would have the power of preservation. Still others attempted to keep the body from decay by immersing it in a container filled with some composition that, upon hardening, would render its contents impervious to all forces of decomposition.

PLATE 42

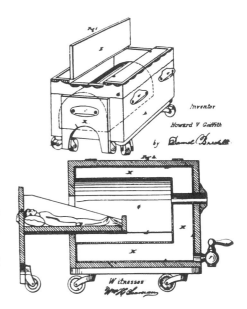

ROBERT FREDERICK,
Would inform his friends and the public generally, that he continues the business of manufacturing

FURNITURE,

As well as repairing and painting, in superior style and at cheap rates.
At his warehouse an assortment of various sizes

COFFINS

are constatly kept, and those requiring would do well to call before purchasing elsewhere, as they will be sold very cheap for cash.

THE CORPS PRESERVER

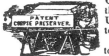

Can be had by applying to the advertiser or any of the Undertakers on moderate terms.
All concerned are invited to give a call at my place of business.

CORNER OF MONUMENT AND ENSOR STREET.

42A. (Left) Advertisement of Co-inventor of Corpse Cooler, 1847.
42B. Refrigerator-type Corpse Cooler, 1870, Patent Sketch.

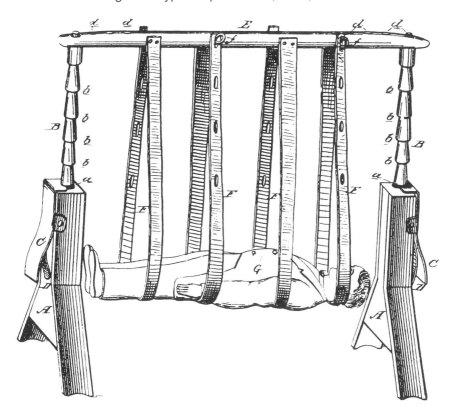

42C. Body-lifting Device, 1880, Patent Sketch.

Possibly most arresting of all (outside of a never-patented proposal to preserve the body by electroplating) was a portable, oval-shaped elastic receptacle with a funnel-like top, handles at the side, a grooved back, and a tube for deodorizing purposes, patented in 1863 by Dr. Thomas Holmes, a resident of the District of Columbia and about whom much more will be said later. (*See Plate 43*.)

This invention, by no means Holmes' first (though one of the five he got around to patenting), was designed specifically for battle use in "the carrying of badly-wounded dead bodies hurriedly away that could not otherwise be quickly removed for want of proper conveyances..." Deodorizing substances were introduced by way of the aperture and tube for the purpose of preserving the body for a short time. After the body was inserted, a large drawstring drew the opening together, and what amounted to an early version of the modern flexible rubberized body carrier was ready to be borne away.[5]

Chemical Embalming by Injection and Its Innovators: In conjunction with the aesthetic and material upgrading of burial receptacles, and especially the casket with its "jewel-box" emphasis, there followed a corresponding disposition to keep the body on display for a longer period.

Although the corpse-cooling devices that depended upon the principle of ice-refrigeration undoubtedly predominated from the 1830s through the 1870s, if not later, the problems attending this method of preservation, including the difficulty of keeping the corpse on display, were sufficiently pressing to induce a certain amount of receptiveness by undertakers for a better mode of delaying the onset of bodily putrefaction.

At the same time, two other parallel developments, one in sanitation and the other in medical pathology, coalesced to give added impetus to the search for better methods of preserving the dead.

The first of these traces back to the early popular concern over the ravages of pestilence and plagues in American cities. From the time of the earliest Colonial settlers, the ravages of sickness and disease contributed a tragic overtone to an otherwise heroic tale.[6] Smallpox, diphtheria, scarlet fever, yellow fever and lesser infectious diseases had repeatedly swept settlements and towns. By the beginning of the 19th century, attention had begun to turn, albeit very slowly, from medical treatment toward the general bettering of health, and the prevention of disease, through improvement of sanitary conditions.

The progress made on the European continent arrested the attention of those who were constructively concerned about the recurrence of epidemics in America. One step forward in the early 1830s resulted from a trip to Europe by Dr. Richard Harlan, professor of comparative anatomy at the Philadelphia Museum and a member of the city health council. As early as 1818, he was in charge of Dr. Joseph Parrish's anatomical room, where anatomical dissection was taught. Dr. Harlan was thus already familiar with chemical preservation of bodies for anatomical purposes by embalming.

His trip to Europe, however, was to study methods of epidemic-disease control. While there, he became acquainted with some of the leading figures in medical and sanitary science, including several pioneers in the development of techniques and fluids for the preservation of the dead.

PLATE 43

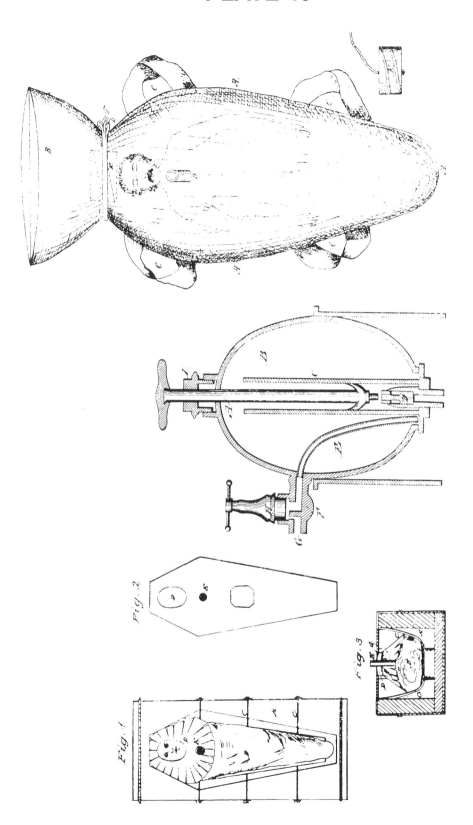

43C. Portable Elastic Receptacle for Shipping Body, 1863, Patent Sketch.

43B. Apparatus for Filling Blood Vessels of Dead Bodies, 1861, Patent Sketch.

43A. Cement-filled Corpse-preserving Coffin, 1867, Patent Sketch.

Embalming as a sanitary measure apparently impressed Harlan. Upon his return he translated from the French Gannal's *History of Embalming* (Paris: 1834) and had it published in Philadelphia in 1840. This work provided Americans with the first treatise dealing entirely with embalming and containing actual instructions on how to embalm. A second edition was published three years later. Harland died during the same year.[7]

In retrospect, it cannot be doubted that through his efforts, a substantial interest in the subject was awakened in this country, not only in medical and sanitary circles, but among undertakers, as well. For a considerable period thereafter, this book was the standard reference on matters pertaining to the preservation of the human body. It also provided the inspiration and material basis for numerous articles in early mortuary trade journals.

It is interesting to note that at least one member of the medical profession saw the possibilities offered by injective embalming for purposes of funeralization. Dr. Valentine Mott, one of the great American physicians and surgeons of his time, indicated this view in a pamphlet descriptive of the renowned Fisk Metallic Burial Case, published in New York in 1850. "...If you connect in your meritorious plan, the practice of Mons. Gannal of Paris, of injecting blood vessels with an antiseptic fluid, the whole system of preservation will be more fully carried out."[8]

Turning specifically to developments in the production of embalming fluids, one has good reason to believe that, between 1840 and 1860, experiments in their production were being carried out more or less independently by physicians, anatomists, chemists and others interested in embalming as an adjunct to the field of funeral service.

On the medical side, as has already been intimated, the preservation of anatomical specimen material in American medical schools demanded a working knowledge of chemical preservatives. Specimen preservation, as examined in Chapter 4, traces back to the end of the 17th century, with great advances in both arterial and cavity embalming taking place in the course of the 18th century as the Hunter brothers, among others, worked toward perfecting injection techniques for preserving human remains. Significantly, the French Gannal, who comes later, was a chemist.

Long before the turn of the 19th century, American anatomists had been preserving human specimens and tissues with chemical preservatives. Bi-chloride of mercury, zinc-chloride and various arsenic-based compounds were well known and used by anatomists on both sides of the ocean. Thus, it was difficult to accept the report, for example, that Ellerslie Wallace, demonstrator in anatomy at Jefferson Medical College in 1846, *originated* a zinc-chloride-based compound for the preservation of dead flesh. It is almost certain that this substance had already been in use abroad, as had arsenical and mercurial compounds.

Notable in this latter respect is the fact that, in England in 1836, an embalming process involving arterial injection of an arsenic compound was patented — 30 years before the first embalming-process patent using arsenic was granted in America. Moreover, poisonous embalming compounds based on arsenic and other metallic salts were outlawed in France in 1846, more than a half-century before the same was done in America.[9]

Thomas Holmes and the Eruption of Civil War Embalming: Until the outbreak of the Civil War, methods to delay body decomposition included ice cooling, encasing in airtight receptacles, sanitizing temporarily with external applications of antiseptic compounds, and, following the practices of anatomists, embalming by chemical injection. (The last would occur only occasionally since undertakers, as yet, knew almost nothing about the method and had very limited access to embalming instruments and fluids.)

Given the earlier developments in medical and chemical research in Europe, it is not surprising that the rise of arterial embalming in the United States is associated with sanitation-minded physicians and surgeons, and preservation-minded anatomists. What is arresting to the student of occupational and social movements is how rapidly American undertakers, compared with European countries, adopted the practice to make it a significant addition to the bundle of funerary tasks they performed, and — correlatively, perhaps antecedently — the social demand for embalming that developed during the course of the Civil War.

The story is inextricably linked with the vocational biography of Thomas Holmes, mentioned earlier, who, in popular history, has been cast in the role of "The Father of American Embalming." Considerable research[10] in the past several decades has more fully revealed the complexity and ambiguities associated with Holmes as a man whose interests and ambitions intersect with the opportunities afforded by the internecine slaughter during the War Between the States.

Thomas Holmes, son of a well-to-do merchant, was born in New York City in 1817. Early on, he developed an interest in the study of medicine and, according to a statement made in 1944 to embalming historian Edward C. Johnson by the registrar of admissions of the College of Physicians and Surgeons of Columbia University, Holmes was enrolled in that institution during the years 1844-1845. Records of these early years are incomplete, but it is not beyond reason to suppose that Holmes did graduate from this school, or from some other New York medical college.

In any event, the name of Thomas Holmes, physician, 103 Chatham Street, New York City, appears for the first time in the 1847-1849 edition of *Doggets New York City Directory*. In the 1853 edition of *The Reynolds Williamsburg City Directory*, Thomas Holmes, physician, is listed for the first time as having a hospital at South 6th Street; and the *Hope and Henderson Consolidated Brooklyn Directory* describes Holmes as "Physician and Surgeon." Holmes also practiced pharmacy and experimented eclectically with a variety of drugs and compounds.

Holmes relates later that during his medical college experience, the preservation of cadavers for anatomical study was neither well understood nor perfectly performed. As a result, many bodies were dissected unembalmed, and others improperly embalmed. He criticized the use of the then-common preservatives arsenic, mercury and zinc — poisonous compounds, the vapors of which were generally believed to be injurious to the health of students during dissecting.

Holmes also studied for three years under the phrenologists O.S. and L.N. Fowlers of Nassau Street, New York City. His experience in examining heads of embalmed mummies from Thebes led him to believe that embalming without the use of poisonous substances was possible. His own experiments, which covered a variety of subjects, turned toward the production of an efficacious embalming fluid he might sell to embalming-surgeons, anatomists and, later, to undertakers, who often would have learned the art of arterial embalming under his tutelage.

Holmes also served as coroner's physician for the city and county of New York. He wrote, "In 1850 Dr. E.G. Rawson was coroner and I was his examining physician."[11]

News stories of the day attest to this service by items such as:

> "The Late Murder on Leonard Street: The coroner held an inquest yesterday... on the body of John Murray... who was beaten to death by the lunatic, Peter Howland... Dr. Thomas Holmes made a post mortem examination of the body of the deceased."[12]

Service as coroner's examiner provided added opportunity for Holmes to pursue his investigations into embalming. After eight successful embalmings, Holmes wrote that he was ready to demonstrate that he "could check decomposition in any stage, and as evidence of my assertion, I embalmed a body and placed it on exhibition in Mr. Edward H. Senior's Undertakers Store, 75 Carmine Street (New York City). The press of the city noticed it, and thousands went to see the body, amongst whom was General Winfield Scott."[13]

At the time of, or soon after, the outbreak of the Civil War, Holmes traveled to Washington, D.C. Arriving there, he distributed thousands of circulars among the soldiers who crowded into the capital, informing them that he would embalm at no charge. For publicity purposes, he exhibited embalmed bodies at the undertaking establishments of Anthony Buckley in Washington, George Burch in Georgetown, and Benjamin Wheatley in Alexandria. Not everyone reacted positively to these exhibitions (and there might have been others) inasmuch as Holmes was once arrested in Washington on the charge of creating a nuisance for his embalming activities in the heart of the city, and he was held on bail of $300. There is no record of the disposition of the case.

Holmes' reputation as an embalmer, however, skyrocketed after he embalmed the body of Colonel Elmer E. Ellsworth, who had been a national figure even before the war. He had served as a clerk in Lincoln's Springfield office. He had organized Zouave (light-infantry) regiments in Chicago and New York, and their exotic uniforms and precision drilling attracted national attention. Ellsworth had also accompanied the Lincoln party as a security guard during the president-elect's much-publicized inaugural trip to Washington. And then, on the morning of May 24, 1861, Ellsworth was shot in Alexandria while defending the flag — the first ranking casualty of the Civil War, and a time when an individual death might still be national news.

Lincoln, distraught, invited the Zouaves to take the body to the White House for the funeral service, but it was Holmes' good fortune, through the intercession of Secretary of State Seward, to receive permission to embalm the body.

The successful embalming took place at the Washington Navy Yard, and cabinet members, leading officers of both services, senators and representatives, and distinguished citizens in large numbers paid their respects. Mrs. Lincoln viewed the body in the East Room in company with a Mr. W.A. Kelley, who found Ellsworth's classic face "natural, as though he were sleeping a brief and pleasant sleep."[14]

Washington newspapers echoed Kelley's favorable judgment, and the reputation of Holmes as a successful embalmer was established in the nation's capital.

As a result of this success, and as the war progressed and casualties mounted, Holmes' services were in great demand. Through his own efforts, and those of several undertakers and aspiring embalming-surgeons with whom he was associated (and whom he might have trained), his operations took on substantial proportions. Benjamin Wheatley, for example, an Alexandria undertaker and the first Virginian to practice embalming, describes his business relationship with Holmes: "In 1861 I associated with me Dr. Thomas Holmes... and during four years of partnership we embalmed and shipped about 1,500 officers and soldiers... who were killed in this vicinity."[15]

Setting the Holmes narrative temporarily aside, it is important to sketch the broader context of Civil War activities, particularly battlefield casualties and care of the fallen, in order to understand the rise of embalming in America at this time. At the outset, in order to understand the virtual plague of body-handling opportunists that descended upon the theaters of war, one must realize that there were no official pronouncements on care of battlefield war dead until 1862, when General Order (No. 33) made it the duty of commanding officers to "lay off lots of ground in some suitable spot near every battlefield so as... to cause the remains of those killed, to be interred with headboards to the graves bearing numbers, and where practicable, the names of the persons buried in them."

This War Department order by no means settled the matter of handling casualties. Francis Lord, Civil War historian, writes:

> It was the practice of new regiments in the field to send home the first of its members who died. This became too expensive and impractical after the regiment embarked on its first campaign. Occasionally the more wealthy families would send for or go in person and recover their sons' bodies and ship them home at their own expense. But the vast majority of Federal soldiers were hastily buried and, if time and circumstances permitted, the burial places were marked with crude headboards. But due to the lack of means of identification and the proclivity of the enemy to remove all valuables and even clothing from dead Federals, it was often impossible to identify the dead after a battle. As a result, almost one half of all Federal dead are in graves marked "unknown."[16]

When feasible, officers on both sides nevertheless attempted to return the dead, along with the injured and dying, to points of medical care or shipment. Field expedients centered on the use of litter, lorry (truck), wagon and, if possible, train in making removals.

The demand by wives, parents and other relatives for locating and returning their dead to their communities did not slacken as the war progressed. If anything, it increased and, alongside the occasional parent found in mournful search for a son whose remains he or she hoped to find and return home, were substantial numbers of undertakers, assistants, "embalmer-surgeons" and possibly slaves performing their sometimes contracted-for, sometimes freelance, services.

Lord (*Ibid.*) is sharply descriptive:

> An important part of the soldiers' life in camp was the burial of their comrades who were killed in battle or died of disease. Some regiments refused to permit strangers to bury their men, hoping for similar treatment if their turn should come. Soldiers killed in battle were buried in their blankets unless comrades saw fit to get old boards and make coffins, which was seldom done. The government sent no coffins to the front but at large assembly points and at the general hospitals coffins were furnished. Metallic caskets, "air-tight, indestructible, and free from encroachments of vermin or water" were advertised by commercial firms who indignantly disclaimed any connection with rival companies using sheet iron and similar materials.[17] Embalmers did a thriving business during the war their "ghastly advertisements" met the eye of visitors in Washington[18] and other large centers as well as at the front. A visitor to the Army of the James noted the roadside dotted with the "neat prospectus of the Embalmer-General to the Army, whose suggestive notices had greeted the eyes of each soldier as he marched to the front." When a staff member pointed out their demoralizing influence, General Butler ordered the embalmer to desist from this method of advertising.[19] At times rival embalmers would send their teams along the front handing out handbills with the heading "Honorable Dead" and containing "an incongruous mixture of the claims of sentiment and the cash cost of caring for a dead comrade."[20] One firm attempted to get a bill through Congress which would have given the firm exclusive right to embalm bodies; this firm also attempted to have Congress authorize a corps of embalmers for each division. The firm charged $50.00 for an officer and $25.00 for an enlisted man. A correspondent had to admit that the bodies looked as lifelike as if they were asleep.[21] Later these prices were raised to $80 and $30 respectively. The embalmed bodies were placed in long boxes, lined with zinc, on the lid of which was written the full name of the deceased and the address of his parents. In the box, beside the body, were placed the papers and other personal effects. Many of these boxes were to be seen on all trains and transport ships.[22]

Returning again to Holmes now, whatever judgment history reserves for his rectitude in performance, salesmanship and merchandising, it remains indisputable that he was in the thick of things from the beginning, and that his influence in training undertakers and aspiring "cmbalming-surgeons" in developing techniques, instruments, and in compounding and merchandising fluids for embalming cause him to stand out as the renowned personage in matters dealing with dead bodies during the Civil War. He possibly made a fortune, although there is no evidence that he took any significant portion of it back to Brooklyn after the war.

Finally, the body of myth and legend that has developed around Holmes and his place in funeral directing and embalming history needs attention. He was said to have joined the "27th Brooklyn Fire Zouaves," but such an organization never existed.

He was reputed by various "myth destroyers" never to have begun embalming military dead until 1863, but the evidence is overwhelming that he was doing this very thing in and about Washington, D.C., in 1861.

His claim at age 76 to have embalmed, through the course of the war, some "4,028 soldiers and officers, field and staff" has been termed excessive. But if one includes all of the embalmings done by and under Holmes' tutelage, and by his associates — such as the aforementioned Wheatley; by his brother-in-law William Bunnell, who kept a journal of his Civil War embalming activities[23]; by Dr. Lewis, his pupil who embalmed for Cornelius; and of perhaps dozens of others trained to use his instruments and who purchased his embalming fluid (at $3.00 per gallon, also sold by the barrel) — the total figure would far surpass the number that Holmes personally claimed to be of his own doing. Proof, one way or another is virtually impossible to obtain through documentation. Holmes' credibility, however, in light of recent decades of research on Civil War embalming, seems measurably to have improved.[24]

Also, as part of Holmesian mythology, it has been claimed, and the claim even supported by Holmes' widow in her later years, that Holmes embalmed the body of Abraham Lincoln. While Holmes himself never made such a claim, the facts are clear on this matter: Lincoln's body was entrusted to the firm of Brown and Alexander, Surgeons and Embalmers, of Washington, D.C., but the actual embalming was performed by an employee, Henry D. Cattell — thought to be the stepson of Brown and one of the many men brought into embalmer service by the war without prior anatomical or medical training.

Finally, the charge that Holmes claimed to have received a commission as an embalming-surgeon is subject to the linguistic equivocation surrounding the term "commission." The U.S. Army never commissioned Holmes as a medical officer, or any other kind of officer. Despite this, he was unquestionably one of the embalming-surgeons "commissioned," i.e., designated or officially permitted by military authorities to prepare, coffin and ship military dead, be they battlefield casualties, wounded who died in hospitals or other medical installations, or those in military service in a particular theater of war dying from disease or other causes.

On the Confederate side of the Civil War, there is no counterpart to Holmes, although similar functionaries, i.e., undertakers and possibly embalming-surgeons (evidence is weak), were to be found in Richmond, as well as Washington.

Undertakers or their assistants can be found accompanying the troops in campaigns that stretched from the Red River of the West across nearly half of America to the East Coast. Undoubtedly, however, the concentration of functionaries — approved, "commissioned," freelance, and camp-following — was in the Washington-Richmond area.

The case of W.R. Cornelius is instructive as a man who both expanded his business to meet opportunity and an undertaker who took no sides when offering his services to military authorities. Born in 1824 in Union County, Pennsylvania, Cornelius learned as an apprentice carpenter to make coffins, as well as cabinets, and assisted his employer in burying the dead. After working in several states, he found employment in Nashville, Tennessee, with the cabinet firm of McComb and Carson.

By 1849, he was foreman of the undertaking and cabinet division of that firm. In June of that year, he conducted the funeral of James K. Polk.

Cornelius later bought a partnership in the firm and, in 1861, when he seems to have become sole proprietor of the firm, he sold off the factory and furniture inventory and continued to maintain only the undertaking business. He states:

> I took a contract to bury the Confederate dead and I continued to bury them — about 1,800 in all — until the arrival (in Nashville) of the Union army, when I took a contract from Captain Gillam, then in charge of that (Quartermaster) Department, basing my prices on what I had received from the Confederate government; and I continued to bury the dead during the remainder of the war, having houses, (branch establishments) at Murfreesboro and Chattanooga, Tennessee; and at Stevenson, Huntsville, and Bridgeport, Alabama; and at Rome, Georgia. During the War I buried and shipped to their homes something over 33,000 soldiers, employees, etc. of which I kept record. It was during the year 1862 that one Dr. E.C. Lewis came to me from the employ of Dr. Holmes and proposed to embalm bodies. It was new to me, but I at once put him to work with the Holmes fluid and Holmes injector. He was quite an expert, but like a great many men, he could not stand prosperity, and soon wanted to get into some other kind of business, which he did.[25]

Thomas Holmes adds to this account:

> In the forepart of the war, a young doctor named Lewis called at my headquarters in Washington and wished me to instruct him in the embalming profession, and sell him an outfit to go to the Western Army and locate at Nashville, Tennessee. He offered as security a property-holding in Georgetown, D.C. for any amount of fluid I would trust him for. I made a bargain with him and he used many barrels of fluid. I was often surprised at his large orders. Dr. Lewis' headquarters were at Mr. Cornelius' undertaking establishment in Nashville.[26]

Cornelius continues his account:

> I suppose I embalmed and had embalmed some 3,000-3,500 soldiers and employees of the U.S. Army. Embalming was not introduced until after the Confederate Army left, so I did not embalm any Confederates. I embalmed and shipped General McPherson, General Scott and General Garesche (actually Colonel Julius Garesche, chief of staff of the Army of the Cumberland). The latter had his head shot clear off. I shipped nearly all of the Anderson calvary to Philadelphia, at one time. After the fight at Stones River, I shipped colonels, majors, captains and privates by the carload some days. I had no trouble with embalming by the Holmes process, using the femoral artery. The only trouble was that the subject would become discolored, but would keep any length of time. We had a great many exciting scenes during the war, and I had but little trouble with either army. I worked for both armies all the time they were here. Both armies treated me properly and paid me promptly.[27]

By recording his own record as a Civil War embalmer, Cornelius thus rendered another service: He memorialized his assistant, Prince Greer, who probably was the first black embalmer:

> When Lewis, the embalmer, quit, I then undertook the embalming myself with a colored assistant named Prince Greer who appeared to enjoy embalming so much that he became himself an expert, kept on at work embalming during the balance of the war, and was very successful. It was but a short time before he could raise an artery as quickly as anyone, and was always careful, always of course coming to me in a critical case. He remained with me until I quit business in 1871.[28]

Dr. Daniel H. Prunk offers another example of turning a service into business success. After serving as a physician with the Union Indiana troops until 1863, he reconstituted himself as an embalming-surgeon, settled in Nashville and there established his embalming headquarters. Prunk eventually operated branches not only in Tennessee, but he also sent embalming-surgeons, whom he trained, to open establishments in Georgia and Alabama. When the war ended, he sold this extensive embalming practice and returned to Indianapolis, where he resumed the practice of medicine.[29]

There was little stability, standardized quality or continuity of performance among these practitioners. Many were jacks-of-all trades; more than a few, outright opportunists. For example, Dr. C.B. Chamberlain, believed to have practiced in Philadelphia, came to Washington to engage in embalming, instruction in embalming procedures, and in manufacturing embalming fluids. In 1862, Chamberlain formed a partnership with F.A. Hutton, but when this arrangement broke up, he formed a new partnership with Benjamin A. Lyford, and the two of them joined the ranks of the many giving service to the slain on the Gettysburg battlefield.

All did not go easily, however, as Lyford was admonished by the provost marshal of the Army of the Potomac for his practices as an embalmer, and Hutton likewise was rebuked by the authorities.

In 1863, Hutton patented an embalming fluid but, somewhat paradoxically, he was arrested that same year by the Washington provost marshal, Lafayette C. Baker, and charged with attempted fraud in the return of a dead body. He was later released, and although he attempted to re-enter practice as an embalming-surgeon, permission was refused by the military authorities.[30]

Obviously, as this example indicates, not all embalmers in Washington, D.C., and elsewhere were sufficiently astute or fortunate enough to keep out of trouble with the authorities. The Civil War was the first conflict to see embalmers waiting and working in camps, on battlefields, in government hospitals, and in nearby railroad centers to serve the needs of the military and the families of the fallen.[31]

In addition, the disruptions produced by army operations and the lack of definite, full and uniform regulations governing embalming personnel and practices (as noted previously) led to abuses. These finally grew in sufficient magnitude to attract the concern of general headquarters.

The dubious distinction of being the embalmer whose conduct of business brought an end to abuses was Dr. Richard Burr, an embalmer who served on the eastern front throughout the war. When Burr was charged with fraud and attempted extortion, the provost marshal of the Army of the Potomac, after a hearing on November 14, 1864, forwarded charges and Burr's defense to Grant's headquarters before Richmond. On January 9, 1865, Grant returned a bill of particulars with the endorsement: "All permits for embalming-surgeons within the lines of the armies operating against Richmond have been revoked and the surgeons ordered without the lines."[32]

The Burr incident resulted in the issuance of a War Department General Order in March 1865 titled "Order Concerning Embalmers."[33] This landmark order established a system for determining, through examination, the qualifications of those who sought to embalm military dead and provided for the licensing of successful candidates — the license to be issued only upon their furnishing a bond to ensure faithful performance of their duties. Another section of this order established a uniform fee for services and prices for merchandise.

Even though the war ended a month after the issuance of this order, and it therefore could not have had much effect on embalming services to battlefield casualties, it was still a milestone in the history of embalming. It represented the first major effort in the United States, and perhaps the world, by an established public agency to define professional requirements for embalmers and to end the chaos of an unregulated field. It would take the individual U.S. states 30 years or more to duplicate these far-sighted regulations.

Embalming Devices, Fluids and Techniques: While Holmes was experimenting in his Brooklyn pharmacy's basement years before the Civil War, others interested in preserving flesh — whether for food, use as anatomical specimens, or in conjunction with the burial of the dead — were conducting similar research. Interestingly, the U.S. Patent Office included devices and compounds for preserving animal flesh for food under the heading of "Embalming" until at least 1885.

In 1856, the first patent (No. 15,972) for a process of embalming the body by a method depending primarily, but not wholly, on injection of a chemical compound went to J. Anthony Gaussardia of Washington, D.C. Incredibly, the process involved injection of an arsenic-alcohol mixture, electrically charging the body, successive washings with various chemical compounds, anointing with oils, and then placing the body in a coffin filled with "an alcoholic mixture of arsenic."

Notable in this case is the lesser importance of display of the body. Permanence of preservation might have been assured, but beyond the utility for transportation, there was little to this mode of preparing the dead that would commend it to the funeral director. A chemical laboratory would have been required to perform the embalming, and the funeral director would have been restricted to hermetically sealed metallic coffins. (*See Plate 44*.)

Undoubtedly, Holmes had been compounding embalming fluids at least a decade earlier than the date of Gaussardia's patent, but such compounds as he was able to produce before the Civil War never got to the U.S. Patent Office. One of the reasons, seemingly, was that the basic ingredients (arsenates and various poisonous metallic salts, chlorides and the like) were fairly commonly known and had been in use for preserving flesh (as noted above) in England and on the Continent for many decades before. Thus, in order to market an embalming fluid made of such derivatives, it was better for him to keep the formula secret and manufacture it himself.

This, precisely, is what Holmes did. Even though he manufactured and sold a prepared fluid, "Inominata" at $3.00 per gallon, he did not patent it. Of his three major patents,[34] two were for embalming by exposing the body to disinfectant gases (1877 and 1891), and the third (1861) for an "Apparatus for Filling Blood Vessels of Dead Bodies." (*See Plate 43*.)

PLATE 44

UNITED STATES PATENT OFFICE.

J. ANTHONY GAUSSARDIA, OF WASHINGTON, DISTRICT OF COLUMBIA.

METHOD OF PRESERVING DEAD BODIES.

Specification forming part of Letters Patent No. **15,972**, dated October 28, 1856.

To all whom it may concern:

Be it known that I, JOHN ANTHONY GAUSSARDIA, of the city and county of Washington, in the District of Columbia, have invented a new and Improved Method of Preserving Dead Bodies, of which the following is a full, clear, and exact description.

The body or subject to be preserved is first placed upon a table or other suitable place in a horizontal position and then injected with a strong mixture of acidum pyroligneum arsenicalis, a gallon of the mixture being sufficient for a grown person of ordinary size, this mixture being prepared by the addition of four ounces of white arsenic to one gallon of pyroligneous acid. The body thus prepared is then gradually charged with electricity from an electric machine until the liquid matters and humors have become congealed or coagulated, this being ascertained by the body becoming firmer or more solid to the touch or pressure of the hand, this part of the process, as a general thing, being effected in the course of from two and one-half to five hours, according to the condition of the body, one of the conductors of the machine being applied to the mouth and the other to the anus. The body is next washed in a strong mixture of arsenic, nitrate of potash, chloride of lime, and alcohol, this mixture being composed of about four ounces each of the arsenic and nitrate of potash, with two ounces of the chloride of lime to one gallon of alcohol, three successive times, a few hours being allowed to intervene between each to permit the mixture upon the body to become thoroughly dry, after which it may be anointed with aromatic oils and placed in a metallic coffin so constructed as to be capable of being hermetically sealed. In this condition the coffin is then filled with an alcoholic mixture of arsenic. The specific gravity of the alcohol in no case should be greater than .285, the quantity of arsenic required for this purpose being about the one-fiftieth part of the whole weight of the body thus treated, or at the rate of about two ounces of white arsenic to the gallon of alcohol, about eight ounces of the oils of cicuta and caryophyllus aromaticus being then added, after which the coffin is hermetically sealed and the process complete.

It may be here observed that the quantity of the mixture of the acid pyroligneum arsenicalis is increased or diminished according to the condition of the body being preserved. If partially decomposed, then a greater quantity is required than if it were in a good condition. Such being also the case where it is large and gross, these conditions being also dependent upon the age of the person whose body is being prepared and the season of the year in which the operation is being performed; but bodies once prepared in this manner will keep in all climates and for almost any length of time.

Bodies can, if desired, be so prepared as to preserve them but for a short time to enable them to be transported from the place where death intervened to the spot where their friends may wish to have them interred, this being effected by merely lessening the quantity of acidum pyroligneum arsenicalis to be administered and the quantity of electricity.

Having thus described my improved mode of preserving dead bodies, what I claim as new, and desire to secure by Letters Patent, is—

Injecting the body with a mixture of arsenical pyroligneous acid and then charging it with a current of electricity for the purposes described, and then filling the coffin in which the body is placed, and which is afterward hermetically sealed, with an alcoholic mixture of arsenic, together with the oils of cicuta and caryophyllus aromaticus, substantially as described.

J. A. GAUSSARDIA.

Witnesses:
P. HANNAY,
ARTHUR C. WATKINS.

44. Facsimile of First Patent for Embalming Process, 1856.

The latter was by far the most significant, and it was Holmes' intention (which seems to have met with some success) to sell the apparatus to undertakers for $100 and the "right" to use it, which might have included instruction for an additional $200.[35] The principle of the force pump was familiar enough and, from later accounts of undertakers concerning their initial ventures into chemical embalming by injection, it appears that many, including John Epply and Hudson Samson, made, or had made, their own.

Cavity embalming appears to be a post-Civil War development. The arterial-injection method was relatively quick and easy to perform, and the poisonous salts-in-solution seemed sufficiently effective in retarding body putrefaction.

Between 1856 and 1870, a total of eleven patents were granted for embalming fluids, related media, and processes, as noted in the following table:

EMBALMING PATENTS IN AMERICA: 1856-1870[36]

Date	Patent Number	Patentees
ARSENATED COMPOSITIONS		
1856	15,972	Gaussardia, J.A.
1860	30,576	Iddings, Warren
1868	81,755	Crane, E.
SULPHUROUS ACID AND SULPHITES		
1863	38,749	Hutton, F.A.
1867	67,170	Granja, Edward
1868	75,992	Sickel, James C.
OTHER DISINFECTANT GASES		
1867	61,472	Scollay, G.W.
MISCELLANEOUS NON-FORMALIN COMPOSITIONS		
1864	44,495	Morgan, John
1867	69,312	Brunetti, L.
1868	74,607	Seely, C.A. & Eames, C.J.
INNOVATIONAL		
1867	67,145	St. Clair, Colin C.

It is obvious that a diversity of approaches to the problem of preservation of the dead characterizes this 13-year period. The two earliest patents specified arsenic as the basic element in the embalming compound, and the third, sulfurous acid. John Morgan's compound, patented in 1864, called for common salt, potassium nitrate and powdered alum. All of these were mixed with water.

St. Clair's patent, on the other hand, as impracticable as it was innovational, required immersing the corpse in a mixture of plaster of Paris and hydraulic cement, with parts of the cadaver temporarily perforated with tubes to permit the escape of gases! (***See Plate 43***.)

The listing of these patents during this short span not only serves to indicate the multiplicity of innovations and inventions for preserving the dead, but also, to some extent, underscores the *futility* of attempting to determine "the first embalmer," "the first embalming fluid" or other equivalent "firsts."

What seems of greater importance is the fact that (as made clear previously) the earliest center of embalming was rather precipitously created in Washington, D.C., at the onset of the Civil War and — within what might be called "the fertile context of ideas" created by the exigencies and necessities of the war — innovational techniques and methods for the care, preservation and shipping of the dead emerged as collective products.

In 1861, we recall the "undertaker's stores" of Buckley in Washington, Burch in Georgetown, and Wheatley in Alexandria. In 1862, the Washington, D.C., city directory lists an advertisement by "Joseph Gawler, Undertaker," offering all conventional funeral items and "bodies embalmed if required."[37] Although the person who actually did the embalming for Gawler might be lost to history, it would be a safe guess that this person was in some, perhaps remote, way connected with the medical profession.

By the following year, this same directory had added three more "embalmers of the dead": Brown and Alexander, Surgeons and Embalmers, 523 D St., North; the above mentioned Holmes,[38] Thomas, 80 Louisiana Ave.; and Hutton, F.A., Dr., 451 Pennsylvania Ave. This Hutton, incidentally, is the inventor of the 1863 variety of "improved embalming fluid," and, undoubtedly, the competition he and others provided Holmes was substantial, in spite of Holmes' statement that he had more work than he could perform.

In fact, in the 1863 directory, Hutton ran a full-page advertisement announcing that Dr. Hutton & Co. had established themselves in the city. The advertisement was designed to convince the public that their method of embalming "exceeds anything of like nature in the world."

<blockquote>
Bodies Embalmed by Us

NEVER TURN BLACK!

But retain their natural color and appearance; indeed, the method having the power of preserving bodies, with all their parts, both internal and external.

WITHOUT ANY MUTILATION OR EXTRACTION,

and so as to admit of contemplation of the person Embalmed, with the countenance of a one asleep... Surgeons and all interested are cordially invited to call and examine specimens after Embalmed...[39]

N.B. Particular attention paid to obtaining bodies of those who have fallen on the Battle Field.
</blockquote>

(Below this advertisement is listed the undertaker E.A. Williams, who was associated with Dr. Hutton. In his portion, he offers both his services and a line of metallic, zinc, rosewood and mahogany coffins.)

The final line of the Hutton advertisement brings again to mind the fact that several of the best-known undertakers of the late-19th century established themselves in the business of caring for the dead directly as a result of receiving army contracts for soldier burial.

In addition to others discussed above, there were Collins H. Jordan of Chicago, who contracted for the burial of soldiers who died in the vicinity of that city; Lewis Jones, engaged by the government for the same services in and around Boston; John C. Rulon, who was one of the many that handled the dead at Gettysburg; John P. Epply, Cincinnati, who buried many of the soldiers who fell in the Shenandoah Valley; and, again, E.A. Williams of Washington, D.C.; and still others.

Jacob Gish, who was engaged as coffin-maker by the Quartermaster Corps during the war, returned afterward to Omaha to enter the undertaking business. Still others, such as George W. Murphy of Quincy, Illinois; John Reade of Milford, Massachusetts; and Robert F. Atkins of Buffalo served as soldiers in the army and returned to set up undertaking establishments at the close of hostilities.

It bears repeating that if undertakers were engaged to bury the war dead by the government, embalming bodies was not apparently specified in such official actions, or by official order. One exception, however, appears to have been the U.S. General Hospital in Armory Square, Washington, D.C., where embalming was routine during the war. Quoting from a letter (actually a form letter with blank spaces filled in) that the surgeon-in-charge sent to the family of J.J. Smith, a Union soldier who died of a "gun shot wound around of right arm... The body has been embalmed and the grave numbered and registered, so as to enable the friends to disinter the remains for transportation, on and after Oct. 1st, (1864) should they desire to do so." (*Johnson Collection*.)

Whatever embalming had been done before the Civil War seems to have taken place more within the context of medical pathology and was based on such non-aesthetic considerations as sanitation, previously mentioned specimen preservation, and other uses in connection with anatomical studies.

Coroners, whose background and orientation were medical, likewise had reasons to seek better methods of preserving bodies.

Thus, it should not be considered unusual that, at the outbreak of the Civil War, chemical embalming by injection would first be performed by those with medical training, since only they were familiar with the process. Their operations in the care of the dead, consequently, were technical and specific.

Undertakers, in traditional fashion, *undertook* the multiple tasks of removing, transporting and "funeralizing" the dead, whilst medical embalmers either associated themselves with undertakers in establishing the business of dealing with the dead, or, as was more likely the case, offered their special embalming techniques professionally, for a fee.

In brief, during the four-year period between Thomas Holmes's 1861 invention of an effective injection pump for arterial chemical embalming and his entry into the Washington, D.C., scene, and the 1865 embalming of President Lincoln, substantial socio-technical change had been effected. A medical science-based procedure, hitherto almost unknown to American undertakers, had become insinuated into the cultural pattern defining appropriate behavior toward dead bodies.

The remainder of the century, as will be seen in the following pages, will prove one for the diffusion of the new pattern by practitioners, "professors," commercial fluid-house representatives, and a few "true believers" — all convinced that a body properly funeralized and buried must be, first, a body properly embalmed.

"Schools," Fluid Houses and the Spread of Embalming: From the Civil War to the end of the century, the story of embalming in America is best seen in three dimensions: first, the resistance to chemical preservatives; second, the rise and decline of the medical specialist as embalmer; and third, the development of a commercial enterprise in the compounding and distribution of embalming fluids, with the attendant rise of the "embalming school."

Resistance to the use of embalming fluids came from two sources: the public, and undertakers themselves. Preservation by ice or "conserving the remains," as was usually the phrase, was somewhat awkward, but it had the virtue of simplicity and it yielded a modest profit. Ten dollars was not an unusual charge for such a service.

The earliest chemical embalming was the specialty of the physician, the embalming-surgeon, and while the fee was usually higher — Holmes charged $100, including casket dressing, cartage, and railway express charges — in many cases, it was a simpler matter to use conventional ice cooling than to bring in the "expert," whose skill was often suspect, and whose finished product was not always satisfactory.

Public resistance to the mutilation of the remains, moreover, had the sanction of Christian tradition that the body is the temple of God, and that the remains are always sacred and must, in every case, be treated with reverence. In an attempt to dispel this objection, advertisements such as Dr. Hutton's, stressed the "humaneness" of the new process.

Important also was the need to embalm chemically without evisceration, which the injection pump and the use of injection needles and arterial tubes had met. There was little, if any, cavity embalming until the mid- or late-1870s, but a significant step was taken with the 1878 patent by Samuel Rogers of the "trocar" — an elongated, "sword-like" hollow needle through which fluids might be injected into, and throughout, the trunk cavity of the dead.

If the opening of the Civil War found embalming and the compounding of embalming fluids monopolized by physicians, surgeons, physiologists, anatomists, chemists, pharmacists, druggists and others connected with the rising medical profession, its close saw changes that would eventually bring these processes and preparations almost completely under the control of pharmacists, undertakers, and wholesale chemical-compounding concerns.

The decade following the war, then, found the surgeon-embalmer playing a less-important role and less eager to make a career out of embalming than certain others outside of, or peripheral to, the medical arts. While Holmes returned to New York and practiced medicine, compounded drugs, and sold his own fluid, pump and process, other medical practitioners dropped out of sight in the mortuary field or, in a few notable cases, shifted to the compounding and sale of fluids, to the teaching of embalming techniques, or to a combination of merchandising and teaching.

As medical practitioners retreated from the field, undertakers advanced into it until, as noted earlier, the period became for them one of great opportunity, during which they experimented with new practices and ideas, and reviewed the developments in the funeral field, as augmented and accentuated by the Civil War. Men such as the above-mentioned Thomas W. Bothick of New Orleans; Robert Atkins of Buffalo; George W. Murphy of Quincy, Illinois; James Taylor of Trenton, New Jersey; and Jacob Gish of Omaha, Nebraska (to mention only a few), could, as a result of their war experience, establish undertaking establishments or shift to undertaking as a full-time occupation.

Embalming, no longer unknown and untried, had already gained a toehold, and these men were willing, along with many others who had known or learned the rudiments of embalming during the war, to add this technique to their services. One of the foremost was Hudson Samson of Pittsburgh, Pennsylvania, who, as early as 1870, embalmed the dead as part of his funeral services. (***See Plate 45***.)

The receptiveness of many undertakers to this innovation had its counterpart in the willingness of druggists and pharmacist-physicians to experiment in the compounding of various fluids. As noted earlier, between 1856 and 1870, roughly a dozen patents were granted for various kinds of embalming fluids and processes emphasizing chemical embalming by injection. Other concoctions, such as Holmes' and Hill's, were marketed but not patented.

It is also interesting to note that the earliest compounders of embalming fluids, whether medically trained or not, chose to call themselves "professors." Although this term had somewhat more validity later, when "schools" of embalming first got underway, it is likely that its original use was due to undertakers and other non-medically trained individuals who felt the need to legitimize their interests and experiments in embalming techniques, the compounding of fluids, and the building of embalming apparatus.

Thus, a good decade before the appearance of any type of formal instruction, "Professor" E. Crane had patented, in 1868, and sold "Crane's Electro-Dynamic Mummifier," a preparation composed mostly of salts of heavy metals, to be forced in all bodily cavities. His customers were undertakers in and around Michigan.

In 1876, "Professor" George M. Rhodes bought the rights to this, or a similar compound, from Crane, heavily advertised it in *Casket* and marketed it as "Professor Rhodes' Electrical Balm."

The advertising in the same magazine in the 1870s shows that Holmes was still marketing his own fluid. Also, Samuel Rogers' "Fluid Allekton" was advertised in an 1879 pamphlet. It is also interesting to note that several advertisements in the 1870s claim that, by *external application only*, an effective preservation of the body could be achieved.

By 1880, at least four concerns were compounding embalming fluids commercially: The Hill Chemical Company of Springfield, Ohio, which had started in 1878 and shortly afterward became The Champion Chemical Company; The Clarke Chemical Works; and Mills and Lacey, of Grand Rapids, Michigan, who were compounding Prof. Rhodes' formula. The fourth company emerged when Crane went to Kalamazoo, Michigan, and interested O.M. Allen Sr. in a similar enterprise. "Crane's Excelsior Preservation" was prepared and sold as a sideline by the Globe Casket Manufacturing Company.[40]

September 1870

John T.
Walnut Casket & box 20.00
Name Plate 3.00
13½ yards of Crape 8.10
18   "   " Ribbon 4.50
4 pairs   " Gloves 1.00
Merino Wrapper 6.00
10 Carriages 50.00   98.60
1 Hearse 6.00
                            $98.60 $98.60

20 Estate of Hannah
    fine O.C. Rosewood Coffin .. 80.00
    Name Plate 3.00
    14½ yards of Crape 7.25
    25   "   " Ribbon 6.25
    13 pairs " Gloves 2.50
    20 Carriages 120.00
    Hearse 9.00
    1 Carr all day 4.00
                              $230.00 $230.00

20 Estate of Hon. P.L.
    fine Rosewood Casket 150.00
    Name Plate 5.00
    12 yards of Crape 7.20
    2 bolts " Ribbon 6.00
    14 pairs " Gloves 8.40
    Embalming & Services 30.00
                              $206.60 $206.60

    Harper & Co
    Mary
    7 yds Crape 3.50
    12 yds Ribbon 3.00
    4 pairs Gloves 1.00

PLATE 46

GREATLY IMPROVED
COOLING BOARD!

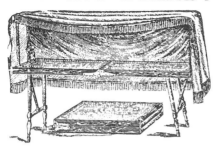

B. F. GLEASON,

A PRACTICAL UNDERTAKER of long experience, submits this **COOLING BOARD** to the profession as combining all the essential qualities to meet every requirement for the proper care of dead bodies. The simplicity of this Board recommends it over all others in the market, and its price places it within the reach of every Undertaker in the land. It is manufactured of the very finest materials, nickel plated, &c.

For prices, apply to the Manufacturer,

B. F. GLEASON,
Brockport, N. Y

James G. Van Cleve,

Successor of DISBROW & VAN CLEVE,

MANUFACTURER OF THE

Improved Patent Felt-Lined
COMBINATION

Corpse Preservers,

15 SOUTH WARREN STREET,
TRENTON, N. J.

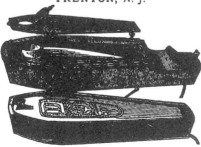

The most perfect, best tried, and the most convenient.

Improved May 1st, 1880.

J. C. TAYLOR & SON'S

Patent Improved

COLD AIR ICE CASKETS

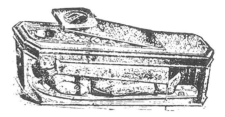

Some of the many reasons why it recommends itself: It is the **Original**; superiority of construction; strength; lightness; freezing qualities; beauty; most popular; most perfect; *most tried*; most reliable; most convenient; most *cleanly*; most *imitated*; most used (over 3,000 in use, more than all other makes combined); sold by most first-class houses; constructed by and under the supervision of *mechanics*; manufactured of best western walnut, finished throughout; three times the space to gain cold air, from bottom, sides, ends and top of Ice Chamber. The Ice Chamber *not* being stationary, it can be filled with ice if desired and placed in the Ice Casket without the least danger of making the ice casket *top heavy*; the water can be retained in the pan, but is of no advantage; the pan can be removed in a second for emptying of ice without the loss of time of picking it out with the hands, or turning the entire lid upside down for that purpose; our pan can also be removed for repairs (if needed), washed, aired or painted. We do not line our Ice Caskets with felt, as it is an objection, as dampness and the unpleasant smell of a corpse penetrates felt and it is impossible to rid the presence of the same, nevertheless if any person should so desire, we will line with felt, but know it would not give satisfaction. The application of felt to corpse preservers has *never* been patented. Cold air does not rise, but *falls*. Our ice caskets being so simply constructed, quickly refilled, does not give the cold air a chance to escape, thus avoiding all possibility of dampening the clothing. A feature that *exist* in our Ice Caskets: each Ice Casket contains a handsome carved or Gardner perforated chestnut Cooling Board, with adjustable head rest, chin support, straps for keeping arms and limbs in proper position, self measurement, the finest and most convenient cooling board in existence, in fact many *original* advantages that do not exist in any other make.

The Cheapest.	PRICES FOR CASH.	The Best.
3 feet 10, $35.00	5 feet 10,	- $50.00
4 feet 10, - $40.00	6 feet 4,	- $50.00

For sale by the following well-known houses: Hamilton, Lemmon, Arnold & Co. Pittsburgh, Pa.; Metallic Burial Case Company, 406 Pearl St., New York City; L. Hornthal & Co., 290 and 292 Bowery, New York City, and 235 Fifth Ave., Chicago, Ill.; Paxson, Comfort & Co., 523 Market St., Philadelphia; W. W. Wagner, 26 N. Sixth St., Philadelphia; Chappell, Chase, Maxwell & Co., Oneida and Rochester, N. Y.; Warfield & Rohr, 62 S. Sharp St., Baltimore; Crawfordsville Coffin Co., Crawfordsville, Ind.; Miller Bros. & Co., Jermyn, Pa.; F. C. Riddle, 700 N. Fifth St., St. Louis, and the only manufacturers,

46. Cooling Boards and Improved Ice Caskets, Late-19th Century.

PLATE 47

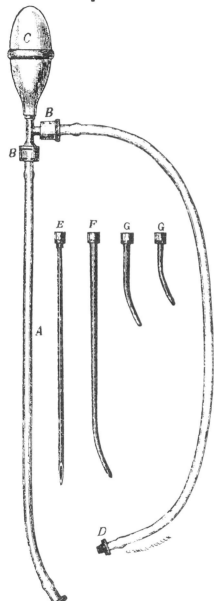

47. Advertisement for Embalming Supplies, 1880, *The Casket*.

The Champion Chemical Company (now The Champion Company) provides an interesting example of the early making and selling of embalming materials. The formula was provided by Ed. Hill, a druggist in Springfield, who had developed it in connection with his interest in the funeral industry and first tried marketing his product with George W. Boyd, of metal grave vault fame. Although Hill did not seem to have success in this venture, he was able to interest Dr. A.A. Baker, a physician in Springfield, and his son Scipio, in developing his formula and presenting it to the funeral industry. Ultimately, the operation of the company fell to the son, who remained its chief executive well into the 20th century.

The multiplication of chemical compounding concerns in the early 1880s created the need for wider markets and expanded distribution. Salesmen were sent on the road, some of them also representing lines of caskets, fluids and other funeral paraphernalia, while others promoted the sale of fluids alone. The sale of embalming fluid was assisted by the wave of humanitarianism then sweeping the country. Here, they claimed, was an answer to the mutilation of the body, to freezing the corpse with ice, or to encasing it in a heavy metal receptacle wherein decomposition might be arrested but not necessarily stopped.[41]

The bugaboo of "poisoning the body" — and perhaps poisoning the embalmer — remained, even after the introduction of the less-toxic formalin (about 1894).

Nevertheless, as late as the 1900s, attempts were being made to compound and sell embalming fluids that contained neither formaldehyde-in-solution nor any of the more violently poisonous metallic salts. According to its advertisements, one company, The Embalmers Supply Company, had for sale four kinds of fluid: "The Non-Poisonous Big Four" that "have shown conspicuous strength in successfully preserving every kind of a case." (***See Plate 48***.)

Joseph H. Clarke's pioneer role in setting up possibly the earliest embalming "schools" or "institutes" is interesting because it reveals the interdependence of the selling and promoting function with embalming instruction. Brought up to be a druggist, he first became interested in the preservation of dead-animal tissue as a young man. Later, he studied medicine privately and was in medical school when the Civil War broke out. His only war service was as a civilian assistant hospital steward.

With the return of peace, he became a "house and road" salesman for the White Water Valley Coffin Company of Connersville, Indiana. While on the road, he met the erstwhile "Professor" Rhodes, who sold Clarke six bottles of embalming fluid and gave him a modicum of advice on arterial and cavity embalming. Using the cadavers of his casket-buying clientele, Clarke experimented with the art of chemical embalming by injection and soon satisfied himself that this skill would not only add a new dimension to the service of the undertaker, but also held out promise for commercial exploitation.

In the fall of 1881, Clarke suggested to Dr. C.M. Lukens, a demonstrator of anatomy in Pulte Medical College, Cincinnati, Ohio, that an embalming school should be set up at that institution. Agreement was reached in March 1882, and the first session opened in the amphitheater on March 8 and ended March 31. This brief course marks one of the earliest attempts to carry out embalming instruction under institutional or quasi-institutional auspices.

PLATE 48

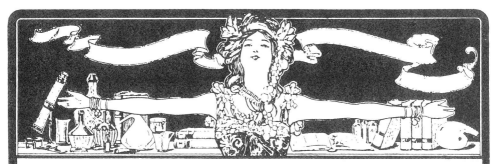

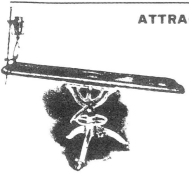

48. Early Advertisement for Non-Poisonous Embalming Fluid, 1909, *Western Undertaker*.

Although the Champion College of Embalming claimed to trace back to 1878, it had a nebulous existence at best.

Another claimant for the "earliest" title was the Rochester School of Embalming. Dr. August Renouard, who, in the minds of many, was the "dean" of early embalming instruction and who had been instructing privately for some years, opened the school in 1882, in time to make it available for demonstration and instruction during the first meeting of The Funeral Directors' National Association of The United States (later NFDA).

It is difficult to determine if these two schools — one organized by Renouard, the other by Clarke — were truly "institutions of learning" locked into one physical setting, or were quasi-institutions with only somewhat more permanence than the many traveling "schools" that would last three or four days to, at most, a week, and end with an "examination" and an embalmer's certificate of "graduation."

No attempt will be made here to determine which "school" (in the modern sense of the word) must be accepted as "first." Rather, as will be seen, the institutional process stretched over a number of years, with no one school having been in *continuous* operation at one site from the time of its inception. In point of fact, the early teachers, in the last analysis, are more important to understand than the "schools" they organized.

One in particular, F.A. Sullivan, stands out (as do Clarke, Renouard, C.M. Epply, and a few others) for his influence in the early field of embalming instruction. A somewhat distinctive figure, Sullivan, who was already an experienced embalmer, attended Clarke's first class in New York City in 1882 and, soon after, opened his own traveling school. This school had the largest attendance of any and continued to flourish until the end of the century.

From 1901 through 1903, Sullivan operated an embalming school in London, England, under the auspices of Oskar K. Buckhout, owner of a chemical company in Kalamazoo, Michigan. Again, Sullivan's venture prospered, and it was reported in trade journals that he had considerable influence in introducing chemical embalming to English undertakers.

Returning to Clarke, the first year of the Cincinnati School of Embalming (as it became known) saw six classes given in Cincinnati in medical schools and in Dr. Lukens' office, and four others in Philadelphia, Boston and New York. These ten classes graduated approximately 122 undertakers, many of them well known in the field. Dr. Lukens acted as principal, while Clarke and C.M. Epply, son of John Epply, assisted as lecturers and demonstrators.

Although Lukens and Clarke attended strictly to embalming matters, Epply instructed and demonstrated lining and trimming caskets, funeral conduct, and practical undertaking. When circumstances permitted, students were given cadavers to embalm and, at the close of a week's instruction, had usually mastered the rudiments of the embalming process.

Clarke tells of one student who ran and hid in a closet at the sight of two dead bodies, but "was brought out of his hiding place, put to work and became a good student and operator."[42]

The proponents of preservation by ice, however, were not always easily convinced. Among the doubters was Major Hulfish of Hulfish and Crans, Newark, undertakers. According to Clarke:

PLATE 49

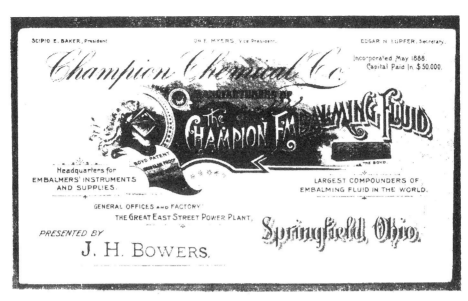

49A. Embalming-supply Salesman's Business Card, About 1900.

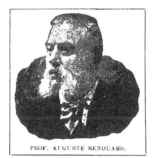

49B. Advertisement of Pioneer in Embalming, Auguste Renouard.

> (Hulfish)... told me I was a fraud and humbug to... say I could teach anyone not a physician how to embalm and preserve dead bodies without ice, and invited me to leave the office, which I did not do until I had an interview with his partner, Mr. Crans, who invited me to call again and have another talk with the major, which I did on my next visit to Newark, and Mr. Crans saw me embalm the body of a lady for Mr. Ormsby, and knew the body kept beautifully without the aid of ice for several days and was convinced. In our next trip east Mr. Crans came to New York to be humbugged, and said that ten times the cost of tuition had been received during the course.[43]

The early tours of Clarke and his associates occasionally met with disbelief and misgivings. In one instance, there was doubt voiced that an embalmed body would ever get to heaven; in many others, the demand for the use of ice was strong. However the demonstrations almost always were convincing, the $30 fee was usually considered money well spent, and recipients prized their certificates.

By the end of the 1880s, numerous embalming-fluid companies had entered the commercial field. In 1886, a manufacturers' directory published in *The Casket* listed 10 companies as manufacturers of embalming supplies. Most companies hired demonstrators for classes, or "schools," of embalming.

One of the foremost teachers of his day, and undoubtedly one of the best embalmers of this period, was Dr. Auguste Renouard, already mentioned and a competitor of Clarke. Each represented a different brand of fluid — Clarke his own and Renouard, for some time, that of the Brooklyn Embalming Fluid Company. Likewise, Dr. Eliab Meyers demonstrated for The Champion Company.

Another pioneer whose family name remains prominent in fluid manufacture, A. Johnson Dodge, was trained in St. Louis, Missouri, medical schools, where he served in the dual capacity of demonstrator and student. In 1893, at age 45, he became actively engaged in teaching embalming and was appointed the original principal of the Massachusetts College of Embalming, where he served until 1904. At that time, he became the active head of the Barnes School of Anatomy, Sanitary Science and Embalming, serving alternately in New York City and Boston.

Some three years later, he succeeded in establishing the Dodge School of Embalming in Boston, which was superseded in 1910 by the New England Institute of Anatomy, Sanitary Science and Embalming — a non profit educational corporation, with Dodge again as principal.[44]

Given its history, it is interesting to review some of the names of the various fluids. An identification with the past, especially with Egypt, is noticeable, such as the Egyptian Chemical Company; the Egyptian Embalmer Company; and such fluids as "Utopia," "The Oriental," "Egyptian" and the like. Later, embalming-fluid terminology tended in the direction of pseudo-scientific imagery, with combinations drawn from the symbol storehouse of modern chemistry.

Techniques of embalming slowly improved. Arterial embalming, as noted earlier, was by far the preferred technique during and after the Civil War, particularly among the embalming-surgeons. The introduction of the trocar in the late 1870s, as also noted, produced a simple, but probably somewhat less-effective method, of cavity embalming when used alone. Many undertakers who were unwilling or unable to learn the modicum of anatomy used in arterial embalming used the latter technique.

For a time, arterial embalmers, who usually possessed a certificate or diploma from a traveling "school" of embalming, considered the practitioners of cavity embalming as their professional inferiors — many of the latter referred to disdainfully as "belly puncturers."

While cavity embalming was, by itself, obviously far less-effective than arterial embalming, it was eventually adopted by arterial embalmers as the final phase of embalming treatment.

Clearly, the spread of the more-perfected arterial embalming techniques coincided with the increased commercialization of fluids and their promotion by the demonstrators of the various "schools" and classes.

By 1886, there was only one company, J.C. Taylor, listed in *The Casket* directory under the category of "Cold Air Preservers."[45]

By the end of the succeeding decade, the battle of "ice vs. arsenic" was definitely over, and arterial and cavity embalming, promoted and popularized by manufacturers of diverse embalming fluids, not only had overcome the resistance of undertakers but had also allayed public fears to such questions as mutilation and other forms of inhumanity on the embalming table.

CITATIONS AND REFERENCES IN CHAPTER 8

1. Charles L. Wallis, *Stories on Stone* (New York: Oxford University Press, 1954), p. 240.

2. *Ibid.*

3. *Ibid.*

4. Ralph H. Gabriel, *The Course of American Democratic Thought* (New York: The Ronald Press Co., 1940), p. 4.

5. These receptacles, first tested at the Battle of Gettysburg (July 1-3, 1863) in and around Gettysburg, Pennsylvania, proved useful to Holmes and possibly other undertakers who flocked to the battlefield. Their light weight (eight pounds, six ounces) made for easy carrying and handling. The rubberized-canvas interment sack, Holmes suggested, could also be rolled up as a knapsack and used as a waterproof sleeping bag during forced marches and in bad weather. It could also serve as an improved stretcher for hurriedly moving the seriously wounded from the field of battle. Holmes himself employed the receptacle wherever possible, quickly embalming the dead, marking and inflating the sack and shipping it north. Later, the Goodyear Rubber Company placed a similar sack in production and made it available to undertakers, but, by and large, the latter considered it a novelty and rejected it for peacetime use. (Rephrased communication from Edward C. Johnson).

6. For an excellent study of epidemic sickness in this period, see John Duffy, *Epidemics in Colonial America* (Baton Rouge, La.: Louisiana State University Press, 1953).

7. *History of Embalming and of Preparations in Anatomy, Pathology, and Natural History: including an account of A New Process for Embalming.* By J.N. Gannal (Paris: 1838). Translated from the French with notes and additions by R. Harlan, M.D. (Philadelphia: Judah Dobson, 1840).

8. "Fisk's Patent Metallic Burial Cases. Airtight and Indestructible. For Protecting and Preserving the Dead, for Ordinary Interment, for Vaults, for Transportation, or for any other desirable purpose." 1850. Sixteen pages. In the Edward C. and Gail R. Johnson private collection.

9. There are two dates given for the outlawing of arsenical compounds. Benjamin Ward Richardson, whose "Art of Embalming" appears in "Woods Medical and Surgical Monographs," Vol. 3, 1889, pages 595-641, writes on page 614: "The government of Louis Phillipe decreed in 1846 that the sale of arsenic and all solutions containing it, was prohibited for soaking grain, for the destruction of insects and for embalming bodies... Later the use of Corrosive Sublimate was similarly interdicted." P. Conil sets the date a decade earlier, writing in *Etudes Historiques et Comparatives sur les Embaumements* (Paris: 1856) on page 40, "Aussi une ordonnance Royale du 31 Octobre, 1836 a-t-elle interdit l'emploi de l'arsenic et de ses composes clans les embaumements. Cetle defense aurait du etre entendu au Sublime, dont l'action est tout funeste que celle de l'arsenic." Exactness of date is less important than knowledge that American anatomists and embalmers, and later embalming fluid-compounding houses, continued for at least a half century to make use of arsenic and a variety of other poisonous metallic salts until the states, beginning with Michigan in 1895, made their use illegal.

10. Nearly three decades of research into the origins of chemical embalming, its use in and after the Civil War, and of other aspects of 19th-century treatment and care of the dead have been conducted by Edward C. and Gail R. Johnson, Chicago, Illinois. Portions of their unpublished work "Alone in His Glory," dealing with Civil War embalming, have been drawn upon in bringing Chapter 8 in line with historical fact. Their work takes the biography of Holmes far beyond the facile "The First Embalmer" by Trentwell M. White and Ivan Sandorf in the November 7, 1942, issue of *The New Yorker*, and the more critical "Who was the Father of Modern Embalming?" by Seabury Quinn in *The American Funeral Director*, May 1944.

11. *Sunnyside*, October 1884.

12. *New York Daily Tribune*, October 15, 1850.

13. *Sunnyside*, October 1884.

14. *Graphic News*, (Chicago), July 24, 1886.

15. *The Casket*, December 1896.

16. Francis A. Lord, *They Fought for the Union* (New York: Bonanza Books, a division of Crown Publishers, Inc., by arrangement with The Stackpole Press, 1960), p. 328. Not only the wealthy sought the return of the war dead. Also, it was not above fellow soldiers to collect and reuse the equipment of fallen comrades.

17. Advertisement in *Army and Navy Journal*, Vol. 2, September 24, 1864, p. 79, as quoted in Lord, *ibid*., p. 256, footnote #122.

18. Julia Ward Howe, *Reminiscences*, Boston, 1889, as quoted in Lord, *ibid*., p. 256, footnote #123.

19. "A Visit to General Butler and the Army of the James," *Frasers' Magazine for Town and Country*, Vol. 71, April 1865, p. 438, as quoted in Lord, *ibid*., p. 256, footnote #124.

20. H. Clay Trumbull, *War Memories of an Army Chaplain*, New York, 1898, as quoted in Lord, *ibid.*, p. 256, footnote #125.

21. "Miscellaneous" (contributions by a Washington correspondent), *Frank Leslie's Illustrated Newspaper*, Vol. 14, May 3, 1862, p. 30, as quoted in Lord, *ibid.*, p. 257, footnote #126.

22. Princess Agnes Salm-Salm, *Ten Years of My Life*, Detroit, 1877, as quoted in Lord, *ibid.*, p. 257, footnote #127. In his reference, Lord lists the name as "Salm-Salm, Felix Princess."

23. William J. Bunnell (1823-?) of Jersey City, New Jersey. A copy of the journal is in the private collection of Edward C. and Gail R. Johnson.

24. Holmes' veracity is strongly attested to in the writings of Edward C. and Gail R. Johnson. See footnote #10 above.

25. *The Casket*, July 1892.

26. *The Casket*, May 1892.

27. *The Casket*, July 1892.

28. "Prince Greer, America's First Negro Embalmer," *Liaison Bulletin*, International Federation of Thanatopractic Associations, April 1973, by Edward C. and Gail R. Johnson.

29. "A Civil War Embalming Surgeon, The Story of Dr. Daniel H. Prunk." *The Director*, April 1973, by Edward C. and Gail R. Johnson.

30. Dr. C.B. Chamberlain is found in the 1862 Washington city directory, and in various connections in the Hutton letters in Baker #363, file (below) in Clarke's *Reminiscences of Early Embalming*, (see reference 40), and *Sunnyside*, March 1886.

F.A. Hutton is centrally figured in File #363, National Archives, Case Files of Investigations by Levi C. Turner and Lafayette C. Baker, and in the *Washington Star*, April 21, 1863.

Benjamin A. Lyford's case is reviewed in the diary of Major General M.R. Patrick, Provost of the Army of the Potomac, Rare Book Room, National Archives.

31. See later section in the chapter quoting from a form letter used by the Armory Square Hospital indicating routine embalming practiced in that hospital. The bodies were buried but could be disinterred by friends or relatives at a later date. See also *Harpers Weekly*, February 27, 1874.

32. National Archives, Record Group #94, Order of Lt. General U.S. Grant, dated January 9, 1865, at City Point, Virginia, as endorsement on complaint against Dr. Richard Burr.

33. General Order #39, War Department, Adjutant General's Office, March 16, 1865.

34. As noted elsewhere, Holmes, despite his penchant for experimentation and invention, received only five patents: #33885, December 10, 1861, *Improvement in Embalming* (Pump), Williamsburg, New York; #39291, July 21, 1863, *Corpse Receptacle* (Bag), Washington City; #48659, May 10, 1864, *Improvement in Coffins* (Deodorizing), Washington City; #188014, March 6, 1877, *Improvement in Process of Preserving Dead Bodies* (Preserving Coffin), Brooklyn, New York; and, #450017, April 7, 1891, *Embalming Mixture* (Gaseous fluid), Brooklyn, New York.

35. Despite the fact that many barrels of the fluid were sold, there is no way to estimate the success of this venture.

36. Adapted from Mendelsohn, *Embalming Fluids*, *op. cit.*, pp. 110-111.

37. Quoted in Quinn, *op. cit.*, p. 28.

38. Holmes had now his own establishment, which was listed in 1863 and 1864 in the Washington city directory at 80 Louisiana Avenue; and in 1865 at 451 Pennsylvania Avenue, where across the front of the building there was announced in large letters, "Embalming by Dr. Thomas Holmes."

39. Quinn, *op. cit.*, p. 29.

40. Joseph H. Clarke, *Reminiscences of Early Embalming* (New York: *The Sunnyside*, 1917), pp. 3-5. This is an important early reference dealing with early embalming education in America. Written in an interesting first-person narrative style, it conveys the way in which embalming was first taught, embellished with many anecdotes. Full lists of all students in each class session are included.

41. Embalming, by a combination of arterial injection and cavity treatment, became not only certain to produce the desired results — natural appearance and freedom from odors and decay — but gradually became desired, if not demanded, by the relatives of the decedent. With the advent of formalin-based embalming fluids, the old dangers of exposure of embalmers and relatives of the dead to the poisons of arsenic, bichloride of mercury, and similar lethal solutions ended, as was any medical or legal question concerning the presence of a poison in the body tissues. The transition from the "poisonous" fluids to the formalin fluids was not without incident. The practicing embalmer quickly learned that he had to ensure blood removal, something he previously had not been concerned about. This gave rise to the need of pre-injection fluids to exsanguinate the body. The strength of the formalin fluid had to be carefully computed, as too strong a solution hardened the body to the point where dressing or positioning of the limbs was nearly impossible. Jaundiced bodies, when embalmed with a formalin compound, turn from yellow to green. The problem still vexes modern embalmers, and special fluids and opaque cosmetics are required to counteract this effect.

43. *Ibid.*, pp. 13-14.

44. Personal communication from Arnold J. Dodge, December 28, 1961.

45. *The Casket Directory of Manufacturers and Jobbers of Funeral Supplies*, 1886.

Chapter 9

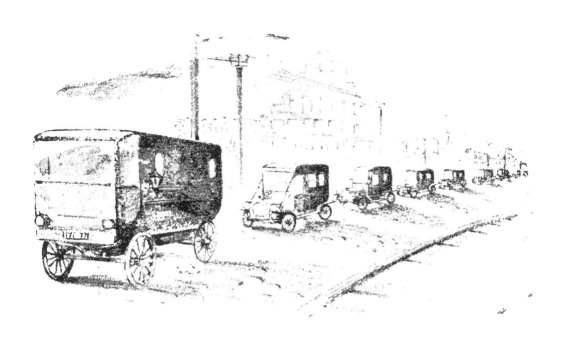

Transportation: Carriage to Gas Buggy

The death of a human being universally interrupts ordinary routines and calls for new modes of physical and emotional behavior. One of the most inescapable needs created by death in an organized society arises from the fact that the corpse must be moved from the point of death to other places for preparation and disposal. Those involved with the dead therefore face a transportation problem that broadens itself to include the mourners and others connected with funeralization.

In addition, with the social, physical and economic development of society, transportation is likely to assume new functions and forms and to take on new meanings and importance.

Although the funeral history examined in preceding chapters has generally moved forward to the end of the 19th century, this chapter begins with a brief glance at early American transportation usages and paraphernalia. Special attention is directed to the changing meaning and form of some of the *terms* that have now become associated with funeral transportation.

Funeral Processions and the Hearse: Whether the point of sepulture be a grave, tomb, pyre or, as an extreme example, a coffin-laden boat to be set afire and set adrift on the outgoing tide, the procession to it is a solemn social act that imparts importance, dignity and profundity to the ceremonial disposal of the dead.

The funeral procession is a dramatic movement involving many actors, whether it takes the form of pageantry; of mournful, simple silence; of noise and expressive behavior; or of mock gaiety or real gloom. Although the performance might have its basis in an indispensable physical act, social participation in it cannot help but produce significant ceremonial overtones.

So important is the collective act of bearing the dead to the place of sepulture that it has tended historically either to be incorporated into religious organization or to come under religious control. Even when the inspiration for them is secular, parades have the power to stir, and when a parade is joined to the intrinsic solemnity of death and burial, that power is increased.

"Of all processions," says Rech, "the funeral procession is the oldest. It starts at a period antedating wheeled vehicles, and it has continued down to the present. The character and form of the procession, or to use the modern term, the funeral, varies widely in different countries. Regardless of variety, it is one of the most universal human acts."[1]

Also note that the word "funeral" is derived from *funeralis*, Latin for "torchlight procession."

One of the standard pieces of equipment, and the most common symbol of the funeral procession, has been the hearse. This term has its origin in the French word *herse*, which, in turn, is taken from the Latin *hirpex*, meaning a rake or harrow. The resemblance that originally existed is clear when it is considered that the first hearse was a stationary framework of wood to hold lighted tapers and decorations placed on a bier or coffin. In this form, it must have looked much like a huge, rectangular rake lying with its teeth or prongs pointed upward.

This early simple frame later evolved into an elaborate, pagoda-shaped erection of wood or metal for the funerals of royal or other distinguished persons. It held banners, candles, armorial bearings and other heraldic devices. Complimentary verses or epitaphs were often attached to the hearse.[2]

Hearses were also used to enclose the tomb or grave. This type varied from the simple iron stand over which the pall might be draped during the ceremony to highly stylistic devices resembling miniature Gothic churches, with iron or brass spikes on which candles were impaled. (***See Plate 50***.)

A simple forerunner of the hearse (in the sense we use today) was a bier or "bear" in the form of a hand-stretcher on which the uncoffined body was carried to the grave. (***See Plate 50***.)

As coffins were brought into popular use, they were likewise borne on a bier, but the additional weight — especially in the case of lined or multiple coffins — necessitated an adaptation to the problem of long carries. One solution was to have two sets of bearers. Four of the oldest or most prominent men were called the "bearers"; another four, whose duty it was to relieve the bearers, were called "underbearers."[3]

As long as bodies were buried in churches, the stationary nature of early hearses is understandable. Once intramural burial became limited or restricted, and cemeteries were established outside of cities, however, the need for some better form of transportation than that provided by "bearing," or by hand or shoulder carrying, became urgent. Moreover, as burial grounds were laid out at a greater distance from thickly populated districts, carrying the body on a hand-bier grew too laborious, and some sort of a horse-drawn vehicle became necessary.[4]

PLATE 50

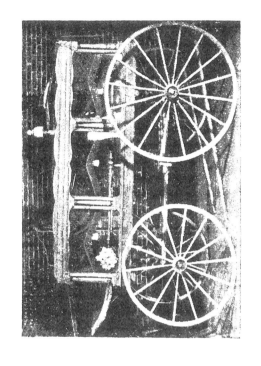

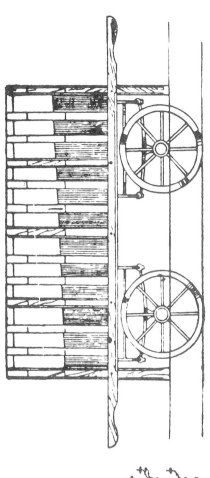

50B. (Top) Drawing of an Early English Bier on Wheels.
50C. Hand-built Early American Hearse, 1787.

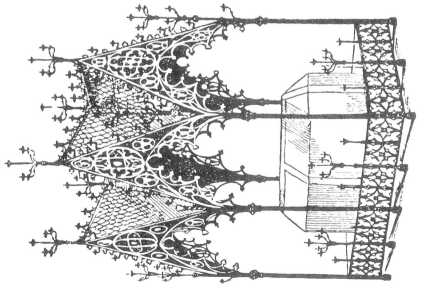

50A. Wrought Iron Hearse of Renaissance Era.

Rech notes that the first instance of a hearse on wheels is found in the burial of Colonel Rainsborowe in 1648, and that, in 1673, Anthony Walker, a preacher, said: "More friends attend a hearse to the Town-end than will drive through with it the whole journey." Also, by 1690, the hearse had become a necessity in England, and advertisements appeared in the *London Gazette* offering hearses for hire.[5]

Despite this, the term "bier" remained in use with conveyances strictly limited to carrying the dead, and, as late as the mid-19th century, "hearse" and "bier" were commonly interchangeable.

Because the roads leading out from early towns and villages were often narrow, rough and muddy, and sometimes little more than paths, the earliest movable hearses were of necessity much smaller than the stationary hearse that preceded them. In some instances, these hearses were so short that the coffin would come up under the seat of the driver, who would either have to straddle it or sit to one side of it. To increase maneuverability, the wheels would cut under the body of the vehicle. Later, the carriage part was made a distinct unit.

Colonial Hearses: In early Colonial times, rural and village funerals undoubtedly lacked the convenience of the hearse, or horse-drawn bier, specifically intended for funeral purposes. Bodies might be transported simply by wagon, although the funeral procession, whether to the family grave or the community churchyard, would more likely be on foot and the body borne by hand.

As cities appeared along the seaboard and in the wilderness behind it, commercial successes fostered more-elaborate forms of social organization, and funerals for prosperous and important people often took on a character reminiscent of upper-class English usage. As early as 1687, Judge Sewall wrote in his diary that, at the funeral of Lady Andros (a Church of England woman, not a Puritan): "The corps was carried (from the church) into the Hearse drawn by Six Horses..."[6]

When Colonel Shrimpton died of apoplexy in 1697 and was given a military funeral, Sewall noted cryptically, "Ten companies, No Herse nor Trumpet, but a horse led. Mourning coach also & Horses in Mourning, Scutcheons on their sides with Death Heads on their foreheads."[7] (Some 27 years later, Sewall noted the surviving use of escutcheons on the hearse carrying Katherine Winthrop's body.)

Nearly a century before the Revolutionary War, a few horse-drawn hearses were in use by several of the richer families in towns in New England and the Middle Colonies. Although well-appointed livery was relatively scarce before 1700, and most funeral processions were on foot, the use of carriages and coaches in making the journey to the grave was no novelty. "Glass coaches" had already made their appearance in England, and until the Colonial craftsmen of a later period could assemble the materials, men and know-how, carriages, coaches and chaises were necessarily imported.[8]

The making of gentlemen's coaches, such as were used in funeral processions, involved considerable skill. Bridenbaugh points out that coach-making was an urban luxury craft:

> One of the most spectacular symbols of colonial affluence and gentility was a gentlemen's carriage, and as men grew richer in town and country the business of coachmaking prospered. It was a trade requiring the careful combining of talents of wood and metal workers, as well as the skills of other artisans; the blacksmith and the ornamental iron worker assisted the joiner or coachmaker, the carver, the upholsterer, and the leather worker in building a vehicle upon which the painter, japanner,

and perhaps the heraldic-device liner placed the finishing touches. An elaborate industry such as this, moreover, demanded a large investment of capital, and not until after the middle of the century (18th) did American coaches begin to compete with carriages imported from London and Dublin.[9]

Another category of workers grew involved as problems of transportation expanded along with the growth of towns and cities. These were the liverymen, who imported and sold hearses to the well-to-do, or rented to the less-well-off who desired the prestige of a coach-and-four.

Bridenbaugh again notes:

> Most of the Boston gentry kept coaches, and carriage makers like John Lucas had orders enough to keep them constantly at work. Gentlemen and their "virtuous consorts" reclined on cane seats or sank comfortably into the green plush of their equipages, while Negro coachmen drove them to church or to social gatherings, for all to see and for laborers and tradesmen to envy. Those with pretensions, but without the means, could hire of George Hewes, "a Handsome Chair Chaise on Reasonable terms," while Samuel Bleigh and Alexander Thorpe kept coaches and black horses to rent for funerals.[10]

In the New England Colonies, the preliminary steps by which the role of undertaker came into being usually involved work as a sexton, cabinet-maker or coffin-maker. In the Middle Colonies, the carriage master or livery-stable operator was more likely to extend his function beyond merely supplying hearses and carriages to that of *service* in the care and disposal of the dead.

Thus, one short step from providing transportation would be directing the funeral procession and taking charge of the order of the proceedings. In Baltimore, Maryland, where the move of the carriage master toward the undertaker had an early start, this announcement appeared in an 1824 city directory (*see Figure 28*). Three types of conveyances appear, of which one of them is definitely a hearse.

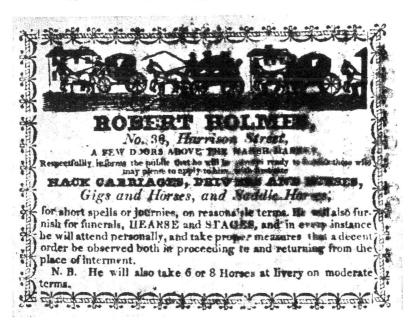

Figure 28. Early 19th-century Ad of the Liveryman-Undertaker.

Examples of American funeral hearses much earlier than those found in livery-stable advertisements exist, however. One such conveyance still in good condition (*see Plate 50*), although reputed to have been built in 1787, has glass panels, ornate exterior cabinetwork, a narrow lined interior, and drapes on either side.

Another fine, substantial example of an early pioneer hearse (*see Plate 51*) shows simplicity itself: large hind wheels; smaller front wheels that turn under the body; a narrow body with the coffin fitting up under the driver's seat; and the only non-functional objects — six wooden-turned "urns" spaced across the top of the vehicle.

Hearses with Horses, 1850-1910: Until the Civil War, the field of hearse manufacture was a somewhat stable sideline for several carriage manufacturers. A few concerns engaged in the manufacture of these transportation specialties, such as the Merts and Riddle Coach and Hearse Co. of Ravenna, Ohio, established in 1831; The James Cunningham, Son & Co., carriage and hearse manufacturers of Rochester, New York, established in 1838; and Brownell's Hearse Repository, founded in New Bedford, Massachusetts, about 1843.

The stability of this sideline arose from the fact that, until the Civil War, fashion had little effect upon hearse design or materials. Advertisements in city directories show that, from 1825 to 1850, hearses changed only slightly, although it is possible that in the largest cities, undertaker demands for improved vehicles were beginning to make headway among hearse manufacturers.

The slowness of change in the next 15 years is evident in the fact that, with only slight modification, the hearse already in use in 1853 appeared in the advertisement of Lockhart and Seelye, Coffin Manufacturers, in the Cambridge, Massachusetts, 1866 city directory.

In spite of the conservatism that resulted in little change in the styles and materials of hearse-making from year to year, the outbreak of the Civil War in the spring of 1861 was beginning to play a more important role in funeral equipage. By the end of the war, the styles had changed to such an extent that older hearses were rapidly becoming outmoded.

The hearse of the 1840s and 1850s might linger in use during the 1860s, but from that point on, styles in hearses changed with cyclical regularity at intervals of about 15 years. Reasonably enough, fashion seemed to have joined hands with the amount of use a manufacturer built into its hearses, for, during this period, the wear and tear occasioned by hard driving, frequent trips and constant washing made it necessary either to replace a hearse or to have it substantially rebuilt.

As explained by a "Cincinnati Expert"[11] in an unsigned article reviewing the history of style changes in hearses:

> After about fifteen years... the owner thinks it time for a change; time to have a new hearse, and something as different as possible, in order that its newness be apparent for purposes of advertising.
>
> So the undertaker buys a new one... (which) creates a sensation; so altogether different; so bright, sparkling and new; and with a new team — a fine pair of young horses, most likely, and with a new livery for the driver, a new silk hat, etc. Everybody notices it. There is a "write-up" in the newspapers, probably, and, all else being right as it should be, there is an increase in business.

PLATE 51

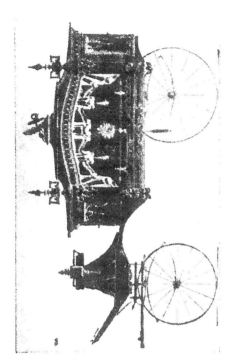

51C. Hearse Used During and After Civil War.

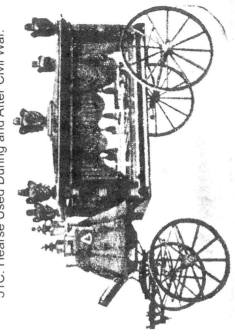

51D. The Return to a Rectangular Design, About 1884.

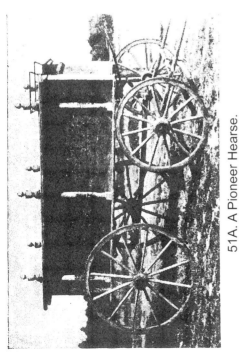

51A. A Pioneer Hearse.

51B. American Hearse of the 1850s.

Competitors "sit-up and take notice." Their own hearses now appear to be a little out of date, not to say back numbers, and pretty soon there is another hearse in town... (In) about eight or ten years there is not one of the previous styles of hearses in town; neither in that town nor other towns, for the new style has spread all over the country.[12]

After all of the local undertakers had put new hearses into use, there followed a period of a few years when the hearse style remained relatively unchanged.

Then, the earliest to make the change found his hearse the oldest of the new, but now aging, style. As before, he wanted something so different that it would be quite evident that he had made another change. Perhaps he had thought of a few innovations of his own, which he would be able to persuade the carriage-maker to incorporate into the newly ordered hearse. Or, perhaps, the carriage-maker himself modified his product in order to keep and enlarge his market.

Although the 15-year cycle naturally operated to their advantage, it does not follow that this cycle was a simple creation of the hearse manufacturers. Had they been able to control the style change, obviously it would have been profitable to exploit annual models, as does the modern automobile industry. But the spread of a new style was slow, and the decision to change by undertakers was a product of a calculation in which the utility of the old vehicle was balanced against the advantages to be gained by getting ahead of competition, or keeping up with it, by purchasing a new vehicle.

For this reason, the style cycle in hearses operated seemingly in terms of a number of distinctly economic and social factors reflective of forces and conditions, many of which were outside the control of hearse manufacturers. Hence, the "Cincinnati Expert" notes:

It is not true, as a rule, that the factories get up the new styles and start them on their way faster than buyers can be expected to purchase them. It does not pay them to do so. The factories do not wish radical changes to come too often. They prefer that the changes come just about as they have come — gradually, and in cycles of about fifteen years.[13]

The hearse of the 1850s (*see Plate 51*) was basically a long, rectangular box with windows of double-thick French glass and skimped curtains along the side. Shafts usually were for one horse only, and the driver's seat was on top.

By the time of the Civil War, the style had already changed (*see Plate 51*) and the hearse had become longer and higher, with full plate-glass sides, fancy scroll-work along the top, metal columns and a scrolled iron neck — a "goose neck" — that connected a fancy seat for the driver with the body of the hearse. Some hearses of this type had plated-metal Corinthian columns.

Although this style was roomier than its immediate predecessor, its inner dimensions only afforded space for an extra-size casket, and it was still called a "hearse," as opposed to a "funeral car." (The latter title did not come into use until the conveyance was later considerably increased in size.)

At the close of the war, in response to a general change in fashion that touched many items of the living, there was a call for something different, more imposing, that finally resulted in building the really large and massive, bent-glass, full-circle end, or Clarence front, hearses. These remained in style for a little more than 15 years, until the New Orleans Cotton Exposition, about 1884.[14]

At least until 1875, no hearse was considered completely trimmed without plumes waving from the urns that usually decorated its top. After this period, deck ornaments and emblems replaced the plumes, and, later, these too were cleared away and smooth, undecorated tops became the fashion.

The James Cunningham, Son & Co. exhibit at the New Orleans Cotton Exposition in 1884 featured a "funeral car" radically different from the prevailing style. (***See Plate 51***.) It was rectangular — reverting back to an earlier form — and had a hip roof, five urns and, at each corner, a gilded column "around which there climbed an ivy vine in green."

Shortly after the Civil War, hearses for children came into use, and the beautiful white child's hearse sold by The Stein Patent Burial Casket Works met with immediate popular approval. Throughout the last quarter of the 19th century, children's hearses were standard equipment for all undertakers and funeral directors. (***See Plate 52***.)

In 1884, the rectangular "four poster" fairly revolutionized the hearse-building industry. As a result, for a few years and in certain restricted localities, the term "hearse" soon became almost an epithet that applied to an out-of-style funeral vehicle. Undertakers either bought "funeral cars" or admitted their hearses were out of date. (Obviously, the word "hearse" has since returned to accepted standard usage for the vehicle used to transport the dead at funerals.)

In 1889, Hudson Samson's special eight-poster, oval-decked funeral car, and a similar vehicle with six columns ordered by James Lowrie and Sons of Allegheny, Pennsylvania, signaled the arrival of a new style and the death knell, after roughly a quarter century, of the ornamented deck. By 1898, all funeral directors of any pretension had an eight-column, oval-decked funeral car, no matter what the price.

At the 1893 World's Fair in Chicago, Crane & Breed Mfg. Co. exhibited the most elaborate and outstanding funeral car of the 19th century. (***See Plate 53***.) Designed for West Indian and South American trade, its features included extraordinary size; church-like design; massive carvings in bold relief; gildings; heavy gold fringes and tassels; and lamps of gold.

Weighing 2,400 pounds (versus a standard weight of about 1,600 pounds), it was laden with golden angels and cherubs; crucifixes and statues; and a processional scene over the middle glass depicting the Savior bearing the cross and preceded by the two thieves, the two Marys, a throng of Roman soldiers and others. Other sculpture over the quarter lights showed the adoration of the Christ child and the Ascension.

As noted earlier, this awe-inspiring vehicle, designed to be drawn by eight horses, was not intended for use in America but, by happenstance, it was used immediately after the close of the fair for the funeral of Chicago's assassinated mayor, Carter H. Harrison. On this occasion, the temporary axles with which this funeral car was equipped sustained the load, although they later bent under the heavy weight. Probably no other American funeral of state has featured so imposing a funeral car; certainly no similar vehicle was ever adorned with an equal profusion of religious scenes and symbols.

PLATE 52

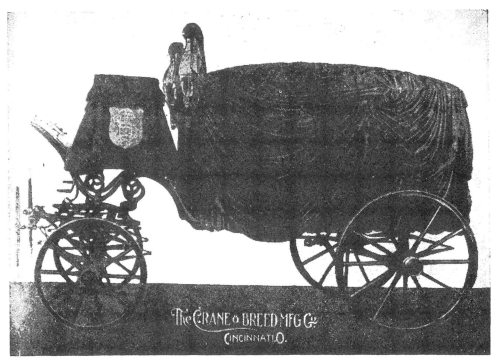

52A. Hand-carved Wooden Drape Hearse, About 1898.

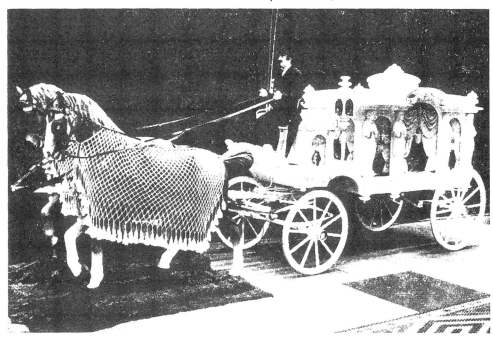

52B. Model of Ornate Child's Hearse, Late-19th Century.

PLATE 53

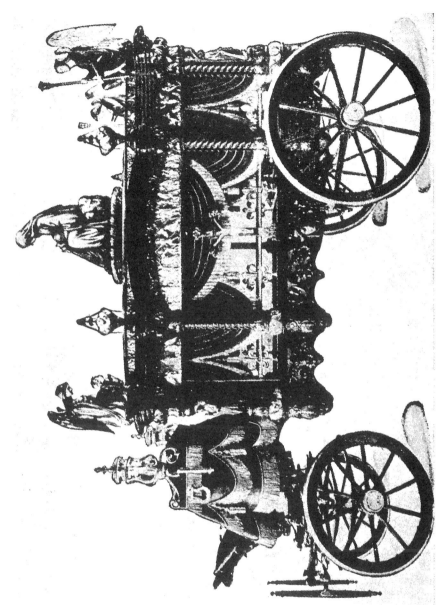

53. Processional Hearse, Exhibited at Chicago World's Fair, 1893.

Afterward, instead of being shipped directly to South America as intended, this equipage was sold to M. Raoul Bonnot of New Orleans for $5,000. A year later, he sold it to Messrs. Infanson and Sons of Havana, Cuba, where it was used for state funerals for many years.

Although the eight column, oval-decked funeral car definitely dominated the style-cycle by 1898, in that year, Hudson Samson, one of America's most famous innovators in funeral fashions, proposed the most radical change in funeral car design ever to find its way into actual general use. His idea was a funeral car, the body of which should be *entirely obscured* by gracefully draped imitation of cloth — an immense pall, held in place by cords and tassels so as to form the draperies, the whole to be carved out of solid wood. (***See Plate 52***.)

This funeral car was finished in February 1898 at a cost of $4,000 and, from the builder's standpoint, was the greatest triumph ever achieved in the art of hearse-making.[15]

Despite the fact that Samson tired of this creation in three years and moved on to other specially designed funeral cars, the seed had been planted for the development of the style of closed, columned hearses with carved wood draperies. Within a decade, these represented the dominant vogue.

Meanwhile, other changes had taken place. During the 1890s, the funeral car with squared ends and an oval or "mosque deck" (***see Plate 54***), in vogue since 1884, began to lose favor, and undertakers demanded a return to the elliptical-ended vehicle, or to modified versions thereof.

By the early 1900s, this feature had been combined with Samson's wood-carved drapery to produce a style that, again, was quite different from that which it gradually displaced.

Summing up the style-cycle pattern, the chronicler of hearse patterns remarks:

> Thus, in 1853 the style was for very small and inferior square hearses with plumes, that were gradually and greatly improved upon until 1867, when the full circle end, or Clarence fronts, came in. From 1867 the style was for full circle ends, with large plumes, gradually improving and substituting deck ornaments for plumes, until 1884, when the square end, 4-columned "funeral car" came in. From 1884 the style called for a strictly square end, with hip-roof, four columns and five urns, gradually improving, until 1893, 94, and 95 (the Chicago World's Fair period) when eight columns and the oval or mosque, deck came in. From 1895 to 1910 the best style was the Mosque deck without any urns at all; 6 columns or 8 columns, but finally settling down to 8 columns, and gradually improving to the beautiful carved-wood draperies, carved woodhammer cloth seat, and other styles of ornamented seats.[16]

In 1909, the answer to "What's next in hearse style?" would have to take into account a major technological development that impacted funeral-car design far beyond simple variations in body style. Already, the gas buggy had become more than a mechanical curiosity, and the broad field of human transportation was experiencing the effects of technological advances that eventually set the entire nation on fast-rolling wheels.

Electric cars had coursed through city streets and plied interurban expanses since 1885, when the first electric street railway in the United States was christened in Baltimore, Maryland.

PLATE 54

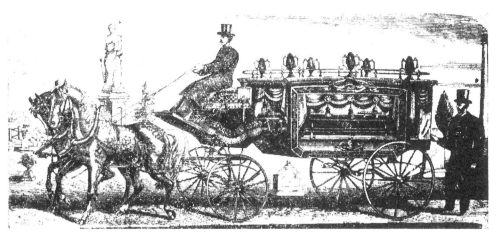

54A. "Ready for the Funeral," a Well-appointed Hearse of the Late-19th Century.

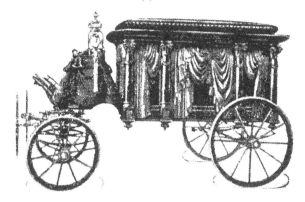

54B. Mosque Deck-style, Popular Through the 1900s.

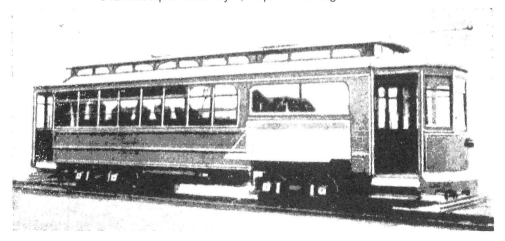

54C. Chicago Funeral Trolley Car, World War I Period.

Four years later, the street railway company of Atchison, Kansas, began operation of a trolley funeral car to nearby Mt. Vernon Cemetery. The car was only eight feet long with a table in the center fitted to hold the casket. Extending lengthwise through the car were seats for the undertaker and the bearers, while, at the back, one large folding door opened wide enough to permit casket entry and egress. Above the side panels were plate-glass windows and, at the end, were movable windows. The car was finished in black and gold within, and cherry without. Fees ranged from $8 to $10, varying according to the distance traveled and the time consumed. Additional cars for mourners were available but these were of the conventional trolley car variety.

The use of funeral trolley cars, most of which were of conventional trolley car size, spread through the 1890s and into the early years of the 20th century. Most of the major cities put them into use, and many were operated on a regular schedule to the larger cemeteries. As late as the 1920s, the somber funeral trolley car could have been seen in Cleveland and Chicago, carrying casket, flowers and mournful passengers out to suburban cemeteries. (***See Plate 54***.)

Yet the use of funeral trolleys was limited to the larger cities, and, even there, public acceptance was short of enthusiastic. The cortège or funeral procession seemingly lost some of its dignity as iron wheels creaked and screeched on turns and rumbled over intersections. The public seemed unable to repress a feeling of repugnance at the spectacle of a funeral "shooting through the streets at a high rate of speed."

In 1896, the first gasoline-powered automobile laboriously and slowly felt its way through the streets of Detroit, Michigan.

Some dozen years later, Fred Hulberg of New York City specified in a letters-patent eight innovations that formed a "new and improved combined hearse and passenger vehicle." (***See Plate 55***.) The drawings displayed a large, boxlike passenger section of a truck-like vehicle, in front of which, and directly above the motor, was a rectangular container for the casket. The driver sat in the open, much like the driver of a fire truck. This compound vehicle amounted to a combination of a horse-drawn hearse, a funeral trolley car, and an automobile power plant. Sixteen feet long, selling for about $6,000, Hulberg's invention was designed to replace three carriages and a hearse. No records exist to show how this innovation fared, and it is doubtful if any were actually produced and placed in operation.

It is quite probable that within the next 10 years, individual funeral directors with a mechanical bent and a flair for innovations made, or had made for themselves, combination carriage and gas-buggy hearses.

For many years, mobile-minded funeral directors had felt concerned with problems of getting around more rapidly. An editorial in the October 1894 issue of *The Casket*, anticipating the advent of rapid transportation, raised the question of the possibilities of the bicycle in the undertaking profession and wondered, editorially, if it might ever be considered proper for an undertaker to head a funeral procession on such a vehicle.

PLATE 55

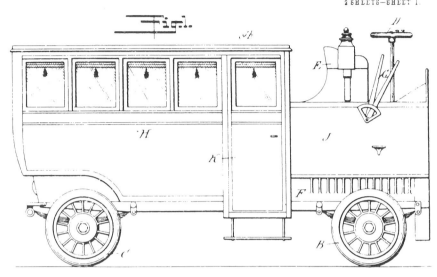

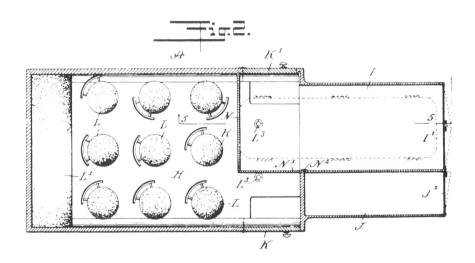

55. Patent Sketch of an Early Auto-Hearse Passenger Vehicle.

By 1905, at least one member of the profession had an "undertaker's auto" (*see **Plate 56***) used for business purposes and, within the next few years, more than one auto chassis had its crudely mounted hearse body. (***See Plate 57***.)

In 1909, at least two companies were producing motorized vehicles for funeral service. From Rochester, New York, early that year came news that the Cunningham factory had produced a model motor ambulance fully equipped with a 32-horsepower motor, rubber tires, a heater, and a gong. The interior consisted of one suspended cot, two seats for attendants, and a system of electric lighting. Inside trimmings were stained mahogany, and the outside was painted silver-gray, striped with gold. First displayed at the local auto show early that spring, the Cunningham Motor Ambulance (*see **Plate 56***) was first advertised for sale in December 1909 in *The Western Undertaker*.

By this time, the Crane & Breed Mfg. Co. already had its first auto-hearse (*see **Plate 56***) in production. This equipage was put on the market in June 1909 and was followed by a more-ornate model in two months. (***See Plate 56***.) The company's first advertisement of this innovation presciently remarked about the revolution that would take place in funeral service as a consequence of the introduction of the automobile hearse. The advertising pointed out that the public was already used to riding in automobiles and was beginning to object to the long and (to them) uncomfortably close and slow carriage journey. The public wanted speed — the smooth glide to the cemetery, the same as downtown or anywhere else — especially in the larger cities.

The first commercially produced auto-hearse was enclosed, painted black, and had little decoration except a rather grotesque replica of the famous Tomb of the Scipios carved in wood atop the otherwise flat roof of the rectangular coach. The second model reverted somewhat to the prevailing style of conventional four-posted, wood-carved, draped-window, horse-drawn funeral car, but still kept the Scipios motif.

By November, Crane & Breed Mfg. Co. had added an auto ambulance to its rolling stock.

Emil W. Hess, a veteran hearse manufacturer, in a personal communication suggests:

> With the advent of automobiles, the first or early motor hearses were bodies from old horse-drawn hearses mounted on lengthened passenger car chassis, or on truck chassis. This was done before hearse and ambulance bodies, suitable for automobiles, could be designed and built.
>
> It may also be of interest to note that the principal demand and sale of our motor ambulances and motor hearses did not come from the larger cities, but from the better class medium-sized cities. This was due to the fact that in the big cities, some of the largest Funeral Directors had a large investment in horse-drawn equipment and they were naturally slower to change to motorized equipment.
>
> For your information, I would like to cite a case in New York City where we had a customer who was a livery man and served some 30 or more funeral directors. This man had both horse-drawn and motor hearses. On one occasion when I visited this customer, he told me he was buying used carriages very cheap (including harness) and he said he was buying these carriages for less than what he formerly paid for the harness alone. I told him at the time that I thought he should not invest any more money in horse-drawn equipment as the demand everywhere was increasing for motorized

PLATE 56

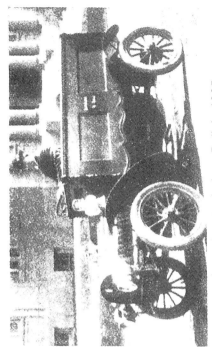

56C. Undertaker's Auto Built in 1905.

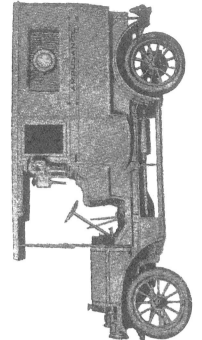

56D. An Early Motor Ambulance, 1900.

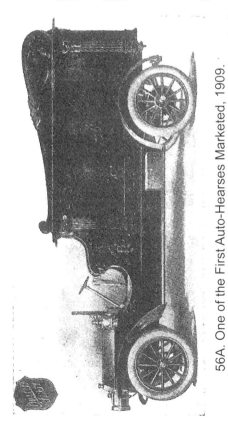

56A. One of the First Auto-Hearses Marketed, 1909.

56B. Improved, More-ornate Version of 56A.

equipment, and that his business in horse-drawn funerals may suddenly discontinue. When I called on this customer a few months later, he said I was right. He further stated that he had over 75 horses to feed and no work for horse drawn equipment. He was shipping his carriages to Cuba and selling them for any price he could get.

It will no doubt be of interest to know that New York City had horse-drawn funerals for sometime after most of the country had adopted motorized equipment.[17]

Public response to these funeral-service additions was at first mixed, and many arguments indicated the non-feasibility or undesirability of automobile transportation for funerals. For example, "Timber Awl," a constant contributor to the "Letter to the Editor" section of mortuary journals, enumerated — at the same time that ambulances and auto-hearses were going into commercial production — five compelling reasons why the "auto funeral" would be slow in coming: first, auto-hearses would involve a high outlay of cash, $4,000-6,000 apiece for vehicles that would be lucky to last three years, versus an average of $1,500 for a longer-lived horse-drawn coach; second, auto-hearses could go no faster than horse-drawn carriages, so if speed were wanted, there would necessarily have to be auto-carriages as well; third, upkeep and the cost of trained chauffeurs would be excessively expensive; fourth, the cost of operation would be so high that undertakers would have to cut costs on some other item — most likely the casket; and, lastly, sentiment militated against rushing people to their grave, and old people would still prefer the slow, leisurely and more dignified trip to the cemetery.

Thus, it would take a new, speed-minded generation to give acceptance to the use of the automobile for funeral purposes.

"Timber Awl" made no mention of ambulances, a type of transportation in which the principle of speed had been accepted, if not demanded, by people.

Events, however, soon settled the argument and proved "Timber Awl" unduly pessimistic. Between 1910 and 1920, the automobile came to dominate the field of funeral transportation and eventually replaced all other types of vehicles used in funeral service. Not only was the hearse replaced, but casket wagons, casket and ambulance wagons, embalmer's buggies and other service vehicles were also superseded in short order by gasoline-powered conveyances serving similar functions.

Through World War I, auto-hearses tended to become increasingly ornate. Martin notes that the peak in elaborate adornment was reached in 1920 when one company marketed a hearse on the body of which was a statue of Gabriel blowing his horn.[18]

Although patents were granted as early as 1909, it was not until after World War I that limousine hearses made their appearance. Apparently tiring of ornately carved vehicles, funeral directors and the public turned toward the longer, smoother lines of the limousine. First conceived as an automobile having an enclosed compartment for passengers and a driver's seat outside, but covered by a roof, the limousine was beginning to set a new standard in style and luxury for passenger vehicles. Reduced height in the new style also made loading and unloading easier.

Limousine hearses thus mark the start of blending the hearse and other conveyances in the funeral procession in a uniform, harmonious and aesthetically pleasing style. (*See Plate 58.*)

PLATE 57

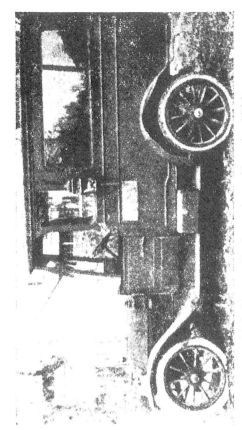

57C. Hearse Body on Auto Chassis, 1908.

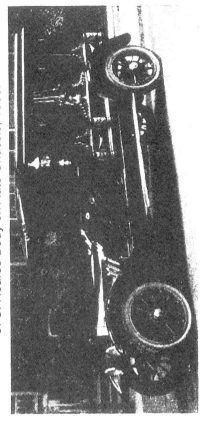

57D. Post-World War I Hearse Showing Persistence of Black in Funeral Vehicles.

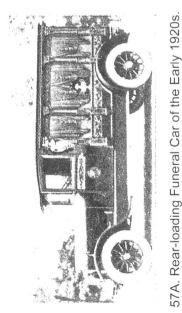

57A. Rear-loading Funeral Car of the Early 1920s.

57B. Two-tone-finish Funeral Car, 1922, as Lighter Colors Gain Favor in Succeeding Decades.

Along this line, the invalid car, as distinct from the emergency-suggesting ambulance, was developed in the early 1920s and followed the limousine pattern. (***See Plate 58***.)

In like manner, passenger limousines, specially built to carry eight passengers, came into use by funeral directors and were rented out for the pallbearers, or as a family car. Larger funeral homes might rent these cars to competitors.

The side-servicing feature for hearses was introduced in 1926. This innovation added greatly to the convenience and dignity of the funeral service by making it possible to load the vehicle without the necessity of the pallbearers' walking out into the street and, as sometimes was the case, into the mud.[19]

Chassis: The first motor-driven hearses were generally mounted on truck chassis that, in many cases, were of the open driver's-cab type. The next change was to use a heavy-duty, passenger-car chassis, usually of the seven-passenger variety, in which case the wheelbase was generally lengthened to accommodate the longer hearse-body requirements.

The extended spliced-chassis has been used intermittently for many years. However, no manufacturer has ever achieved any great degree of success in merchandising the extended-chassis cars because of the high upkeep and poor handling characteristics of the final product. Because of the unsatisfactory operation of the extended chassis, it soon became apparent that a full-length commercial chassis, designed specifically for the purpose for which it was to be used, was the final answer.

In regard to this latter development, Hess remarks:

> Through the efforts of the body builders in the ambulance and funeral car industry, we finally prevailed upon the large manufacturers to engineer and build these commercial, specialized units, and as a result today, the spliced frame or converted passenger car chassis has dropped to a low of only about 3% to 5% of the total volume of the industry.
>
> Down through the years, there were other types of conversions that proved unsatisfactory because of the fact that they were not designed specifically for the service requirements of the funeral car. Among these were the deluxe panel delivery, the station wagon, and the common suburban type vehicle.
>
> Because of the necessity of keeping a commercial vehicle for a greater number of years than the average passenger car, it was found that the larger, higher prestige-type of car was a better overall investment because of its low depreciation over its life span.[20]

Hearse Sizes and Colors: Until the Civil War, hearses were nearly always painted black. After the war, as they increased slowly in length and width, they began to exhibit some variation in color.

Children's hearses, introduced within a decade after the war, were nearly always white, while the larger funeral cars kept to the darker colors.

The most popular color combinations were basic black, with fine lines of silver or gold. Light grey, however, became a favorite for carved hearses and, during their vogue, possibly half of all funeral cars were finished in some shade of this color.

A light purple hearse was exhibited at the 1893 World's Fair in Chicago but the popular consensus was that this color was too delicate and too likely to fade or show wear and tear.

PLATE 58

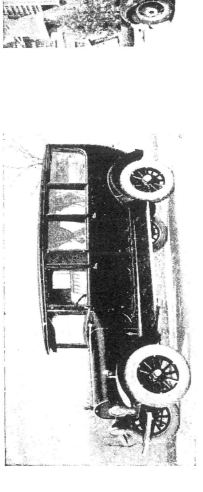

58A. Funeral Limousine, c. 1922.

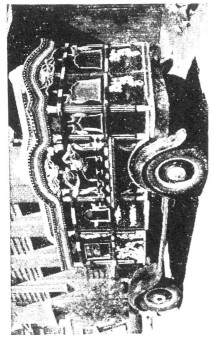

58B. Funeral Hearse Used by Chinese in America.

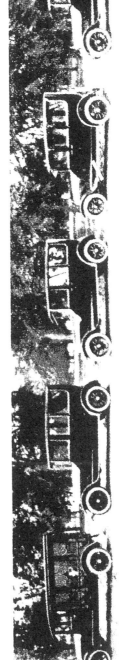

58C. Matched Funeral Vehicle Procession, Early 1920s.

Motor hearses were first black and, later, around the time of World War I, were also offered in various shades of grey. (**See Plate 57**.)

Because hearses were always scrubbed and polished after each funeral, maintaining a fine finish proved a real problem. To meet it, some companies included in the purchase of a new hearse a repainting service every six months during a stipulated period.

Changing fashions, however, provided another solution because it was common for an undertaker to tire of his hearse long before it became unserviceable. In the classified section of the March 1909 edition of *The Western Undertaker*, for instance, the following advertisement indicates the variety of types of funeral vehicles then in use, their different styles, and their inevitable depreciation:

> FOR SALE — Fine 5-glass landau in maroon leather. Very light weight. $650. Fine full leather landau, almost new, drab cloth, $700. Four passenger broughams, $350 to $700. Embalmers buggy, $275. Panel wagons $300 and $400. Very elegant Crane & Breed car, cost $2,500 and not hurt, for $1,200. Six column white car, 6x4 table by Cunningham, $500. Four column white hearse by Cunningham, $450. Side door 6-passenger pall bearer's coach, like perfect order, $475. Ambulance, silver gray, full size, complete $500. Address William Seymour, 381-387 Wabash Ave., Chicago, Ill.

The transportation of flowers to the gravesite called either for special arrangement or separate vehicles. Earlier, flowers were transported in regular hearses equipped with special trays or receptacles attached to the sidewalls of the hearse body above the casket. When it was necessary to handle an extra-large quantity of flowers, a second car was put into use to transport them.

With the advent of the automobile, the first flower cars put into service were the large seven-passenger phaeton type, or open-touring cars on which the top was let down. After this type had been in vogue for a few years, an entirely new style of flower car was designed and built. These new cars were used principally in the larger cities.

Just as the automobile effected a great change in the life of individuals, so too has the development of the motor hearse, with its constant technological improvements, helped revolutionize the burial of the dead. For one thing, as the journey to the grave grew longer, providing a means of transportation for both corpse and mourners became an integral and necessary part of the development of modern funeral service.

Thus, while the undertaker who entered coffin and casket production on a mass scale found himself further removed from the bereaved, the funeral director who gave up production of burial receptacles and turned toward families, including taking over transportation responsibilities, received closer professional interaction with those served. While interpersonal relations alone do not guarantee services will be of a professional character, a requisite of professional service is that the interaction between professional and clients is based on an understanding of the latter's personal needs.

This involvement of the funeral director with problems of transportation did more than increase the number and closeness of contacts with the bereaved, however. It also added to the complexity of the task and further helped shift it toward a professional status. As funerals became more involved, and the process of funeralization was carried with the procession to increasing distances, the task of

PLATE 59

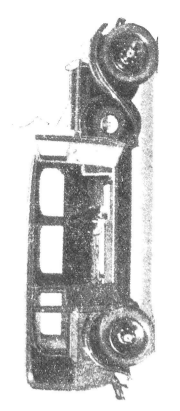

59C. A Side-servicing Car of the 1920s.

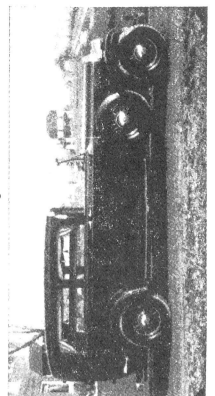

59D. Style-setting Funeral Car, 1932.

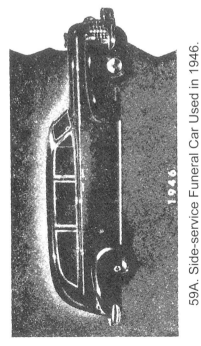

59A. Side-service Funeral Car Used in 1946.

59B. An Ambulance Used in 1934.

directing this extended service — of arranging the procession and successfully moving it, of leading it to the burial ground, and assisting in the committal service — naturally fell to the funeral director.[21]

One of the more important concepts called to mind by the term "funeral director" defines this person as skilled in the management of the funeral procession. To produce a coffin or casket upon demand involved a relatively simple business transaction with responsibilities attuned to the ethics of a tradesman-customer relationship. To move people about in a vehicle is a service relationship. But to organize and direct a procession that must be profoundly ceremonial, cannot be rehearsed or repeated, and in which mistakes are always magnified by a high level of emotional intensity, defines and fixes a responsibility that, by conventional standards of occupational recognition, elevates a funeral director's work beyond and above that of the craftsman, tradesman or purveyor of petty personal services.

CITATIONS AND REFERENCES FOR CHAPTER 9

1. Edward H. Rech, "Glimpses Into Funeral History," unpublished ms., prepared under the auspices of The Hess & Eisenhardt Co. of Cincinnati, Ohio, n.d., n.p.

2. *Ibid.*

3. Edward Martin, "Hearses and Funeral Cars," unpublished ms., 1947. Archives of NFDA, Milwaukee, Wis., n.d., n.p.

4. *Funeral Customs Through the Ages*, *op. cit.*, n.p.

5. Rech, *op. cit.*, *passim*.

6. Sewall, *op. cit.*, p. 54.

7. *Ibid.*, p. 147.

8. See Bridenbaugh, *The Colonial Craftsman*, *op. cit.*

9. Bridenbaugh, *Cities in the Wilderness*, *op. cit.*, p. 90.

10. *Ibid.*, p. 412.

11. "Concerning the Evolution of Styles in Hearses," *Sunnyside*, March 15, 1913, pp. 14-15. The authors have followed this excellent sketch in their discussion of the influence of fashion in hearses.

12. *Ibid.*

13. *Ibid.*

14. *Ibid.*

15. *Ibid.*

16. *Ibid.*

17. Personal correspondence to Howard C. Raether from Emil W. Hess, president, The Hess & Eisenhardt Co., April 29, 1955.

18. Martin, *op. cit.*

19. *Ibid.*

20. Personal correspondence to Howard C. Raether from Emil W. Hess, Oct. 9, 1953.

21. Cf. Martin, *op. cit.*

Chapter 10

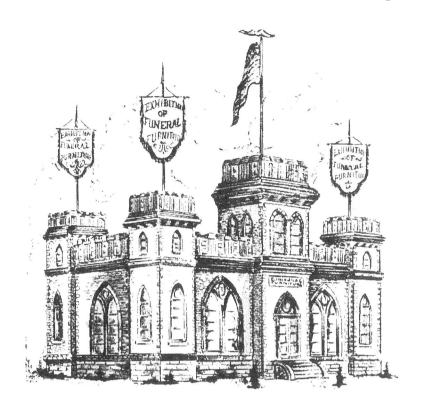

The Pattern of Late-19th-Century Funerals

As the previous chapters examined the functions, mortuary goods and paraphernalia of the 19th-century undertaker and funeral director, it was difficult to avoid a certain amount of discontinuity in the narration. This chapter, however, provides a balanced, continuous account of the numerous items explored in the previous chapters, and adds additional material that will help provide a typical illustration of funeral service, and the care of the dead, centering around 1880. The actual time span of the example will be brief, covering only the few days beginning with death and ending with burial.

In addition, because America at this time showed wide variations in funeral thoughts and customs between the rural areas (frontier, farm, village, town) on one hand and the urban areas (the larger cities) on the other, the characteristic problems of death behavior of these two social groups will also be compared.

While necessary at times to survey a field in which there is some uniformity in the midst of many variations, and to collect these common elements into broad generalizations, this can prove hazardous, especially when dealing with nearly contemporary or contemporary society. If the practices of funeral directors at any period exhibited complete uniformity — if statutory law or some necessity defined and regularized the practices — it would be easy to describe these patterns accurately.

But here is a field in which room for many variations still exists, and in which there are some contrasts set by custom and law. For instance, during Catholic funerals in some Ohio cities (among them Cincinnati, Cleveland and Youngstown), it has been long customary to seat mourners on the right or "Epistle" side of the church. In Brown County, Ohio, however, which is only 30 or 40 miles from Cincinnati, mourners have been seated on the left or "Gospel" side.

No comprehensive survey of the practices of funeral directors was made in the 1880s; nor is one available that carefully describes practices today.[1] Thus, as we approach the nearly contemporary or contemporary scene, the likelihood increases sharply that for every general statement, someone, somewhere, will be able to point out exceptions he or she knows from personal experience or hearsay. From region to region, place to place, and person to person, there are differences. In spite of such variations, the limited evidence available indicates that, in the latter part of the 19th century, there are broad patterns of development that can and will be described.

First Responses to Death: In an American home in 1880, the coming of death brought with it the same shattering of human bonds and the resulting confusion that, in any society, everywhere and at all times, have attended the death of a human being.

In addition to this fundamental, universal reaction, the atmosphere of anxiety and emotional strain was heightened by the general tone that characterized the death customs of the period. The frontier was passing, and some new and challenging, or traditional but satisfying, theme of social existence was needed to give meaning and support to a way of life that was in rapid transition from fundamentally rural and agricultural to predominantly industrial and commercial.

Large numbers of immigrants were continuing to pour into the country during what historians have since named the "Great Migration." These new arrivals brought with them diverse backgrounds of race, religion, language, manners, customs and ways of making a living. In the large cities, and to a lesser extent across the whole country, they were thrown into "the melting pot" with descendants of earlier arrivals, and without the benefit of a common and unifying basis in tradition, culture or morality except in the most general terms.

Under such conditions, a society — in the sense of an enduring and competently cooperating social group firmly held together by custom or tradition — could not be built overnight. Likewise, a young nation making astonishing growth even while it was being assembled out of highly diverse elements could not be expected to do so.

The prevailing funeral mood of the time was one of stiff formality, overlaid heavily with gloom. This mood, strangely enough, did not originate in this lusty period of brawling American growth, nor did it express the irreverent matter-of-fact spirit of the day. Instead, it was borrowed from abroad, specifically England, from an earlier period and a different type of social organization. In other words, the pompous, elaborate, rigidly prescribed, prolonged, morbid, feudal-type funeral of the 1880s was a transplant in America.

Despite this, the sense of rugged individuality generated in frontier living, and the preoccupation of the early 19th-century American with his fellow man as a person, could not help but leave its mark on the developing and changing pattern of American mourning behavior. Something of the simple sincerity, the primitive neighborliness, of the frontier was never lost in the folkways of American funerals, no matter what imported fashions were mixed with it.

Looking back on her mother's girlhood in Delaware County, Ohio, in the 1810s and '20s, Mrs. A. Baldwin, chronicler of the Midwest, reckoned that although her father and mother did not like funerals, they always went to them.

> In those days, every man within ten miles was a neighbor and every neighbor was a friend and when anyone died, a boy was sent on horseback from house to house to tell the sad tidings. On the day of the funeral, all the men and women in the country round laid aside their work, however important, and attended it. Rough wagons, with boards across for seats, perhaps with a chair for some old grandmother, formed the procession, followed often by men on horseback with their wives behind them. They had no hearse and the best wagon of the settlement held the coffin, and a homespun blanket answered for a pall. I have seen many grand processions since then. Once I saw a city hung with mourning and thousands of soldiers marching with muffled drums and all the people mourning a great man. But I have never seen anything that seemed to me so solemn as those wagons winding through the forests and over rough roads to the half-cleared graveyard of that new country.[2]

Beneath the external pomp and show that marked late-19th-century funeral customs, the practice of giving way to grief and anguish — a reaction well supported in earliest Hebrew and Christian funeral behavior — indicates that Americans were modifying the imported fashion. By the same token, this element of unfiltered emotional release grew more pronounced as one moved from the cities to the towns and villages, from the urbanity of the metropolis to the expressiveness of the frontier.

A final contribution to a developing pattern of mourning behavior in late-19th-century America was a growing desire to provide a setting that was beautiful to see and feel despite the facts of death and burial. This all-pervasive tendency was in strong contrast to the mood of gloom and somberness imported from the mourning style of feudal times. It is this tendency, often alluded to, that in its unfolding has done most to set American funeral behavior apart from other Western cultures.

The composite form of response to the operation of these, and possibly other, social forces does not, as possibly might be gathered from the following sketches, crystallize into a uniform and enduring set of conventions, however. For every point designated, it is necessary to make exceptions and qualifications.

But such variations must not obscure the single, simple conclusion: toward the end of the 19th century, a conflict took place in America between the two great themes of death — gloom and formality, and beauty and expressiveness — and the latter won out. In a period of activity, bustle, great opportunity and free competition, Americans chose not to maintain an attitude toward death and certain archaic practices that had come down to them from a feudal society that had flourished 500 years before.

At the House: In late-19th-century America, when a person died, the anxiety and nervous strain that attended the care of the sick or injured might be dissolved in the tears of the immediately bereaved. Most deaths then occurred in the home; if outside, the body was quickly returned there. Thus, the home was, for most people, the central point of mourning. A hush fell over the household, the blinds were drawn and people walked about on tiptoe and spoke in restrained tones.

The first gestures toward the dead would be made by the women of the home, who closed the eyes and straightened the limbs. In cities, the undertaker, as he was called (although a few were already calling themselves "funeral directors"), would be summoned to come and take charge. The decision as to whom to call might already have been made, as it would be natural to look to the same person who had laid out and buried other members of the family.

In the city, the arrival of the undertaker released the deceased's family and friends from many of the responsibilities that rural folk traditionally accepted as their own. Instead of proceeding with the actual preparation of the dead for burial (this presupposed no embalming), the men of the family decided what plans should be followed for the funeral or burial. In such deliberations, the undertaker played an important advisory role.

Although the great majority of funerals were held in the home, the choice of a home funeral or the undertaking parlor service was available in some places as early as 1880. As late as the 1910s, it was often virtually impossible to get permission to remove a body from the home. Indeed, when death occurred in a hospital or other place outside of the home, the family was often most insistent upon bringing it to the house as soon as possible. Even then, funeral parlors were used for people who had no home of their own, or had no relatives or friends who would offer their quarters.

While sentiment and custom at that time dictated home funerals, the impulse to delegate both the care and custody of the body to the undertaker, reinforced by the desire of the latter to do his work, particularly embalming, in more functional surroundings, made the decision of some importance and difficulty. In addition to agreeing upon the place of the funeral, it was necessary to decide how much time would elapse before burial took place. If the answer were more than one day, preservative measures would be needed. Again, the choices were two. Until the funeral, the body could either be kept in a cooler or "corpse preserver" surrounded with ice (*see Chapter 8, Plates 41 & 42*), or the undertaker could embalm it with chemicals.

Although the latter method was widely talked about after the Civil War and had recently become popularized when certain great personages, including several U.S. presidents, had been embalmed, a common fear remained based on Christian and humanitarian concerns that the process involved mutilation of the body. Much of the opposition was based on a fear of the unknown. People did not understand the nature of embalming; many embalmers could not or did not explain it very clearly; and the mutilation question was dragged in by some persons seeking an argument to defend a position.

In rural areas and small towns, news of a death spread rapidly, and many — relatives, neighbors and friends — found themselves somehow involved in the care and disposition of the body. The body was laid out either by the bereaved or by community members with experience in these matters.

Once washed and dressed in the best or favorite suit or dress, the deceased was moved from the bedroom to the parlor, to be viewed even before a casket was obtained.

The mourning behavior of small-town Midwesterners during this period is well described by Atherton, who emphasizes the social participation of the whole community:

> Friends began pouring in to the bereaved home as soon as the news reached them, and the members of the family, seated in the living room, received their condolences. Each caller tiptoed into the parlor to see the corpse, as everyone was expected to perform that rite, and all commented on how natural and peaceful it looked. Cakes and pies and meats began to appear in the kitchen in profusion, the gifts of friends and neighbors.[3]

If an undertaker was trained in chemical embalming, he probably promoted its "humaneness" and pointed out to all its obvious advantages over ice cooling, i.e., sanitation, duration, reliability and simplicity. The possibility of an ice-cooled corpse decomposing rapidly once taken out of the "preserver" and exploding the casket during the funeral ceremonies could not be ignored. (Nor would an astute embalmer-undertaker fail to mention it.)

Prices either way did not vary greatly; chemical embalming, on the whole, tended at the time to be a little more expensive, unless the amount of ice used in keeping the body cool was excessive. Some 20 years earlier, Holmes had charged as high as $100 for chemical embalming; in 1870, a prominent undertaker, Hudson Samson, charged as little as $15. By the 1880s, there was little variance in practice, $10 being a usual charge. (*See Figure 29.*)

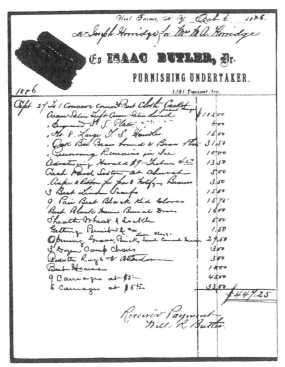

Figure 29. Itemized Bill for Luxury Funeral, 1886.
(Note sixth line: "Preserving Remains in Ice.")

The books of a well-known Cincinnati establishment show that, subsequent to this time, additional charges were made in the case of men for "washing, shaving and dressing," and for women for "casketing and dressing." Having settled these matters, the undertaker would defer consideration of other details until the body had been properly "laid out."

Assuming that the body would be chemically embalmed, the undertaker would have brought along a portable "cooling board" on which to embalm the body, and an embalming cabinet and dressing case containing, essentially, a hard-rubber pump with check valve; arterial tubes; trocar; needles; forceps; scalpel; scissors; eye caps; razor; granite cup for shaving; combs; brushes; shaving soap; chin supporters; surgeon's silk; a piece of oiled muslin; a package of court-plaster; a paper of pins; a dozen collar buttons; cotton sheet; whisk broom; and two half-gallon bottles.

In addition, he carried several bottles of concentrated embalming fluid and an assortment of floral door badges. During the first call, the undertaker would select the appropriate door crepe or badge and attach it in such manner that the doorbell or knocker was covered. Custom decreed black as the color for the old, white for the young, and black with white rosette and ribbon for young adults. Before the end of the 1880s, combinations of purple, lavender and gray were used in connection with mourning, and door badges often reflected this changing choice in color. (*See Figure 30*.)

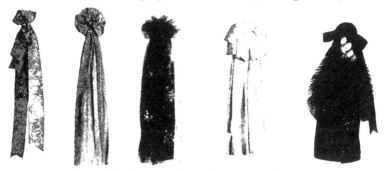

Figure 30. Door Badges, Late-19th Century.

Later, when most funerals were still conducted from the homes of the decedents, and floral wreaths had taken the place of door crepes, the florist in the city often failed to attach the flowers until several hours later. In rural districts, the funeral director carried with him artificial-flower door badges.

Embalming the dead in the family home presented 19th-century undertakers with problems, both physical and social, that have long since been relegated to the realm of historical anecdote among modern funeral directors. If the family raised the mutilation objection strenuously, it was sometimes necessary to permit a close friend or male family member to watch the process.

In addition, many people had the erroneous idea that embalming necessitated the removal of all, or the majority of, the internal organs. When the observer saw the size of the small incision made to raise a major artery, he was generally satisfied and seldom remained to witness the balance of the embalming procedure unless he was curious as to its operation and developing results.

The body was undressed, washed on the bed, and the orifices plugged before it was swabbed with embalming fluid and then placed on the embalming table. After moving the body into the best light in the room, it was shaved (if a man); the eyes were closed over eye caps; the mouth closed; and, if necessary, the lips were lightly sewn together. If the deceased wore false teeth, these would always be inserted and a chin support might be used to keep the jaws closed. An early attempt at "restorative art" might be tried using the new liquid flesh-tint recently marketed by the fluid companies.

Having finished the preliminary work, the undertaker then embalmed the body. If following recent advances in the field, he employed arterial injection, supplemented by cavity injection, with the trocar inserted in the umbilicus and in the corner of the eye, where neither incision would be noticeable.

Having injected the body sufficiently with fluid — being careful to get none on his hands or other parts of his body — he tied off the vessels and sewed up the incision. Some embalmers wore rubber gloves; others embalmed with their bare hands.

Next, he dressed the body, placing a clean sheet under it, and then dusted the face with powder, placed a small pillow under the head, draped another sheet over the body, and placed a small square of white cotton material or a handkerchief over the face. The net effect was the impression of a reclining form. Additionally, he might attach a canopy to the cooling board.

In either case, the body was ready to be placed in whatever room was chosen for it to be viewed, and the first call was completed. The undertaker's next step was a conference with the family to complete the arrangements for funeral ceremonies.

Funeral Arrangements: Although, in the 1880s as now, there were standard services that the undertaker was called upon to perform for the dead and the living, in actual practice, many variations appeared. While the following statement mentions only a few of these, the practices it details are generally quite typical of those of the time.

Before the undertaker departed from his first call, he inquired regarding local notification and asked what telegrams should be sent. On a printed blank, he made a brief record of the earthly career of the departed. Another blank provided for the names of the clergymen who were to officiate, and the singers who were to compose the choir. These persons were promptly notified.

As soon as possible, the following day preferably, the arrangements were completed. Important items included the choice of the casket, the elaborateness of the ceremonies, the selection of the pallbearers, the number of relatives and friends for whom carriages should be provided, and the order of precedence of mourners in the procession. In case the funeral was to be held in a church, the proper authorities and the sexton would have to be notified. Even the floral pieces, if any, were ordered through the undertaker. (At this time, the battle of flowers versus drapes had been well underway for more than a decade.)

The casket was chosen either from a catalog, the undertaker's display room or stockroom, or, in some cases, from the casket showrooms that manufacturers were beginning to set up in the larger cities and to which undertakers might take their clients. The casket selections, in any case, ranged widely in style, composition and price. Although polished hardwoods of oak, mahogany, walnut or rosewood were long the traditional favorite, the bulk of sales was in less-expensive caskets. Metallic burial cases and caskets formerly finished in imitation rosewood were now offered in a distinctive bronze finish; a few styles of metallic-glass combinations were available; and a substantial line of cloth-covered wooden caskets in a somewhat cheaper price range completed the conventional list of alternatives.

As early as 1875, the Stein Patent Burial Casket Works had published a striking catalog of pictures to be shown customers. (***See Chapter 7, Plate 39***.) In addition to conventional black for adults, and white for children, the company made available broadcloth and velvet-covered caskets in combinations of royal purple, aniline blue and lavender, with ornaments and trim in gold, silver and black enamel.

The 1881-1882 catalog of Chappel, Chase, Maxwell & Company contained a line of cloth-covered caskets featuring a variety of color combinations equal to that furnished by the Stein Company. While the variety of styles, colors and material were not as wide in the 1880s as it is today, it still gave people a chance to exercise some refinement of choice. Previous chapters have already explored how fashions and taste at this time were beginning to intrude themselves into areas of life that long had been under the canons of custom and traditions.

The selection of a casket from a catalog, and its delivery in time for the funeral, were made possible by improved techniques of body preservation and by developments in communication and transportation. If a family selected a casket that the funeral director did not have in stock, or made a selection from a catalog, then the question of delivery became an important problem. There were many instances in which the desired casket could not be secured in time without curtailing the hours of visiting; and other instances when it could not arrive for the original date of the funeral itself.

The hours between placing an order for a casket and its delivery, and then its subsequent inspection to see that the order had been carried out in every detail, always harrowed the funeral director. Nor did the fact that this situation occurred repeatedly relieve his anxiety. He was always conscious that there was a whole array of contingencies that might disarrange his careful schedule.

Once the choice had been made, the undertaker immediately dispatched a coded telegram to the factory. When first manufactured in job and mass lots, caskets and burial cases were given names to designate particular styles. These names might indicate a style or form designed or suggested by an undertaker or, on occasion, by his wife, such as the "Emma." Likewise, the "Peltier," "Hogan" and "Curtis" styles of caskets were named for the undertakers who designed them or suggested the style. Others, especially the more expensive, had names descriptive either of important phenomena, such as "The State" (*see **Chapter 7, Figure 17 & Plate 32***) and "Imperial," or of important personages, such as "Monarch," "Princess" and "Grand Duke."

As early as 1876, however, the Stein Company was already using letters and numbers to code their caskets, and as the century came to a close, impersonal and colorless code words and numbers replaced descriptive terms and personal names.

Once the telegram reached the factory or warehouse, the casket ordered was immediately boxed and rushed to the express office for shipment, if it was available. An undertaker in New York City could expect a casket from the Stein factory in Rochester, New York, 20 hours after his telegram had been received; to Chicago, it would take 30 hours; and to St. Louis, 38 hours. Even the

"State" casket, which was "only made to order," was guaranteed delivery at any point within 1,000 miles from the factory within 60 hours. This company claimed to have shipped more than 3,000 telegraph-ordered caskets in the 12 months ending June 1876.

On the other hand, the selection of a casket was a fairly simple matter in rural and village areas. Either the local cabinet-maker was called upon to build one for the occasion, or a ready-made receptacle was purchased from the furniture store. In the latter case, the casket might not yet be lined, or "trimmed," and the furniture dealer, who might also advertise on his signboards that he did undertaking, would, with the aid of his wife, often complete the trimming.

In 1880, the undertaker was not licensed either to practice or to embalm (another 15 years would elapse before states began to pass licensing legislation). But with the establishment of bureaus or departments of vital statistics, it became incumbent upon the undertaker to meet certain legal requirements before arranging for the burial or cremation of the human dead. Certificates authorizing burial or cremation had to be secured from city or township officials. Physicians were obliged to notify these authorities of the deaths of patients they had attended, and the approximate time of death and the causes thereof. Without such notice, the registrar, town clerk or other official authorized to issue burial certificates would not do so.

Consequently, to facilitate matters, the undertaker would take a death certificate to a physician for his statement and signature, and then secure the burial permit. This is still the accepted practice.

In like manner, burial within a cemetery required sanction from cemetery officials. Burial on a particular lot or in a particular location necessitated some evidence of ownership and right of sepulture. This once again became a self-imposed responsibility of the funeral director. Often, he accompanied members of the mourning family to the cemetery to give suggestions regarding the location of the burying place and made arrangements with the superintendent for the bricking up of the walls, if not the bottom, of the grave, or the building of a vault of sandstone slabs to receive the casket. Sprigs of evergreen might be used to trim the grave and soften the harshness of the freshly turned clay. For a child's burial, fresh flowers would be used instead.

The Funeral: In the rural and village areas of America during the late-19th century, the role of the funeral director was considerably different from what it was in the city, and he played a smaller part in the funeralization of the dead.

H.J. Blanton, dean of American small-town newspaper editors, in his engaging reminiscences of youth in the small town, notes the "modest part" of the undertaker who did not "lay out" the corpse, but ordered the casket made by the local furniture factory, helped place the body in it, and generally arranged things so that the preacher could play the dominating role.[4]

News of death traveled fast in small communities and, often, most of the people of the town or village, in one way or another, were involved and, in keeping within the Christian tradition, shared the sorrows of the bereaved. In cities, people received notice of death first by special courier — indeed the position of "Inviter to Funerals" in New York City goes back to the late-17th century — who delivered funeral notices, invitations and mourning cards. (***See Plates 60 & 61***.)

PLATE 60

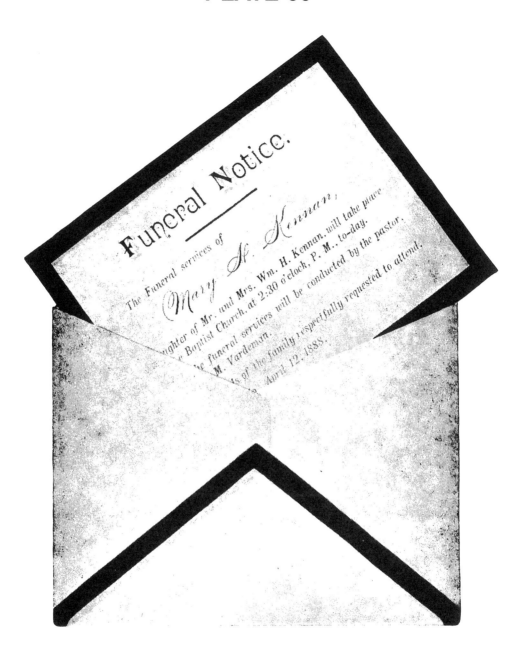

60. Funeral Notice, Late-19th Century.

PLATE 61

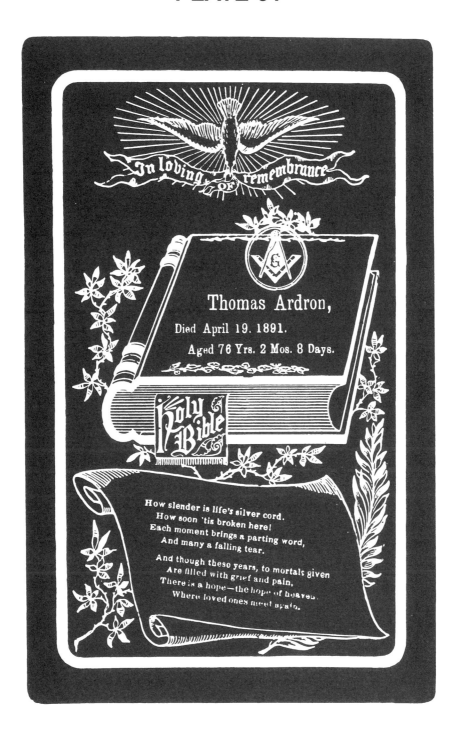

61. Mourning Card, Memento of the Deceased.

But, from the middle of the 19th century, the invitations were often sent out by the undertaker as one of the many personal services that were coming under his direction. Hill's *Manual of Social and Business Forms*, 1879, under "Etiquette of the Funeral," recommended the more traditional usage of sending out invitations to friends of the deceased by private messenger, but, as noted by Landauer, the contemporary Gaskell's *Compendium of Forms* stated that newspaper announcements might "meet the requirements of distant friends."[5]

Before 1900, the mourning card for personal communication had changed into the "letter edged in black," (*see Plate 62*), while for those less touched by the event, a newspaper announcement sufficed.

Before the turn of the century, funerals were most likely held in the home of the deceased, sometimes in the church, and only seldom in a funeral parlor.

In the city, the undertaker generally arrived at least an hour before the service. The casketed body was in view. Taking leave of the remains had already become a custom toward which the undertaker could develop little enthusiasm, but the wishes of the family traditionally governed the procedure.

Otherwise, the undertaker tended to regard his role as one of general supervisor of the funeral, having slowly moved in his occupational duties from a supplier of objects, and an arranger of paraphernalia, to a director or supervisor of a complex set of practical and ceremonial actions.

By the time of his arrival, his assistant would have distributed folding chairs and arranged furniture so that an assembly could take place. As friends came into the house, they were directed to seats, some of which would be assigned to close relatives.

Fraternal orders often participated in the funerals of the time, and it was incumbent upon the undertaker to make arrangements so that participation functioned smoothly and integrated itself with the ceremonies performed by the clergyman.

"Abide With Me" and "Thy Will Be Done," or "Over The Stars There is Rest" and "Christian Hope Beyond," were favorite musical selections of the time.

The arrangements for the several component parts of the funeral service were generally gone over in advance, with the funeral director acting as prompter, if one were needed, and standing by to smooth over any last-minute hitches.

Services at the home were invariably long and delivered in a mixed context of religious awe, hope, fear and gloom. After an opening prayer of some four to five minutes at a Protestant funeral, the minister would, in many cases, read the 23rd Psalm, and possibly short passages from the seventh chapter of Revelations. Following this would be the remarks on the mystery of life and death, the suffering on earth as a prelude to a more glorious life to come, and then would come the eulogy, in which the character of the deceased would be thoroughly reviewed.

Often, a short life history would be included, in some cases delivered by a close friend of the deceased and couched in terms of personal reminiscence.

After a closing prayer and the singing of one or several songs, or possibly the recitation of a favorite piece of verse, the funeral service was completed. The total time consumed was seldom less than an hour.

PLATE 62

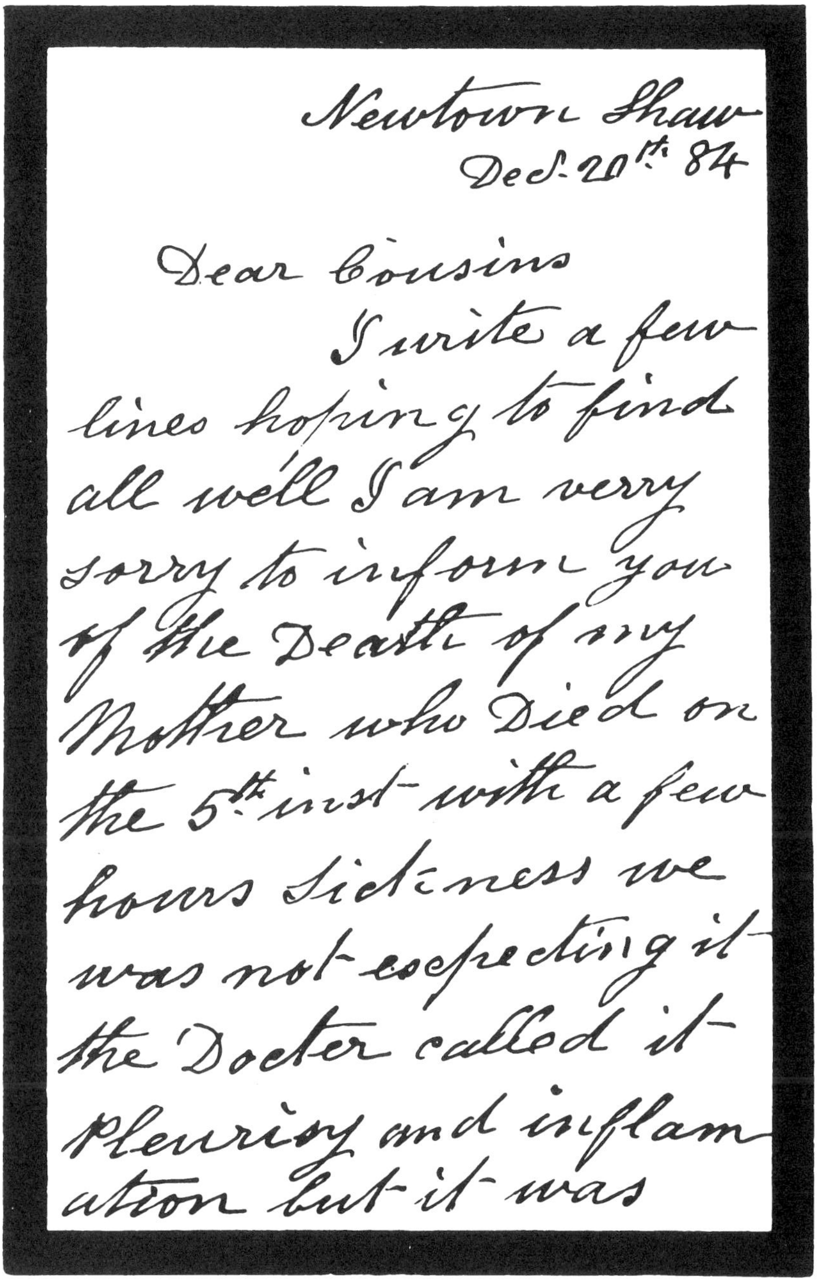

> Newtown Shaw
> Dec 20th 84
>
> Dear Cousins
> I write a few lines hoping to find all well I am very sorry to inform you of the Death of my Mother who Died on the 5th inst with a few hours sickness we was not expecting it the Docter called it Pleurisy and inflamation but it was

62. Harbinger of Death — the Letter Edged in Black.

Home services over, the undertaker would take charge of the pallbearers. Funerals held on an upper floor always posed a special problem, and a long strap or a length of webbing was frequently used to lower the casket, step by step, down the stairs. Doors often were so constructed that egress was impossible without removing the hinges and, in some cases, a part of the framework. (One of the earlier manuals of funeral management advised the undertaker, in extreme cases of blocked passageways, to consult with a safe mover!)

Hearses were seldom backed to a curb unless the mud was prohibitively deep. While the body was being loaded into the hearse, the assistant busied himself gathering up the flowers to be transported ahead of the procession to the church or cemetery, where they would be properly rearranged.

The occupants of the carriages were then seated in rough order of their closeness of kinship to the bereaved. Here, skill in human relations was necessary for, then as now, some relatives might not be on speaking terms with others, and it was imperative for the undertaker to maintain harmony. Immediate consideration, of course, went to the family, who were loaded first. To fill a dozen or more carriages and bring them into proper order unavoidably produced a certain amount of delay.

To the majority of participants, however, the factor of time was negligible because funerals were neither rushed to, rushed through, nor rushed from. The logistics of funeral service were only just beginning to become a matter of concern to the undertaker, yet as his function of *direction* took on depth, it was inevitable that a smooth, well-ordered funeral in which little motion was wasted should become his goal.

Once the procession got under way, its direction was in the hands of the undertaker. Sometimes he rode with the driver on the hearse, and sometimes, but less frequently, he left the procession in the hands of an assistant and drove to the cemetery to make sure that everything was in readiness there. If the undertaker stayed with the procession, he rode with the minister in the front carriage. In cases of very large funerals, his position was in a carriage of his own at the head of the line of march.

As the funeral left the private home, an assistant immediately began to restore order. Folding chairs, rugs, pedestals and door scarf were taken away. Furniture was moved back into position so that the family, upon returning, found nothing to remind them that a funeral ceremony had taken place there only a few hours before.

While the body was ordinarily kept in the family home, in some cases, especially in larger cities, the undertaker might have a "morgue" in his establishment in which the body could be kept until the time of the funeral, or it might be "in state" in the funeral parlor. In 1880, the funeral home, in the modern sense, was just beginning to appear, and for every funeral undertaker operating an independent establishment, four or five others still carried on the trade in connection with some other business.

Thus, the common alternative to a home funeral was a funeral that began in the home with the viewing of the body, was followed by a procession to the church for the main ceremony, and completed by the conventional trip to the cemetery and the committal service. Should the family decide upon a church funeral, then a new complication was added to the work of the undertaker. A church funeral called for further expenditure of time, effort and paraphernalia, and added such problems as were involved in organizing and directing a group of persons in a performance for which there could be no rehearsal and whose complete success could not be guaranteed in advance.

The introduction of the chapel into the funeral home at the end of the 19th century marks no lessening of religious involvement in the funeral ceremonies of the time. Instead, it points up a natural reaction to the problems of transportation, time involvement, and of directing the performance of group ceremony and ritual in physical areas over which the undertaker had little control.

In the typical church ceremony, the clergyman met the undertaker in the vestibule and preceded him up the aisle. The body was placed at the head of the center aisle, and flowers that had been sent in advance or were brought with it were arranged about it in stands or on tables. In the Catholic ceremony, three candles were placed at each side of the bier.

During the rest of the ceremony, the undertaker assumed a vantage point from which he could assist, if needed, and assumed his duties when they arose.

Fraternal escorts were given a special position so that, in leaving, they would occupy the same places as on entering.

The custom of opening the casket in church for a final view of the body persisted strongly during the 19th century despite objection by clergymen and undertakers alike. When such practice was observed, the mourners filed silently by and passed outside to the waiting carriages. Finally, the pallbearers carried the casket to the hearse, and the procession moved slowly toward the cemetery.

Undertakers preferred to have their hearse and carriage drivers dressed in livery. In keeping with the somber-toned tradition, throughout most of the century, the dress followed the gloomy motif: well-dressed liverymen were garbed in black broadcloth or doeskin coats, pantaloons and vest. The coat and vest were single-breasted and buttoned up completely to the neck. With these garments they wore a white linen, garrote shirt collar and black silk tie, black kid gloves and black top hat. (*See Figure 31.*)

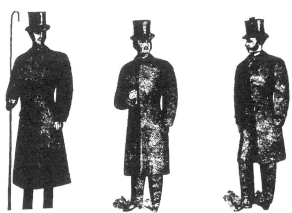

Figure 31. Professional Dress.
Left, Coachman; Center, Undertaker; Right, Undertaker's Liveried Assistant.

Since the independent undertaker of the time could not afford to keep a dozen drivers on his staff, he faced the problem of getting drivers from carriage stables to appear in respectable, uniform livery. This was one of the earliest issues taken up for consideration in the first undertakers' trade journals.

The Funeral Cortège: The long line of coaches and carriages moving slowly toward the cemetery not only presented an imposing spectacle, but also helped generate a sense of the importance the social group attached to the matter of the demise of one of its own. The hearse invariably dominated the procession by its beauty and magnificence, decorated with the classical symbols of grief: the drooping cypress, the reversed and extinguished torch, the cere, and "black plumes awaving."

During the late-19th century, the role played by the plumes atop the hearse was of great importance, for their number and color revealed the station of the deceased. An absence of plumes indicated that the deceased was poor; two plumes, that he was of moderate circumstances; three or four plumes, fairly well-to-do; five or six, well-off; and seven or eight, rich.[6]

For children, the undertaker supplied a miniature hearse, usually white, that would be drawn by one horse. (*See Chapter 9, Plate 52*.)

As flowers came more generally into use, a special carriage was added to the cortège solely to transport them. Customarily, it preceded the pallbearers' carriage, yet was not so far from the hearse that the association of flowers with the body and casket would be lost.

A common arrangement of the procession was as follows: clergymen, flower carriage, honorary pallbearers, active pallbearers, hearse, immediate family and relatives, and, finally, friends. Societies or fraternal orders, if they formed part of the procession, always took the lead. In the funeral procession of a well-known funeral director in 1890, there were in line:

> Ballston Spa Brass Band
> Morning Star Encampment, I.O.O.F.
> Odd Fellows Lodges
> Knights of Pythias
> Ancient Order of United Workmen
> Rechabites
> Union Fire Company #2
> Wheeler Post, G.A.R.
> McKittrick Post, G.A.R.
> Minister
> Bearers and gun squad
> The Hearse
> Relatives and mourners in Carriages

In cases such as this, fraternal and other organizations would precede the carriages on foot. If the cemetery were too far, these marching groups would drop out after several blocks or, possibly, at the city limit.

The number of carriages and, in some cases, the grandeur of the hearse, the appointments, and the size of the escort served as visible index not only of the social status or position of the deceased, but also of his sociability because they depended, in large measure, upon the friendships and social connections he developed during the course of his lifetime. The bereaved felt they had an obligation to ensure that the funeral provided the fullest measure of respect for the dead. And, in a time when the measure of things was becoming increasingly worldly, they were likely to translate this respect into material objects and display.

At the Cemetery: The working relationship of the clergyman and the undertaker was compounded at the cemetery by the presence of another functionary, the sexton, or cemetery superintendent. Here, the undertaker relinquished a portion of the directing function, as either of the latter would direct the procession to the grave.

While the undertaker directed the activities of the pallbearers, the clergyman prepared to lead the way. The pallbearers then deposited the casket over the grave, and the clergyman took his position facing the family and began the committal service.

At his words, "Earth to earth...", either he or the undertaker sprinkled a handful of fine dirt over the casket. Under the supervision of the undertaker, the casket was lowered into the grave, either by the pallbearers — not an easy task for the unskilled — or by trained cemetery attendants. Filling the grave nearly always awaited the departure of the bereaved.

Rural Variations: Although, for rural and village funerals of the period, the treatment of the dead bore a basic similarity to funerals in cities, definite variations were evident. At the home or church, men, women and children turned out in numbers. Atherton remarks that, "while the bereaved family would not have had things otherwise, they were in for a rough hour. A long eulogy by the preacher and doleful hymns by a quartette only served to weaken those closest to the deceased and to leave them defenseless for the final ordeal at the grave."[7]

The funeral sermon provided the minister with a choice opportunity to appeal to the unsaved and to remind others of the fires of damnation awaiting unrepentant sinners: "The time to make peace with God is now."

Special attention was given the family of the deceased. In his remarks on the life of the departed member, a minister would spare no sector of human sentiment, and, until all the members were wracked in uncontrollable grief, minister and community alike could not pronounce the funeral successful.

Blanton notes that in Paris, Missouri, well before the turn of the century, the filling of the grave took the form of a contest, with the masculine friends vying with each other in their ability to manipulate a shovel. Nobody thought of leaving until the grave was filled.

Late-19th-century Mourning Symbols: In major part, the symbols of mourning during this period expressed the gloom and formality, the solemnity and lugubriousness, of the feudal funeral of the late Middle Ages and early Renaissance. That such a pattern of death-response should be incorporated into the mourning of a rapidly growing, ever increasingly industrialized American society is a puzzle for social and cultural historians. For decades, Americans had been enthusiastically writing and reading romantic fiction; certainly, the wave of Romanticism — a backward looking philosophy — would have supported such turning back from the simplicity and realism of American funeral customs of a century before.

Whatever the basic reasons, the solemnity and gloom were obvious enough. The house in which the death had struck not only had its scarf or "crepe" on the door, but it was not unknown for the bereaved to drape the room in which the dead lay, or possibly the whole downstairs of the house, in black or deep shades of gray.

Deeply colored veils were often hung in the doorway, and servants attired in mourning livery were stationed at the doorway to attend the callers. If the household contained a maid, she would wear black, with apron, collars and cuffs of white, and black ribbons attached to her white cap.

For the bereaved, black was considered the color most suitable for the trappings of woe. Its somber effect was reflected not only in the mourning garb but also in the dress of the functionaries, as well as the shroud, the hearse and its plumes, the pall spread over the casket, and even the horses used in the funeral cortege.[8]

Of the fabrics employed, funeral crepe was considered most effective, although black and blue-black bombazines, alpacas, black silks, black kid, and black cotton were used in the making of mourning garments and accessories.

The combination of the shrouding folds of the major garment, the black mourning bonnet with streamers reaching "well below the waistline," and the black crepe of the widow's veil made her mourning garb the most distinctive and lugubrious of any.

Following a death, mourning wear was used to indicate not only degrees of kinship with the dead, but also the several defined periods of mourning. The widow, for example, was clearly labeled by the white ruche that showed as an inner lining along the front of her bonnet. For the first year, the widow was expected to wear everything with a dull-black finish. Her gloves, purse, handkerchief border, ornaments and gown were to show no luster, as if a lack of luster in her appointments declared the lack of luster brought into her entire being by death.

In the first six months of the second year of mourning, the crepe gave way to less funereal materials, such as black silk or crepe-de-chine, and for the remainder of the year, the use of both white and violet was permissible. After two years, the widow again could wear ordinary clothes.

Should a woman lose her husband late in life, she might commonly wear mourning clothing for the remainder of her days. As the 19th century drew to an end, the fashion of wearing all white for summer mourning made its appearance, although white never became a dominant mourning theme, as it had once been in classical antiquity.

The mourning garb for women was varied enough to indicate the nature of the bereavement, whether for a husband, child, grown offspring, brother, sister, parent or even grandparent.

The widower customarily wore a suit entirely of black cloth with plain white linen. Any other coloring was prohibited. Shoes, gloves, cufflinks and hat were all of dull black. A conspicuous crepe mourning-band adorned the hat.

For a widower, mourning might last for a year, with a period of secondary mourning in which he was permitted to relieve his black garb by gray. Wearing a mourning band on the sleeve of the coat was not generally approved, unless the ordinary costume was a uniform that might not be changed.

With some latitude allowed for special cases of attachment, mourning was not generally prescribed or approved for kinfolk living apart from the immediate family, such as uncles, aunts, nephews, cousins and other collateral relatives.

In any event, the first six months after a death, commonly known as the period of "deep mourning," carried with it a proscription against participation in any social or recreational affairs. As the mourning colors during the mourning period grew progressively lighter, so in parallel fashion did the social and personal contacts of the mourners.

By the time all mourning garb was dispensed with, so were all restrictions as to movement and social contact. For the woman, this was more definitely the case; for the man, social activity was resumed somewhat more quickly.

Another phase of social contact, correspondence, fell under the regulation of mourning custom. Stationery was prescribed as to color: for the widow, white or gray with black border, a quarter-inch wide for the first year of mourning, an eighth-inch for the next six months, and a sixteenth for the remainder of the second year. (***See Plate 62***.)

Colored crests were prohibited, as was perfume. Simplicity in the lettering, and even the containment of scrawling handwriting, were advised.

Calling cards were likewise edged in black, the edging's width indicating the degree of relationship to the deceased — the thinner the edge, the more distant the relationship. Propriety and decorum were to be observed in all correspondence, as in all behavior involving others, and in all actions, perceived or private, of the person in mourning. Postcards were decidedly not permissible.

Other classes of people participated in the symbolization of the mourning gloom. Not only was the undertaker's garb of traditional black, but so generally was the garb of all who figured importantly in the funeral: minister, pallbearers, drivers and other functionaries, as well as the bereaved. Friends would don either black or their darkest or most-subdued dress to attend the ceremony.

Other symbols were affected, as well. For example, it was still fashionable in 1880 to wear a funeral sash or a linen scarf, which were worn along with gloves, ribbons and badges. An 1878 ad in *The Casket* for badges lists, "black, white or black-white combination lettered in gold or silver, 'Pall Bearer,' 'Undertaker,' or with Masonic, IOOF, Catholic or other society emblems as may be desired." (***See Plate 63***.)

Music likewise symbolized solemnity, if not gloom. It was considered singularly appropriate at the time to have a brass band precede the funeral procession, and the strains of the "Dead March" from "Saul," with musicians marching in broken ranks, were as much in keeping with the tenor of the occasion as are the strains of "Lead Kindly Light" on the church organ for the funeral of today. These songs were designed to be sung on such occasions. Other intensely religious songs or, perhaps, the favorite numbers of the deceased might be included. In all cases, the emotional character of the situation was enhanced, reserves were further broken down, and feelings were given an opportunity to find full expression.

A church bell tolling to mark the arrival of the funeral procession has been a customary feature of village and city life in America since Colonial days. In rural areas, the church bell played a communicative role — by different modes of tolling, the age and sex of the deceased were indicated.

In some sections of the country, a trombone choir was used to announce the death of a fellow member of the church. The musicians assembled in the belfry and played certain selections that were codes for the members. One piece was used for married adults and another for children.[9]

Aesthetically Pleasing Mourning Symbols: Despite the overwhelming tone of gloom, formality and solemnity with which it was characterized, it would be a mistake to think of the late-19th-century funeral as entirely governed by the pattern of the feudal system of mourning behavior, as developed in the late Middle Ages. Chapter 7, which focuses on burial cases, coffins and caskets, provides an illustration of the breaking away from this pattern.

In addition, well before the Civil War, people were demanding that the receptacle for the dead should do more than indicate social status by its expensiveness (as was the case after the Revolutionary War) or serve as an object of mere utility. The very term "casket" signified a box or container for something precious, and the preciousness of the human body was felt to be best expressed to the world *symbolically* by the aesthetic luxury of the casket, and *dramatically* by the funeral ceremony.

From about 1850 on, the casket increasingly found its meaning in the realm of popular tastes, where sweeps of fad and fashion played across the appetites and dispositions of the 19th-century American mind. The appearance of the casket, its form and composition both subject to the prevailing canons of taste, signaled the beginnings of the breakdown of a system of mourning that was yet to peak several generations later.

By 1880, the enterprising town or city undertaker, selling caskets out of the catalogs of three or four large casket companies, could present a customer with at least a 100 different choices of casket styles, embracing such materials as wood, wood-cloth combination, metal, wood and metal, and metal-and-glass combinations. As noted earlier, colors ranged from the conventional black to varieties of silver, bronze, aniline blue and lavender, in many variations.

Despite the selection, these caskets had a standard form and came in a limited range of standard sizes. The discriminations in style that could be made covered a broad range, but the variations were minor; one chose from a great variety of styles, but seldom were the choices radically different.

The second major breakthrough of the funeral gloom of late-19th-century mourning came in the area of the setting, or backdrop, for the casket. Just as the casket became more an object of beauty, or evocative of aesthetically pleasant feelings or imagery, so eventually did the setting change, and the heavy black folds of the casket drape were replaced by the colorful, warmer or more-striking colors of the casket lining, which, by the end of the century, had come to dominate the casket exterior, especially in the "couch" types.[10] (***See Figure 32, page 300.***)

With the remarkable changes in the burial receptacle and the increasing emphasis upon its aesthetic effect, the traditional "props" of the draped pedestal and, possibly, the bedraped room could only produce an ambiguous or disharmonious effect. A more appropriate setting commended itself in the form of the floral backdrop. Starting with the placing of a small bouquet on a table

PLATE 63

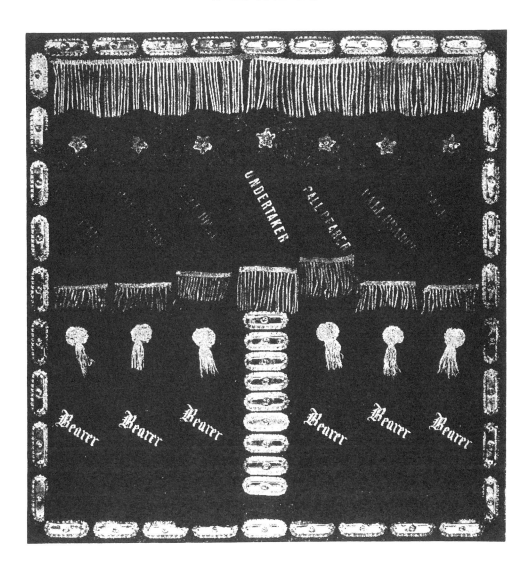

63. Funeral Badges — Indispensable to the Late-19th-century Funeral.

beside the casket — a custom lost in its origins — from the middle of the century on, there was a slowly increasing sentiment in favor of matching the color, beauty and aesthetic appeal of the casket and its striking colored, or white, lining with the natural beauty and color of flowers.

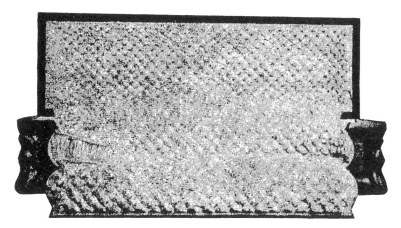

Figure 32. Couch-style Casket.

While this new fashion became popular, or at least gained acceptance, however, questions arose as to whether funeral flowers had pagan associations, and whether a wealth of floral tributes might not be an indefensible waste of money. Although opposition to the use of flowers was never organized, church officials were not loath to criticize excesses in display as a departure from Christian custom.

Another form of religious criticism appeared as early as 1878, when the bishop of Rochester, New York, in a letter to the *Catholic Times* remarked:

> Whatever of sentiment may have been in the use of flowers on and around a corpse when, at first, loving hands placed a few near it was killed by usage demanding that such tributes should be repaid on the first occasion available. Thus, in time, floral tributes for the house of mourning became a question of give and expect: a compliment to a friend with a marketable value attached. No wonder that some families deprecate the invasion of their homes with such tributes and cry out, "Omit the flowers."[11]

It is interesting to note that in the same city, and in a catalog dated the same year, the Stein Patent Burial Casket Works advertised floral offerings, for order by funeral directors, in fresh flowers or "immortelles" in 20 different designs, most of them carrying four or five sizes, and ranging in wholesale price from $1.50 to $25.00. "Immortelles" (non-perishable, artificial, dried, or prepared natural flowers and leaves) generally were 50% cheaper.

Those wishing to order funeral decorations through their undertaker had a choice of set pieces: the Plain Wreath; Cross, flat or standing; Anchor, or Anchor Cross, flat or standing; Faith, Hope and Charity (anchor, cross and heart in one piece); Harp or Lyre, standing; Square and Compass; Crown, flat or standing; Star; Heart; Maltese Cross; monograms, sold by the letter; Three Links; Combinations of Wreath and Cross, Harp, Anchor, Crown, and Star; Crescent; Crescent and Star Combined; Broken Column; Monument; Shield; Sickle; and, finally, Lamb and Cross.

The fact that there was opposition to the use of flowers on the grounds that they were pagan; to their extensive use on the score that it was wasteful; and to the sense of reciprocal necessity because it was worldly indicates that the usage must have been growing. Moreover, the broad choice of styles, forms, sizes and motifs gives further proof, if such were needed, that a shift in popular taste was making heavy inroads upon the tradition of feudal gloom at the very time that the pompous and solemnly formal funeral seemed to be enjoying its greatest vogue.

Victory of flowers over crepe was given striking support by the flower burial of the controversial, widely popular anti-slavery clergyman Henry Ward Beecher, in connection with whose death, in 1887, a virtual "flower funeral" was held. Beecher had always been of the mind that flowers were more appropriate at funerals than black crepe. Thus, when he died, a basket of flowers was fixed at the door of his residence in Brooklyn, New York, instead of the conventional black emblem.

Likewise, the floral theme dominated all the church decorations. The old reading desk, placed to the right of the pulpit platform, was covered with asparagus ferns and pink and white roses. Beecher's chair was lost in a sea of white carnations, pink roses, smilax, and eucharis lilies. Behind the dais, where the coffin rested, was a solid bank of flowers extending to the ceiling formed of azaleas, calla lilies and other blooms. Each post around the face of the gallery was surrounded with clusters of plants, and a continuous bank of flowers covered the gallery ledge. Between the pillars were wreaths of laurel; from the chandelier in the center of the church, ropes of laurel were stretched in every direction to the cornice, where they were met with clusters of evergreen fastened against the walls.

In addition, underneath the gallery, the walls themselves were hung with wreaths of evergreens, and the ceiling was completely concealed by hangings of smilax, caught up with bunches of bright flowers. From each gas bracket in the church were hung baskets filled with cut roses, azaleas, chrysanthemums, and other bright and fragrant flowers. On the Bible stand was a design of ferns in which there were three doves; to the right was a floral cross bearing the words "Our Chaplain," while nearby was a large pillow of white flowers with the letter "B" formed of pink roses in the center. To complete the flower motif, the front of the church was decked with ropings of smilax and evergreen.[12]

In the year before the Beecher funeral, the principal floral offering at the funeral of a fire chief was a large floral fire engine, nine feet high and six feet long, patterned after the old Red Rover #3 and covered with smilax, carnations and roses. Lettered in violets on the boiler were the words, "Our Chief." Another floral piece was fashioned after a fire-alarm box bearing the number "4" in memory of the last fire to which the chief had responded.

During the same year, the custom of writing with white ink on the leaves of natural flowers became popular. In 1888, the International Funeral Directors Association (the title used by NFDA during its affiliation with the Canadian Funeral Directors Association) encouraged its members to use flowers instead of crepe.

Inscriptions were the vogue in funeral flowers. It is recorded that a New Yorker sent an office boy to get flowers for a visiting Cuban friend's stateroom for the steamer-voyage home. The boy returned with two broken columns inscribed, "We mourn your loss" and "Gone to another shore."

When the secretary of the New England Funeral Directors Association died, he was honored with a floral offering of a closed book on a mound of smilax on which was laid his secretarial pen, surmounted by a wreath of roses. Above these symbols was poised a floral crown.

Artificial flowers were widely sold in the 1890s because the distribution of natural flowers was spotty and could not be obtained in some areas and at some times.

By 1892, it was recorded that floral pieces containing sentiments and descriptions were going out of fashion.

Three years later, some concern was expressed over the stereotyped patterns of floral offerings and the suggestion made that supporting bouquets or greens could better be employed than the endless repetitions of "Gates Ajar," "The Broken Column," or the "Unstrung Harp" with its gold or silver wires.

But the fashions were too well established to be terminated by a little criticism. When the elaborate pieces of the Philadelphia Immortelle Co. were criticized, it answered that the business of all florists had increased, and that one florist with a $10,000 annual gross had made 50% of his sales in dried flowers and wheat sheaves.

The floral vogue did not reach Jewish funerals during this period.

Sepulture and Memorialization: In urban communities in the 1880s, burial would most likely take place in a "central" cemetery, that is, in a large burial tract on or beyond the outskirts, in which many families drawn from a wide area of the community owned private lots. Single grave spaces could be purchased also.

Although a large number of such cemeteries were denominational, non-religious corporations sponsored some of them. Most contained remains transferred from older, smaller cemeteries that had been crowded out by the rapid expansion of American cities. In some cases, graves had been so removed several times.

Under the changing fashion that sought beauty in death and burial, cemeteries during this period began taking on the aspect of a park. Perpetual-care plans were still uncommon. The breaking away from the custom of burying in the church graveyard, or in scattered small public or private lots, had been going on for three-quarters of a century.

A movement for burial outside the corporate limits of cities arose in the United States in the beginning of the 19th century. France's example proved a strong influence in the matter. A report of the New York City Board of Health in 1806 advised the removal of all graveyards from the city and recommended that burial places should be made public works.

In that same year, a law was passed authorizing the Corporation of the City of New York to prohibit interment within the city limits. No effort was made to enforce it until the following year.

Nor did anyone show much interest in the problem of intramural burial until epidemics of yellow fever and cholera convinced the public that there was need for cemeteries outside the city.[13] The condition of some of these city graveyards became apparent from the fact that in 1822, quicklime was placed over them to kill the summer odors arising from them.[14]

The first of the new extramural cemeteries was Mt. Auburn in Boston, Massachusetts, established in 1831; Laurel Hill in Pennsylvania opened soon after; and Greenwood in New York City in 1837.[15]

A treatise by Dr. John H. Rauch of Chicago seems to have been influential in later cemetery development. The state of New York passed a Rural Cemetery Act in 1847 providing for the founding of cemetery associations and granting certain privileges. The latter included such things as freedom from taxes, the right to make rules and regulations, and to distribute payment for land purchased for such cemetery uses over the life of the cemetery.[16]

While each town or city had its own cemetery experiences, the problems were generally common, and they were therefore likely to find more-or-less common solutions. Chicago offers a case in point. An 1830 map of Fort Dearborn, Illinois, shows a cemetery on the edge of the small military reservation or garrison. In 1832, a ship sailing into Chicago was ravaged by cholera. The first dead were weighted and buried at sea. Eighteen others were interred on land, not far from the place where the American Temple House was later erected at the intersection of Lake and Wabash. The burial was primitive, without coffins or shrouds, and used blankets for winding sheets, with the earth removed to cover one corpse hollowing a grave to receive the next that died.

By 1835, the village authorities were facing the cemetery problem, and the trustees ordered the surveyor to lay out 16 acres on the South Side, near the foot of 23rd Street, for Catholics, and 10 acres on the North Side (on what is now Chicago Avenue, just east of Clark Street) for Protestants. Burial in any other part of the town was forbidden.

The first recorded gravedigger, a Prussian immigrant named Henry Gherkin, arrived in Chicago in 1836. The laying out of the two cemeteries, Catholic and Protestant, apparently left unsolved certain of Chicago's burial problems, as can be inferred from the fact that only two years later, the city's charter was amended in the interest of public health to permit the establishment of a city burial grounds. The amendment also gave Chicago the right to regulate the burial of the dead.

By 1840, the sprawling town was again in cemetery trouble, and the council decreed the abandonment of the early cemeteries and the establishment of a burial ground farther out. The new location was on the site of Lincoln Park. Three years after this action, the city passed an ordinance providing penalties for burial in the old cemeteries.

In the meantime, Greenwood Cemetery was established in 1842. Oakwood Cemetery, at what is now 107th and Greenwood, had its first burials 11 years later.

But the growing pains still continued and, in 1865, the Chicago Council decided to vacate the Lincoln Park Cemetery as it could not establish clear title to this property. Lot owners were given titles to lots in newer cemeteries. The moving of the bodies took several years.[17]

The celebrated Mt. Auburn Cemetery, where many Boston notables are buried, illustrates some of the influences that changed the American pattern from interment in a church graveyard or privately owned plot to a central cemetery. In 1825, Dr. Jacob Bigelow expressed that a country cemetery should be established to put an end to what he believed were public-health dangers resulting from the church vault and churchyard burial. To put his ideas into practice, he called a meeting of his friends.

Strangely enough, in order to gain for itself a place in which to conduct experiments, the Massachusetts Horticultural Society decided to lend a hand with the project, and a Boston citizen, George W. Brimmer, at no profit to himself, sold "Stone's Woods" to the society. To gain support, public meetings were called and the newspapers were supplied with announcements and articles. Distinguished Bostonians and others lent their names and active support to the project, including Supreme Court Justice Joseph Story; the great Daniel Webster; the eminent statesman and orator Edward Everett; Abbott Lawrence; Samuel Appleton; and Henry A.S. Dearborn, president of the horticultural society.

On June 23, 1831, an act was passed authorizing the horticultural society to dedicate real estate for a rural cemetery. Consecration services, with Justice Story providing the oration, were held on September 24th of the same year.

It was soon discovered, however, that an experimental garden and a cemetery were two distinct enterprises, so, by act of March 31, 1835, the cemetery was placed under separate management.

In 1881, six central cemeteries were available to the citizens of Milwaukee, Wisconsin. The vestry of St. Paul's Episcopal Church established the largest of these, Forest Home Cemetery, in 1850. Three members of St. Paul's vestry served, without pay, as a management committee. Thirty years later, the property consisted of 188 acres. "Thousands of dollars have been expended in cutting and smoothing wide graveled roadways, maintaining beautiful flower beds, planting trees, erecting a fine fountain and otherwise making it a Forest Home — a restful city of the dead. For beauty of natural location and taste in artificial adornment, it has not a superior in the West."[18]

In 1864, under authority of Wisconsin's state legislature, about 1,200 bodies interred in Milwaukee Cemetery, then being surrounded by the growing young city, were transferred to Forest Home.

In 1880, "several lot owners are considering the propriety of bequeathing certain sums of money in trust for the purpose of perpetually providing for the care and maintenance of their lots. The corporation would gladly take charge of such trusts." That same year, recorded interments reached about 14,000.

Catholics could find burial either in Calvary or Trinity cemeteries. Like Forest Home, Calvary Cemetery, a 55-acre tract established in 1857, was the inheritor plot for several earlier graveyards. In the very early days within the original boundaries of Milwaukee, a small, non-sectarian, fenced-in cemetery was developed. Later, this became a Catholic cemetery, and, in 1844, Bishop Henni purchased the "Old Catholic Cemetery," a 10-acre tract on Grand Avenue (now Wisconsin Avenue) in the very heart of the present city.

As the city developed, the First Ward Cemetery was no longer used for burial, and the bodies buried within were transferred to the "Old Cemetery." The first interments at Calvary consisted of remains transferred from the "Old Cemetery," which in turn was abandoned as the city closed in.

In the 23 years from 1857 to 1880, Calvary Cemetery received 10,307 remains. Holy Trinity was a smaller Catholic cemetery originally purchased to provide burial grounds for a single Catholic parish. The graveyard was three or four miles removed from Holy Trinity Church.

Union and Pilgrim's Rest Cemeteries accepted Protestant burials. Greenwood Cemetery, adjoining Forest Home, was "devoted exclusively to the use of Israelites."

Frederick S. Frantz, a third-generation Pennsylvania funeral director, traces, in most general outlines, the history of cemetery development in the Middle Atlantic region:

> In Grandfather's time, there was no cemetery as we know it today. In fact, it was not called a cemetery — it was a "graveyard" or "churchyard" or "God's acre." As our forefathers settled this section of the country, they set aside part of their own land for their own families. It was God's acre, and kept as such. This little tract of ground so hallowed, was convenient and necessary — but later it often became a handicap in the sale of property, for the next owner would not wish the first party's burial lot, and the original owner would not wish to be separated from the dead. One can easily see the complications that would arise from this transaction. The churchyard then became the logical place for burial and this ground was placed in the hands of the church officers, who in turn had authority over the permits. No lots were sold and space was opened for graves as needed. This often meant that husband and wife were separated by as many graves as were used between the two deaths. We have some records where these graveyards were divided into the following groups: married section, single adults, choir, children, and those who were outside the church — not members.
>
> About this time, the duty of grave digging fell upon the shoulders of the pallbearers. They assisted the family and undertaker from the time of the first call to the very end — the closing of the open grave.
>
> The church "graveyard" had its limitations in growing sections, for in many towns of 1,500 people there were at least 15 "graveyards." Ground became valuable and the boundaries of the lot were limited by houses that had been built on the four sides. Therefore, the central cemetery was the logical growth, and the burial lot passed from the hands of the church to organized and chartered groups who developed the beautiful memorial parks of today.[19]

The effort to beautify the surroundings of death had further expression in the memorialization of the dead. In their designs and materials, gravestones themselves responded to the changing funeral mood of the day. Instead of the earlier simple marble or limestone slab, the sculptor went to work industriously to add cornices, fancy caps, arabesques, scrolls, imitation tree trunks, or statuary. Sometimes he combined several types or shades of stone. The peculiar bad taste of the romantic period that produced Main Street mansions faintly reminiscent of German castles or Italian palaces, and furniture that looked to the jigsaw and lathe rather than to the carver's bench, filled cemeteries with a minor vertical forest of petrified and very indifferent art.

But here, again, the impulse to create beauty even in death was strong, although the effect is not always happy to the modern eye, which prefers simplicity and harmony. It has been well said, however, that with the passing of such ornateness, something has been lost as well as gained. The "uncouth lines and shapeless sculpture" of which Thomas Gray once spoke are no longer in fashion. The present tendency toward uniformity and simplicity might add a sense of dignity to cemeteries, but graveyards lack somewhat the intriguing personality of an earlier day.[20]

Something of the changing mood toward death and funerals can be learned from a reading of grave inscriptions. Wallis remarks:

> On these stone silhouettes of bygone days, we may read the hopes and despairs, the joys and frustrations of Everyman. The manner of expression may be ribald and ridiculous, pompous and lugubrious, eloquent, or serenely simple.
>
> The common grave slab probably originated as an effort to safeguard a new grave from wild beasts. Names and dates were inscribed for purposes of identification.
>
> An epitaph, representing pious sentiments consistent with a person's life, or words of advice or caution for the instruction of the living, later made one stone distinctive from another. Quotations from the Bible have long seemed singularly appropriate.[21]

Inscriptions and decorations on tombstones provide additional clues to popular attitudes toward life and death at any period. Early American epitaphs minced no words and used no sweetened or softened expressions to veil or sugar the hard natural facts.

Moreover, through the 18th century and before, and well into the 19th, they spelled out the reality of death. When they told biography, it was unvarnished. They called sinners, sinners, and saints, saints. They did not shun to tell what lay beneath them; not infrequently, they spelled out the message with skull and crossbones to illustrate the point.

After looking into the face of death, some survivors were not beyond making a crude jest or a merry pun. Although the endless variety tempts one to linger here, a few illustrations must suffice. For example, there is the harsh New Hampshire epitaph, written in simplest imagery, which reads:

> This rose was sweet a while,
>
> But now is odour vile.[22]

Some forgotten necrophile uses an undated, nameless Massachusetts tombstone to express his frustration:

> Oh would that I could lift the lid and peer
>
> within the grave and watch the greedy worms
>
> that eat away the dead.[23]

Or the terse:

> Soon ripe
>
> Soon rotten
>
> Soon gone
>
> But not forgotten.[24]

Or the pathetic couplet to the eight-year-old boy who, in 1795, was buried in Milford, Connecticut:

> Christ called at midnight as I lay
>
> In thirty hours was turned to clay.[25]

No one has ever written better "The short and simple annals" of a young wife and mother who died in childbirth:

> Eighteen years a maiden,
>
> One year a wife
>
> One day a mother
>
> Then I lost my life.[26]

Details concerning the manner of death were badly and boldly written:

> Killed by a kick of a colt
>
> in his bowells.[27]

When a four-year-old boy died of burns from an overturned coffee pot, his tombstone commented:

> The boiling coffee on me did fall,
>
> And by it I was slain,
>
> But Christ has brought my liberty
>
> And in Him I'll rise again.[28]

Friends of Thomas Mulvaney were reminded:

> Old Thomas Mulvaney lies here,
>
> His mouth ran from ear to ear,
>
> Reader, tread lightly on this wonder,
>
> For if he yawns, you're going to thunder.[29]

In many old graveyards are found inscriptions and other reminders of the sicknesses that caused untimely, and even timely, deaths. Dropsy, heart disease, consumption, and St. Vitus's dance are commonly mentioned, as are inscriptions that describe the suffering brought on by the several maladies: "severest pains," "body affliction" or "painful illness." Sermons in stone can be found on many an older monument in an old graveyard, at the side of a church, or next to the village green.

While there is no sharp cleavage, it is noticeable that, after 1850, monument prose, verse and art increasingly softened the hard facts, grew less blunt, and grew less inclined to roar with rude laughter. The skull and crossbones gave way to the winged cherub and other symbols of faith and hope.

By 1865, it was not deemed inappropriate, as it would have been a half-century before, to write:

> 'Tis but the casket that lies here
>
> The gem that fills it sparkles yet.[30]

And, by 1880, a wife would comment:

> Stranger call this not a place
>
> Of fear and gloom,
>
> To me it is a pleasant spot
>
> It is my husband's tomb.[31]

Sentiments such as those adorning tombstones in the 1880s conform in mood to that of the four-by-six-inch, gilt-edged, gilt-printed "mourning cards" of the period. These were distributed to friends.

For example, the card of Thomas Ardron (*see* **Plate 61**), who died April 19, 1891, at the age of 76 years, two months and eight days, has a dove at the top holding a streamer that bears the legend

"In Loving Remembrance." Upon the outline of the Holy Bible are printed Masonic symbols and the name of the departed. Below, on a scroll, is the elegiac verse:

>How slender is life's silver cord.
>
>How soon 'tis broken here!
>
>Each moment brings a parting word,
>
>And many a falling tear.
>
>And though these years, to mortals given
>
>Are filled with grief and pain,
>
>There is a hope — the hope of heaven,
>
>Where loved ones meet again.[32]

When James S. Pilling died on March 14, 1889, at the age of eight, his card, "In Loving Remembrance," carried two separate poems: the first reminded the bereaved that:

>"There is no death." What seems so is transition;
>
>This life of mortal breath
>
>Is but the suburb of the life elysian,
>
>Whose portal we call Death.[33]

The second dealt with the small boy himself:

>Sleep on in thy beauty,
>
>Thou sweet angel child,
>
>By sorrow unslighted,
>
>By sin undefiled.
>
>Like the dove to the ark,
>
>Thou hast flown to thy rest,
>
>From the wild sea of strife,
>
>To the home of the blest.[34]

The impulse to memorialize in verse, and the willingness of verse-makers to provide copy for such memorials, have both persisted to our day. Even though mourning cards have long gone out of fashion, the reminders of death and anniversaries of death occasionally appear in the daily newspapers.

The Changing Functions of the Undertaker: We have seen that early in the 18th century, the role and duties of the undertaker were changed by the new emphasis placed upon the coffin as the major item in the funeral, together with the resultant development of the coffin-warehouse, or wareroom.

Later, toward mid-century, other changes were produced by the emergence of the "furnishing-undertaker," whose concentration of necessary funeral paraphernalia in one establishment made it possible for the undertaker to provide increased attention and personal service to the bereaved. Such changes in an occupation would suggest that it was in a state of transition, and that the last 20 or 30 years of the century would produce further change. The facts well warrant the assumption.

As early as 1862, the furnishing-undertakers were issuing professional cards. (***See Chapter 6, Figure 3.***) While it is true that many of these establishments carried lines of other wares, such as furniture and household necessities of many sorts (*see Chapter 6, Plate 25*), there is a noticeable change in emphasis away from undertaking as an incidental or auxiliary service, or from the furnishing of undertakers' supplies as a mere sideline.

True, undertaking in 1875 to 1900 had not as yet crystallized into a clear-cut occupational role, yet the outlines were clear enough, and the general image of the modern funeral director was coming into clearer focus all the time. There were yet activities that he must lose, slough off or delegate to others. And there were new functions, such as counseling survivors, which were still in the future.

Despite the hazards of interrupting this narrative for a circumspective glance at a period marked by transition rather than stability, it seems worthwhile here to pause around 1880 and, in keeping with the general sense of this chapter, to take a cross-sectional view of the occupational role of the undertaker.

In the first place, the undertaker had probably reached a peak in supplying material objects, or funeral paraphernalia, for the care and disposal of the dead. At this time, not only did he provide major items, such as casket and carriage, but also such mourning materials as drapery, door badges or scarves, items of clothing, and caps and neckerchiefs for such participants as pallbearers, ministers, honor guards and others, as well.

He also kept on hand a variety of memorial cards, announcement forms and other stationery upon which he arranged to have pertinent information printed, such as names, dates and places.

He provided flowers, stocking immortelles or other imitations, or ordering such from dealers by telegraph. He also made arrangements with the local florist to supply tributes made of either fresh or imitation flowers.

He provided, likewise, chairs, robes (*see Plate 64*), pillows, nets, gauze, candlesticks and crucifixes, kid gloves and ornaments. In short, the undertaker generally furnished any material object that was likely to be used specifically for funerals.

Yet, at the same time that the peak in furnishing material goods was reached, there were already seeds germinating for the appearance of the new role of the funeral director. Thus, by the end of the century, the undertaker, as dominantly a furnisher of goods, represented an occupation that was fast becoming obsolete.

The new fact in late-19th-century undertaking was the great increase in control that the undertaker was beginning to exert over the whole matter of the funeralization of the dead. Spelled out in detail, this meant that he moved from a merchant, who first provided goods needed by the bereaved in their burying activities; to a seller of service, who actually took part in the preparation of the dead, performing a portion, or all, of the laying out of the body in the home — "conserving the remains" — and transporting body and mourners to places of worship and sepulture; and finally to a director, who took charge of the body and of the proceedings involved in its ceremonial disposition.

Funeral direction as an emerging service occupation grew out of three needs: First, embalming by chemical injection for most dead bodies carried with it the need for a special working laboratory, constructed and equipped along clinical lines. Second, the crowding of cities and the development of small living units in apartments and other buildings, created a need for the establishment of the funeral "home" or "parlor" especially designed for the ceremonial disposal of the dead. Third, in urban communities, the problems attendant upon the transportation of both the dead and living to places of worship added a need for the development of a chapel in such establishments that could be used by those desiring such use, as a setting for the religious ceremonialization of the dead.

As the 19th century drew to a close, consolidation of these three functional areas — the clinic, the home, and the chapel — into a single operational unit gave rise to the modern funeral home and provided the cues for the emergence of the funeral director as we know him today.

Yet, funeral directing — in the sense of managing a complex series of activities, designed, among other matters, to create and sustain a mood — was still in an unformed state. Basically, in 1880, the American funeral undertaker was a merchant, selling goods to customers but, at the same time, he was becoming increasingly involved in taking charge of the management aspects of the care and disposal of the dead. Thus, he still tendered bills that itemized goods and services without discrimination. (***See Figure 29 earlier in this chapter***.)

As a matter of fact, many of the services were profitable, even if small, transactions. These included such things as the opening and the bricking up of the sides of the grave, the arrangements made with sextons and cemetery superintendents, the securing of permits, extra ice for coolers, the provision for carriages, and the like. The undertaker had as yet to conceive of the value of personal services offered professionally for a fee, legitimately claimed. Being "in attendance" was as far as he would concede his services as worthy of such fee. The charge for this item was very minimal, usually only a few dollars, while the profit from the sale of the casket was substantial, and the undertaker sometimes realized his greatest return from providing a number of carriages.

On the other hand, the making of cash-advances, one of the more obviously non-service functions in a private-enterprise economy, was clearly more of a personal accommodation than a financial transaction. This practice had its origin about the middle of the century. Although undertakers might have been merchants, they were never commercial moneylenders. Had they assumed this function as one of their occupational specialties, it is doubtful if the personal-service element, involving professional judgment of what are appropriate actions in funeral service, would ever have evolved out of 19th-century undertaking.

In a word, by the dawn of the 20th century, the undertaker was a supplier of funeral necessities who was, at the same time, on the threshold of becoming a provider of directions, definitions and ideas for appropriate ceremonial actions. To provide humane treatment of the dead, he could (or soon would) be able to: take the body from the home and, in the same physical structure, preserve it and make it available for appropriate viewing as custom dictated; and provide, when and as desired, a religious setting where, with the aid of the clergy, the body could be made ready for burial.

PLATE 64

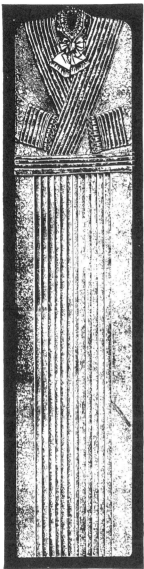 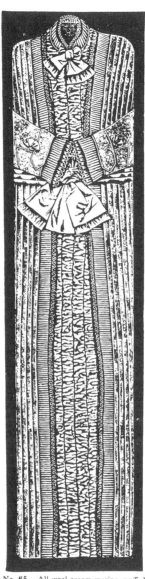 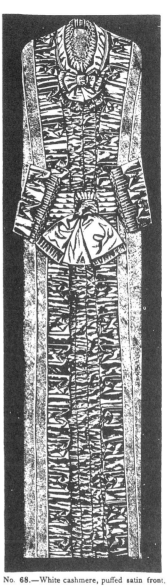

No. 63.—All wool cream merino.

No. 65.—All wool cream merino, puffed satin front, knife plaiting, and crepe lisse trimmed, cream satin sash.

No. 68.—White cashmere, puffed satin front, double point box plaiting.

64. Burial Robes Sold by Undertakers, 1880.

Although the furnishing of goods and paraphernalia has always been part of the business of the funeral undertaker, and continues to be one of a number of functions of the funeral director, its relative importance began to decline before 1900, and it has long since been relegated to one of the numerous specialties of a profession-oriented occupation, centrally based in the performance of personal service.

CITATIONS AND REFERENCES FOR CHAPTER 10

1. The nearest to a modern treatment of contemporary American funeral customs is found in *Funeral Customs the World Over* by Robert W. Habenstein and William M. Lamers (Milwaukee: Bulfin Press, 1974), pp. 729-767.

2. Mrs. A. Baldwin, *When Our Mother Was a Little Girl* (1888), p. 2. From the collection of NFDA, Milwaukee, Wisconsin.

3. Lewis Atherton, *Main Street on the Middle Border* (Bloomington, Indiana: Indiana University Press, 1954), p. 191.

4. H.J. Blanton, *When I Was a Boy* (Columbia, Mo.: E.W. Stephens Publishing Company, 2 vols., 1952). See especially "When the Undertaker Had a Modest Part," Vol. 1, pp. 1-3.

5. Landauer, *op. cit.*, p. 226.

6. Harry A. Weisbord, "Time Stays — We Go," *Hobbies*, August 1940, pp. 10-11.

7. Atherton, *op. cit.*, p. 192.

8. See, for example, Marvin Dana, *The American Encyclopedia of Etiquette and Culture*, 1922, n.p., Part Six.

9. Frederick S. Frantz, "The Funeral Director in Grandpa's Time," in *Clinical Topics*, p. 6.

10. See George S. Herrick, "The Facts About Casket Textiles," *Casket and Sunnyside*, reprint contained in a brochure titled *Casket Manufacturing*, n.d.

11. *The Casket*, July 1878.

12. Adapted from the document "The Beecher Flowers" in the collection of NFDA, Milwaukee, Wisconsin, n.p., n.d.

13. Wilson and Levy, *op. cit.*, p. 21.

14. See F.D. Allen, *Documents and Facts, showing the Fatal Effects of interments in Populous Cities* (New York: publisher unknown, 1822).

15. C.F. Perkinson to Maynard C. Weller, February 7, 1944. Letter in the collection of NFDA, Milwaukee, Wisconsin.

16. *Ibid.*

17. See Paul Gilbert and Charles L. Bryson, *Chicago and its Makers* (Chicago: Felix Mendelsohn, 1929). Also Bessie L. Pierce, *History of Chicago* (1673-1848), Vol. I (New York: Alfred Knopf, 1937).

18. *History of Milwaukee* (Chicago: Western Historical Company, 1881), pp. 953-957.

19. Frederick S. Frantz, *op. cit.*, p. 6.

20. Charles L. Wallis, *Stories on Stone* (New York: Oxford University Press, 1954), p. xv.
21. *Ibid.*, p. xi.
22. *Ibid.*, p. 185.
23. *Ibid.*
24. *Ibid.*, p. 181.
25. *Ibid.*, p. 182.
26. *Ibid.*, p. 173.
27. *Ibid.*, p. 116.
28. *Ibid.*, p. 119.
29. "The American Funeral Director"; loose clipping. Collection of NFDA, Milwaukee, Wisconsin, n.p., n.d.
30. Wallis, *op. cit.*, p. 185.
31. Charles L. Wallis, "Their Last Words Had a Punch," *Saturday Evening Post*, April 17, 1954, p. 44.
32. Mourning card in collection of NFDA, Milwaukee, Wisconsin.
33. *Ibid.*
34. *Ibid.*

Chapter 11

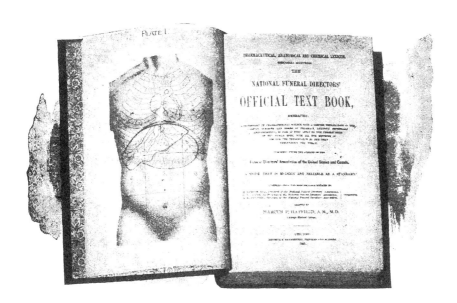

The Associational Impulse

The 19th century produced an economic revolution that shifted the nation's economy from one based predominantly upon an agrarian society to one increasingly characterized by industry, manufacture, urbanism and corporate business.[1]

In the social and cultural realm, this process was paralleled by the emergence of new social movements — some seeking to set the world aright by harking back to the venerable ways of the past, and others with bold ideas hoping to chart new programs of human action.

As the century rolled by, there were few important areas of American occupational life left untouched by these changes and developments. One of the most significant effects of these social and economic forces was the appearance of large scale *associational* activity — the gathering together and organizing of significant numbers of people around a limited set of interests and objectives. Thus, in the world of industry, the laboring man formed his trade union; the industrialist found strength in his trade association; and the practitioner sought colleagueship in his professional organization.

This chapter focuses upon the formal organization of funeral directors into various limited-objective types of associations, and the growth, prosperity, problems, issues and changing forms and functions of these associations.

BACKGROUND FACTORS

Occupational Organization: The modern concept of an occupational or professional association was almost entirely a creation of the 19th century.[2] Before then, professional organization had been limited to the fields of medicine and law, but this period witnessed an astonishing extension of occupational organization among a vast number of vocations and organized forms of personal services.

A partial explanation of this extension is evident in the progress of science and technology, which gave rise to numerous new professions, such as engineering, architecture, chemistry and dentistry. In addition, the resultant social and cultural revolutions created a demand for all types of specialists trained to cope with the increasingly complicated machinery of changing patterns in government, business and education. This furthered the burgeoning of new occupations, such as various types of public administrators, accountants, secretaries, real-estate agents, surveyors, patent attorneys, nurses, librarians, and the like.[3]

In consequence of these developments, there appeared a growing occupational self-consciousness among these and various other personal and service occupations, and in vocations bordering upon traditional or established professions. Two not-unrelated models of association commended themselves: professional and trade. The former was exemplified by the organizations of medical practitioners and lawyers; the latter, although less distinct in form, functioned basically to define and help attain the interests of businessmen.

While the ends of these forms of collective association were not necessarily opposed, neither were they in any sense identical. Professional associations sought not only to formulate standards, control membership, and to enforce an inspectional system, but most of all, to assure their respective clientele of the high personal character and the good moral standards of their members.

While seeking somewhat allied goals in many ways, trade associations subscribed to the proposition that the buyer-seller, or market, relationship, is impersonal and calls for an awareness of both parties of values given and received. The trade association thus turned its attention primarily to the material interests of its special membership. Other matters, such as standards of character and the adequacy of training, were held as definitely secondary in nature.

In those vocations where personal service was emphasized, it was a natural occurrence for associational activities to look to the model of the professions; for vocations involving merchandising transactions, on the other hand, the trade association offered the greatest potential.

As this chapter will later explain, in the case of 19th-century funeral direction, neither of these two associational models commended itself forcefully to the exclusion of the other. Also, to create further complexity, the funeral establishments themselves were often patterned after the guilds, with master, journeyman and apprentice relationships featuring their internal personnel organization.

To assist associations — particularly those of a professional and semi-professional nature — to attain their ends, two instruments have been available. The first is the use of educational prerequisites and training institutions to indoctrinate new recruits into the professions. The system of educational requirements has been used by the occupation to control the supply of new members.

The Associational Impulse

The second, described below, is the regulatory system developed by the state as an outgrowth of its police powers. Systems of this type generally are incorporated into small bodies or boards, which the law empowers to set standards for admission to practice, to license, to establish codes, and, in these and other ways, to exert a significant measure of control over certain vocations.

Internally, the primary method for defining the vocation-wide relationships of the professional practitioner with others in his or her field, as well as with the community, has been the ethical code of the profession. The licensing system marks the next step toward protection of professional status by giving legal status to the codes of ethics and by establishing a legal register of "qualified" practitioners.[4]

Until the Civil War, established professions could scarcely be termed "organized" in terms of associational structure. Moreover, at that time in the service vocations and quasi-professions, associational activities were virtually nil. During the remainder of the 19th century, state, local and national associations representing a wide range of vocations with professional aspirations formed, and, as a matter of immediate concern, pressed for the passage of state licensing statutes.

By 1900, of 38 professional and technical vocations, 21 had been touched by at least one piece of statutory legislation, with a total of nearly 200 statutes passed since 1870.[5]

In the first quarter of the 20th century, occupational licensing reached its peak. Since then, with the rules fairly well set, the rate of enacting new legislation has naturally declined, although the number of different occupations licensed by one or more states continues to increase.[6]

Of the 200 pieces of legislation mentioned above, at least 19 dealt with the funeral director and embalmer, since that same number of states had passed laws licensing one or the other of these occupations by 1900.

Although the subject of licensing and state regulation of funeral direction and embalming will arise later in this chapter, with emphasis on the latter, it suffices here to point out that 1875-1900 marked a period of tremendous growth for professional and trade associations, and that the impulse to professionalize seems to have diffused rapidly through many occupations whose earlier status was something less than that shared by such established professions as law, medicine and the ministry.

Such, then, is a portion of the backdrop of social and economic forces that have impinged upon the groping efforts of undertakers attempting to rise above the traditional status of providers of funeral paraphernalia and factotums of burial.

One other set of broad social factors concerning socio-cultural movements needs to be explored, however, before the specific associational efforts and gestures of these individuals can be taken up directly. Two, in particular, helped shape this associational development: the general public-health movement, and the specific movement in America for burial reform and the cremation of the dead.

Socio-Cultural Movements — The General Public-Health Movement: The general awakening in social reform, humanitarianism and philanthropy of the mid-19th century had its basis in the cardinal tenet of the dignity and worth of human beings. Unique by virtue of a capacity for rational thought, men and women can discover the natural order of things and the laws that govern their behavior. Having discovered these laws, individuals can then initiate action calculated to better themselves and their society. Armed with such knowledge, when necessary, he or she can reorganize political and social institutions with the goal of creating the kind of society that will best realize the worth of all people.

This was the underlying political philosophy for late-19th-century social reform, and it was supported by religious philosophies of disinterested benevolence that turned the mind toward society and away from introspection and concern with self.

It was also supported, albeit in less philosophical fashion, by the exigencies that made themselves drastically felt as America experienced rapid industrial growth, a flood of immigrants, the rise of cities, and the breakdown of customary modes of behavior during this period. In default of clear-cut and universally accepted, traditional rules for handling them, behavior problems were solved by everyday, catch-as-catch-can methods, i.e., pragmatically, with little thought beyond just making the best of the immediate situation.

Yet, the social problems attending the burgeoning of a new industrial society called for more than a simple, pragmatic approach. Themes for organizing human endeavor and responses in terms of large problem-areas emerged at this time. One of the more significant of these, in terms of its relevance to American funeral directing, is the general social movement for the betterment of the nation's health by the use, primarily, of preventive sanitation measures.

The public-health movement in America was formally launched in 1850 with the publication of the "Report of the Massachusetts Sanitary Commission." This body recommended the establishment of a system of sanitary police, with state and local health departments, and a careful collection and analysis of vital statistics. No effective action was taken upon this report until 1869, however, when the Massachusetts State Board of Health, the first of its kind in the nation, was established.

By 1878, 16 other states had set up similar boards, and by 1900, the total had swelled to 30. (It will be noted later that the several associations of funeral directors brought strong pressures to bear for the establishment of such state boards of health and for the setting, within their framework, of special boards to examine and license the members of their own occupational group.)

Since 1789, when John Adams, the second U.S. president, began his second annual message to Congress with a reference to the yellow fever pestilence, urging passage of federal laws to promote the health of persons in the several states, the federal government has been aware of the need for national health legislation.

Quarantine legislation demanded the attention of presidents Jefferson and Monroe. Between 1837 and 1853, presidents Martin Van Buren, John Tyler and Franklin Pierce sent messages to Congress regarding plans and sites for marine hospitals.[7]

Moreover, as U.S. president, both Andrew Johnson and Ulysses S. Grant transmitted to Congress papers relative to an international conference on cholera. Recognizing the importance of quarantine to control the epidemics of cholera and yellow fever that plagued the country, President Rutherford B. Hayes recommended to Congress in 1878 that the use of quarantine should be brought under federal jurisdiction. In April of that year, a weak quarantine law was passed.

Shortly afterward, following a severe epidemic of yellow fever, Congress established a National Board of Health, with a term of four years. Although this board did not become a continuing part of the federal government, the Marine Hospital Service, which succeeded it, grew into the United States Public Health Service. Today, this organization is the principal, but not the only, health agency of the federal government.[8]

At the same time, state governments continued to rely upon their own health organizations in meeting problems of epidemics and plagues. Despite their independent efforts, however, it became increasingly evident that the magnitude of some of these health emergencies was too great for individual states to meet. When the need for federal jurisdiction over matters of quarantine became apparent, the Quarantine Act was passed by Congress in 1893, and amended in 1901. This act forms the basis for present federal authority in this field.

But there were other pressures and forces coalescing to bring public attention, effort and organized action to the matter of the nation's health. Cities such as New York City had been the scene of citizens' organizations or "Sanitary Associations," which pledged to bring under municipal control the sanitation problems that sorely beset them. The "Metropolitan Health Bill," passed by the state of New York, created a Metropolitan Board that was not subject to judicial review. It was submitted to the legislature in 1866, just as cholera was raging in Europe and seemed certain to visit American shores. With its passage, New York was given the most comprehensive and powerful piece of state sanitary legislation in the country.

From the religious leaders of the country came added pressures for better health measures in the name of sanitary reform. Among the New England clergy, literally a score of those best known preached a gospel of health and sanitation. Their words and work were given concrete expression in their efforts during the Civil War, particularly with the Sanitary Commission, a great philanthropic movement organized during the Civil War by Dr. Henry Bellows, minister of the All Soul's Church in New York City.[9]

This commission rendered innumerable services to men in the Armed Forces of the North, and to their dependents. It set better mental and physical health as its great aim and, to promote these, it launched a campaign of education in personal health and spiritual guidance. Most of the influential positions in this organization were held by ministers or prominent laypeople. Through its activities, it set a precedent by the end of the war for both its wide-reaching efforts to better the nation's health, and the spirit in which these social-reform efforts were carried forth.

From this concern with the public health in general, the problem of the disposal of the dead and the menace of the overcrowded urban graveyard emerges as an area of specific focus for those with a social and reformist bent.

Socio-Cultural Movements — The Specific Movement for the Cremation of the Dead: Although articles appeared in American journals and newspapers on the subject of burial reform as early as 1737, when the *Boston Post* published a letter protesting the extravagance in dress and gift-giving at funerals (*see Chapter 5, Figure 2*), and, from time to time (as examined in earlier chapters), legislative bodies in the American Colonies had acted to restrict funeral expenses, the first organization to seek a specific program of funeral reform precipitated out of a movement to introduce cremation of the dead into American funeral customs.

In New York in 1873, the subject was first discussed at occasional assemblages, but no organization was set up. There was interest, however, among physicians and sanitarians and, by 1876, nine articles had been written on the subject — seven of them from the pens of men of medicine and health.[10]

In 1876, Dr. F. Julius LeMoyne, prominent Washington, Pennsylvania, physician, erected in his hometown America's first crematory, constructed primarily for the incineration of his own body and those of his friends. In the same year, the body of Baron de Palm, eccentric elderly German theosophist, was the first cremated in a building dedicated solely to that purpose.

During the next several years, other cremations were performed for the remains of some rather prominent persons, including the wife of the well-known Cincinnati phonographer Ben Pitman, brother of Sir Isaac Pitman, inventor of a phonographic (shorthand) system; and for the founder, Dr. LeMoyne, as well. Quite a variety of religious beliefs held by those cremated is noted, including Presbyterian, freethinker, theosophist, Swedenborgian, and Lutheran.

Augustus Cobb, early historian of cremation, notes the blossoming of collective action for cremation in the early 1880s:

> Between 1881 and 1885 a number of cremation societies were organized in different cities in the United States, and many lectures were delivered, and pamphlets and articles published advocating the reform. Efforts made during the preceding years had met with very little success, and it was only during the years above that a general popular interest became manifest. The work by the different societies was almost entirely educational. The object of all of them was about the same. As expressed in the by-laws of the New York Cremation Society, it was "to disseminate sound and enlightened views with respect to the incineration of the dead; to advocate and promote, in every proper and legitimate way, the substitution of this method for burial; and to advance the public good for affording facilities for carrying cremation into operation." The steady, unobtrusive work of these societies was destined to produce good results, although as late as the spring of 1884, there was but one crematory in the entire country.[11]

The New York Cremation Society was established in 1881, and, as a separate but complementary unit, the United States Cremation Company was organized to build and operate a crematory (although it was not until 1885 that the latter went into operation at Fresh Pond, Long Island). Meanwhile, a second cremation retort had made its appearance in Lancaster, Pennsylvania, built by Dr. M.L. Davis with the support of the cremation-minded citizens of that town.

As the number of crematories increased, so did the number of cremations. Between 1876 and 1884, there were 41 cremations in America; in the next five years, there were 731; the total number of cremations for the five years preceding 1894 was 2,898; in 1899, the five-year total was 7,197; and, with the addition of the year 1900, the grand total for the 15 years was 13,281.[12]

Although the rate of increase obviously was rapid, the percentage of cremations to total deaths did not reach one percent before the turn of the century. By this point, however, 24 crematories were operating in 15 different states, including California, where retorts had been established in both Los Angeles and San Francisco.

Meanwhile, the same number of cremation societies had sprung into existence, with notable organizations in New York City; Buffalo, New York; Lancaster, Pennsylvania, where, in 1886, the local founder of the society, Dr. M.L. Davis, edited and published the first cremation journal, *The Modern Crematist*; San Francisco, California; Davenport, Iowa; Detroit, Michigan; Milwaukee, Wisconsin; Philadelphia, Pennsylvania; Boston, Massachusetts; and New Orleans, Louisiana.

The personnel making up these societies were of several distinct sorts. In many larger cities, German ethnic groups established among themselves burial "assurance" societies, and some of these groups, whose cultural history included acceptance of "flame burial" as a legitimate mode of disposal of the dead, adopted the practice of cremation. In San Francisco, the cremation society was originated by a group of German freethinkers. In New England, Protestant clergymen, basically interested in burial reforms, organized several cremation societies. A third major supporting group was composed largely of members of the medical profession and sanitarians.

It is interesting to note the increasing number of articles written on the subject during the last 25 years of the 19th century, with the peak reached in 1884-1889, when 61 pieces of literature appeared. More than half of these (35) were written by men of the medical, public-health and sanitation professions. During the 1904-1908 period, by contrast, the figure had dropped to four.

While leadership for a burial-reform movement in the east was scattered, among New England leaders, those most active were the Rev. John Storer Cobb; Rev. Paul R. Frothingham; and Charles W. Eliot, president of Harvard. In 1874 in New York, the Rev. O.B. Frothingham was the first to preach on the subject of cremation. In his 28-page sermon on "The Disposal of Our Dead" from the religious-rationalist approach, he strongly advocated cremation, protesting that, "Its significance is in its simple humanity."[13]

Two decades later, in 1894, Bishop Henry C. Potter organized the Burial Reform Association of New York.

Dr. Hugo Erichsen, indefatigable cremation enthusiast, provided the spark of leadership that eventually led to the formation of the Cremation Society of America in 1913. From 1876, when, at age 16, he read accounts of the first American cremation, until his death in 1942, he devoted much of his time and energies to the propagation of cremation as an instrument of social and sanitary reform.

It was Erichsen's idea to form a national association that embraced all who favored cremation, and in 1886, he organized one of the Midwest's first state cremation associations in Detroit, Michigan. But it was not until 1913 that his dream of a national association was realized. At the initial meeting that year of the Cremation Association of America (CAA) on August 27-28 in Detroit, the majority of attendees were operators of the 40-odd crematories in the country under business management, or their representatives.

Under such sponsorship, the question of burial reform received scant consideration. When Erichsen was elected the first CAA president at this meeting, however, his initial remarks to the fledgling organization still emphasized reform:

> Every crematist must be a missionary for the cause, and embrace every suitable occasion to spread its gospel, the glad tidings of a more sanitary and more aesthetic method of disposing of our beloved dead.[14]

But Erichsen was not speaking to his audience but instead to the memory of a social-reform movement that was already rapidly changing. Although cremation was an integral part of the "burial-reform" movement in the latter part of the 19th century, by the time a national organization was formed, the "reform" elements were a definite minority.

19TH-CENTURY ASSOCIATIONAL DEVELOPMENT AMONG FUNERAL DIRECTORS

As indicated in earlier chapters, the close of the 19th century witnessed major changes in the role and function of the undertaker. From an enterprising furnisher of goods, paraphernalia and, occasionally, the rudiments of personal "services," along with items of merchandise, the undertaker moved in the direction of becoming a seller of personal services. This new role involved undertakers closely with the bereaved, whom they now perceived as distraught human beings rather than customers for wares.

In carrying out this new role, undertakers had to exercise not only technical skills in preparing the bodies of the dead, but also administrative skills in the direction and organization of funeral proceedings, and logistic skills in arranging the order and sequence in the transport of both the living and the dead.

Beyond this enrichment of function, 19th-century funeral directing had another major achievement to its credit: the development of strong occupational groups at local, state and national levels. Bear in mind that funeral directors, as well as members of other occupations that were becoming self-conscious and occupationally mobile at the time, had before them the two associational models — trade and profession — from which to choose.

Origins and Early Developments: Insofar as available records indicate, the first formal organization of undertakers occurred in Pennsylvania when the Undertakers' Mutual Protective Association of Philadelphia formed in January 1864. This group adopted a constitution that, among other provisions, called for the establishment of a "Black Book, to keep a register of objectionable and delinquent customers, for use and inspection of members only..."[15] (*See Plate 65*.)

Four years later, Chicago undertakers organized and sustained a city association that functioned in a much broader capacity than the Philadelphia group.

It is probable that in most major cities from 1865-1880, undertakers founded associations for mutual protection, dispensing information and setting preliminary operation standards for their trade.

In New York City at this time, church sextons generally dominated undertaking. Thus, one of the first organizations of undertakers there was designed primarily to harmonize the relations between sexton-undertakers and those who more-or-less made undertaking a full-time occupational pursuit.

PLATE 65

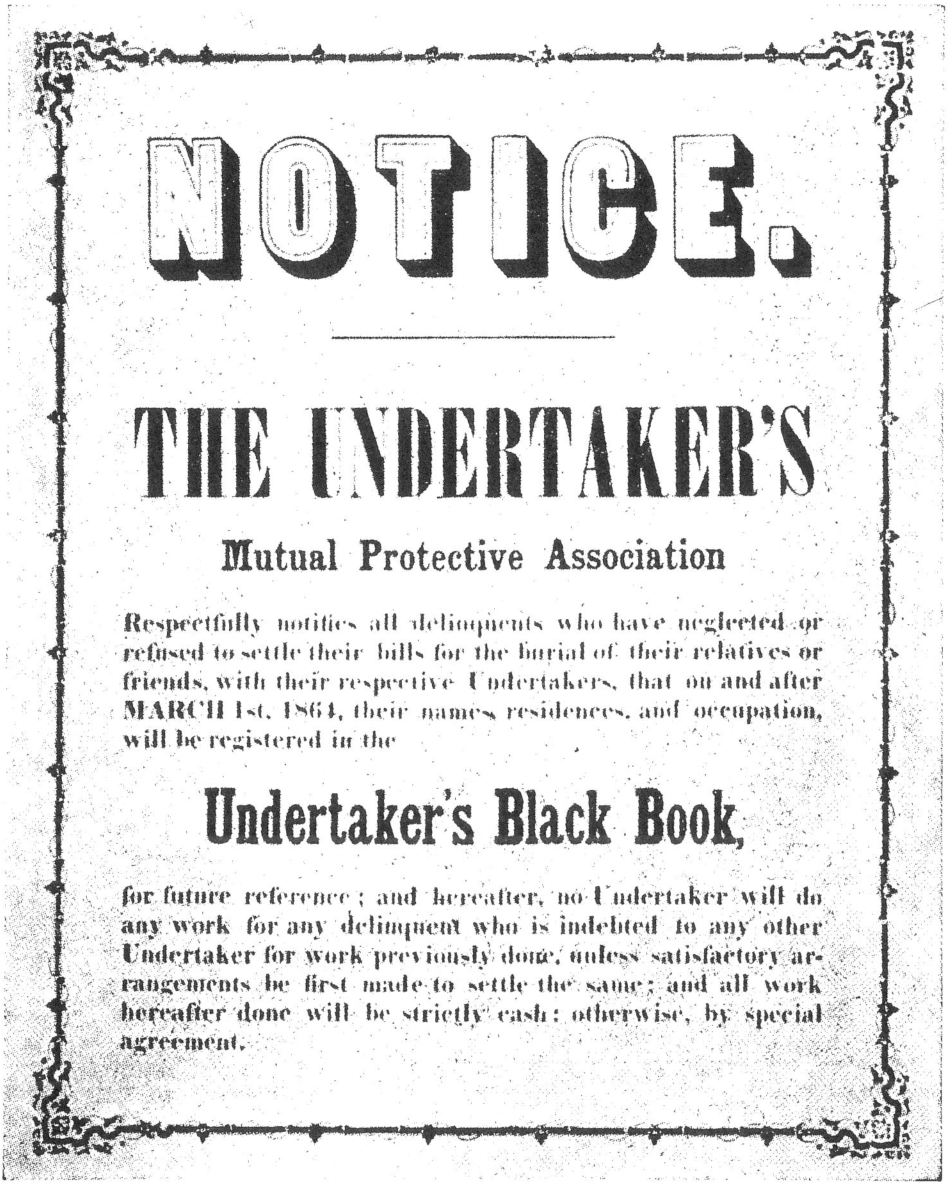

NOTICE.

THE UNDERTAKER'S
Mutual Protective Association

Respectfully notifies all delinquents who have neglected or refused to settle their bills for the burial of their relatives or friends, with their respective Undertakers, that on and after MARCH 1st, 1864, their names, residences, and occupation, will be registered in the

Undertaker's Black Book,

for future reference; and hereafter, no Undertaker will do any work for any delinquent who is indebted to any other Undertaker for work previously done, unless satisfactory arrangements be first made to settle the same; and all work hereafter done will be strictly cash; otherwise, by special agreement.

65. "Black Book" Notice of Early Philadelphia Undertakers Association.

While these early local organizations performed many useful services, association on a wider scale commended itself to many undertakers, and to the editors of the trade journals, as well.

The role of the latter is stressed (and possibly overstressed) by an early funeral director-historian, George L. Thomas of Milwaukee, Wisconsin. In an address at the 28th annual convention of the National Funeral Directors Association, Thomas stated:

> The beginning of the association movement in the undertaking and embalming profession dates back to 1879; and the first faint inklings of a desire for united efforts on the part of those engaged in caring for the dead were apparent in the columns of trade journals, which constituted a definite medium through which the voices of all who were anxious for better things might be heard. The trade journal was undoubtedly the alma mater of the association movement, and due honor and credit must in every history be given to Albert H. Nirdlinger and Thomas Gliddon (editors of *The Casket*), who early recognized the value of associated effort in other lines, and who, always having the best interests of our profession at heart, fostered and encouraged the early growth of the association movement.[16]

In considering the various forces affecting undertakers of the time and motivating the impulse to form associations, it would be fairer to state that the progress of association was certainly accelerated by the actions Thomas credits to the trade journals, which are discussed at some length later in this chapter, and that the point of their being used as a medium for the expression of opinion of practicing undertakers is well taken.

But the associational impulse came from leaders among the funeral directors themselves. An instance of such initiative developing within the occupational group is found in a letter in which William J. Camp of Covington, Kentucky, proposed a "Southern Undertakers' Union." In response to his proposal, many favorable letters reached Camp.

After reading an article on the "Etiquette of Undertakers" written for *The Casket* by Silvanus Hawley of Wyoming, New York, Camp repeated his proposal, adding his hope that "at no distant day would there be organized a grand undertakers' union upon plans similar to those of the 'Knight of Honor' or 'The Ancient Order of United Workmen.'"[17]

Although the idea of a fraternal, benevolent and insurance organization did not fit the undertaking trade, the proposal was not without some effect because it led Nirdlinger and Gliddon to editorialize: "The desire for a more satisfactory understanding between the profession in various towns and cities should promote an immediate convention, even though it should impress those of only a small territory. Who will lead in this movement and carry it to success?"

At this moment, leadership among undertakers themselves seemed to be in the hands of Hawley, who perspicaciously pointed to the need for the formation of legitimate associations, "such as are for the improvement and protection of the interests of any profession or trade." These, he maintained, "are good and worthy... whilst the clan or league for selfish ends is reprehensible..."[18]

Hawley then suggested communicating with profession representatives in the hope that a favorable response would warrant holding a national convention in the middle of August 1879.

The next six months found the editorial pages of *The Casket* filled with comments on this proposal, including many letters written by undertakers from various states pointing out the obvious need for such a convention. Despite this strong support, the plan for a national organization at this time never reached the point of actuality, and it remained for the state groups to form their own organizations first before a coast-to-coast organization could be launched.

In November 1879, Allen Durfee, well-known Grand Rapids, Michigan, undertaker and compounder of embalming fluid, inserted a circular letter in *The Casket* asking fellow undertakers in the state for their opinion on the possibility of holding a "State Convention of Undertakers at some central point, say Grand Rapids, Jackson, or Lansing, for the purpose of forming an Undertakers' State Association, which the rapid advancement in the science of undertaking seems to demand."

Response was immediate and so favorable that an *ad hoc* committee composed of Durfee, E.A. Tompkins, C.A. Conklin, Charles L. Benjamin, T.H. Roberts, and Sammons and Quincy, all prominent Michigan undertakers, was successful in arranging the first state convention of undertakers at Jackson, Michigan, January 14, 1880.

In his opening address, Thomas Gliddon, editor of *The Casket*, who was invited to help with organizational matters, recommended the appointment of several committees. One of these was to look to the formation of a permanent organization; another to draw up and submit resolutions; and a third to gather, edit and publish the convention proceedings, disseminate information regarding professional duties, agree on rules to govern ethical advertising, indicate a policy to be applied to distributing price lists, and finally memorialize (*sic*) the legislature.

Durfee, later elected the first president, outlined the possibilities of the gathering and presented arguments for a permanent association. Moreover, he hoped that, from the state association, there might be born a national organization "as broad as the United States and as imperishable as our national union."[19]

His words were prophetic, and the Michigan association served not only as a prototype for future state organizations, but, in many respects, for the national association, still two years from its birth.

In the preamble of the Michigan constitution, the models of both trade and professional organizations were accepted as undertakers pledged to form "into an association for the purpose of mutually disseminating the most correct principles of business management, the best methods of protecting our own interests in professional practice, and the general good of all recognized legitimate undertakers."[20]

The year 1881 was prolific in the formation of associations. Iowa, under the leadership of W.P. Hohenschuh of Iowa City, later to become an authority in the field of funeral directing and mortuary education, organized early in that year; Indiana, led by S.R. Lippincott of Richmond, was next; then Ohio, with John Sharer of Alliance playing an active role. Before the year was out, undertakers had further organized state associations in Wisconsin and Illinois. California followed suit the next year, along with Kentucky, Missouri, Nebraska and Pennsylvania. Georgia, Kansas and Minnesota made abortive attempts at organization at this time, as well.

By the middle of 1882, even while state organizations were rapidly forming, leaders of the several groups were becoming increasingly conscious of the need for a national organization. The matter emerged from discussion into action when, in January 1882, at the insistence of President Durfee, the Michigan association passed a resolution stating:

> ...the time has come for the calling of a National Convention, for the purpose of forming a National Association, and the opportune time would be the third week in June next, and the place in the City of Rochester, in connection with the New York State Funeral Directors' annual meeting, and the National Fair of Funeral Goods, which is to be held there at the same time, and that the association appoint three delegates, with three alternates, whose necessary travelling expenses shall be borne by this association.[21]

This call was circulated among the various states, and 105 undertakers, many of them leaders in their state associations, signed. Thomas Gliddon volunteered as secretary, pro tem.

The next issue of *The Casket* contained, in large headlines, the following announcement:

1882

THE DAWN OF PROGRESS

NATIONAL FUNEREAL INDUSTRIAL EXPOSITION

Commingling of Inventors, Manufacturers and Professionals

A NATIONAL MEETING

Special Session of all the Embalming Experts

TWELVE PRACTICAL LECTURES

And Operating Lessons in a Special Amphitheater,

Under the immediate charge of

AUGUSTE RENOUARD, at Rochester, N.Y.

Beginning Monday, June 20th and continuing six days

To close with a

Grand Complimentary Banquet at Niagara Falls,

ON SATURDAY, JUNE 24.

Instruction, Recreation, and a Great Reunion

On June 22, 1882, 241 persons appeared at the City Hall of Rochester, were welcomed by the mayor, and addressed briefly by Durfee. He reviewed the steps that led to the calling of the convention, remarking significantly: "The desire for a more rapid educational improvement, led me to believe that through meetings and associations much good might be accomplished, which could not be obtained in any other way."

Robert Atkins of Buffalo, New York, was elected temporary chairman, and the business of organizing the association got under way.

Three significant events took place at this first national convention. First, after rather heated discussion, it was decided that all undertakers present were entitled to votes in the convention, but that, in future conventions, three delegates only from each state were to have a voice.

Opposition to this procedure came heaviest from the delegates of the Chicago Association — a strong city organization that had been continuously operating longer than any other association, state or city. This decision set a pattern for the national association that, in effect, meant that it should function as a parent organization for state associations, and that, henceforth, organization at the state level would necessarily take precedence over organizations at the local level among undertakers in states not yet featured by such associations.

A second development that had significant consequences, not so much for direct action as for the development of a new self-conception by undertakers, was the decision to name the organization "The Funeral Directors' National Association of The United States" (later the National Funeral Directors Association, or NFDA).

This decision was reached only after lively argument, with many present favoring the traditional term "undertaker," and a few the less-familiar, less-frequently used "funeral manager." One delegate, Thomas Blood, had been advertising his services as a "mortorion," but he did not suggest this term as an associational title. No one offered the term "mortician" — later to come into currency as an alternative to "undertaker" and "funeral director." The emphasis in the title of the national organization was on funeral directing and, henceforth, the use of the designation "funeral director" was, as defined by the association, a mark of progress.[22]

The third feature that marked the first NFDA convention was the close relationship manifested between the national convention and the manufacturers of morticians' goods. A precedent was set at this meeting when James Cunningham, Son & Co.; Chappel, Chase, Maxwell & Co.; Stein Mfg. Co.; Egyptian Embalming Co.; and the editors of *The Casket* gave a complimentary banquet jointly.

The meetings of the New York State Funeral Directors Association, held simultaneously with the National Fair for Funeral Goods, likewise tended to make the exposition of merchandise and paraphernalia integrally a part of the national meetings, thus underscoring their associational aspects.

Pressures, Interests and Motives: While in no sense detracting from the important role played by the trade journals in fostering associational activities among funeral directors, it should be noted that the social and economic pressures generating in and around the occupation were such that some form of collective action was almost inevitable.

As indicated at the start of this chapter, the late-19th century was a period marked by a proliferation and tremendous expansion of associations, both trade and professional, or semi-professional. The associational impulse was strong and growing. Physicians and surgeons, pharmacists, civil engineers, architects, dentists and veterinarians had all organized their national societies and associations before 1870, and other similar groups were in the process of formation at the time.

In closer relation to the subject at hand, one notes that, before 1880, there had been formed the Carriage Builders' National Association; the Coffin Manufacturers' Association of the East and West; the National Burial Case Association (later referred to by funeral directors as the "Manufacturers' Association"); as well as the National Association of General Baggage Agents — whose importance will be discussed later.

During the decade following, the list grows to include the Eastern Burial Case Association; the National Cloth Casket Association; the Metallic Burial Case Association; the New England Burial Case Association; the Casket Hardware Manufacturers' Association; the American Association of Cemetery Superintendents; and the Casket Salemen's Protective Association.

A further impetus to group action, and therefore organization, developed out of the fact that other associations and agencies were looking to funeral directors for spokesmen or representatives with whom to transact necessary business on a state or national level. The problem of the transportation of the dead is typical. This problem reached a crisis during the Civil War, demanding general regulations when it became necessary to inspect trains at depots for improperly embalmed bodies, broken shipping cases, bodies bearing the germs of infectious diseases and the like.

The powers of the National Board of Health severely restricted, regulation of the transportation of the dead fell to states and smaller governmental agencies. One exasperated funeral director describes the problem caused by the chaos of uncodified and non-articulatory rules and regulations:

> By the laws of one city the certificate of death is pasted on the coffin or case, there to remain till its destination is reached; but before that, they are stopped just outside of another city with the order to detach it and bring it to their health office, and in return they will issue one. With this a State is traversed, and reaching a third city in the evening, they find though the entrance is easy, exit is denied until a third certificate is obtained, and as it is late there is nothing to do but remain all night, breaking all connections and involving perhaps from twelve to twenty-four hours' delay.[23]

It should be stressed that when railroad officials naturally went to funeral directors for advice concerning the proper methods of handling and shipping dead bodies, they wanted (and their want created a need among funeral directors) a single, collectively made answer that would provide them with a uniform or standard practice. To supply such answer, it was necessary that the funeral-directing occupation itself should be organized to a point where agreement could be reached and declared. To repeat: until such single answer was made, and practice set up nationally in accord with it, funeral directors themselves experienced difficulty in shipping bodies.

While easy to exaggerate the influence of these, and similar, needs upon the development of the associational impulse among funeral directors, the fact remains that, to some extent, occupational associations tend to create situations calling for other occupational associations, although far more compelling than these collective factors were two basic motivating forces impelling funeral directors into associational action. One was the need to protect themselves from excessive, and therefore harmful, competition from within their own ranks, as well as from destructive business practices by manufacturers and jobbers. The other was the urge to bring a sense of professionalism to what had formerly been, for many, a mere trade or sideline.

The need for protection from unfair, albeit legal, competition within the occupation itself was quite evident. Protection was especially needed by funeral directors in Eastern and Midwestern states, where nearly any merchant who sold furniture could also include a line of caskets in its wares, thus threatening the existence of recognized establishments.

In 1888, the first for which statistics are reliable, for every funeral director (representing almost every funeral establishment), there were about 4,700 inhabitants. In the above-mentioned Eastern and Midwestern states, however, the proportion was smaller. Thus, in New York, the ratio was one funeral director for every 3,200 persons; in Vermont, 1 per 2,000; Pennsylvania, 1 per 3,000; Michigan, 1 per 3,800; and Illinois, 1 per 3,600.[24]

Despite the fact that death rates were about twice as high as at present, infant mortality was greater.

Moreover, while the gross average of deaths per funeral director countrywide was about 87, for states in which the first state associations were formed, the figure was lower. Michigan had about 77 deaths per funeral director; New York, about 70; and Pennsylvania, about 60. In these areas, competition was keen from fellow undertakers, the majority of which (nearly 80% of the total number of establishments) were engaged in combination operations in which the sale of coffins and caskets was a sideline.

Thus, from within the occupation, the established funeral director with aspirations toward becoming an independent seller of personal services and funeral merchandise exclusively — apart from any ideas about professionalism — frequently found the going rough. That irresponsible, marginal or unsound competition might have kept within the law, as it then existed, probably offered small consolation to the responsible operator facing it.

From without, the pressures, threats and forces were enough to provide ample material for a speech delivered in 1884 before the Illinois association (and later read to the national association), in which the burden of the argument was that the national association must take immediate steps "in regard to the multitude of jobbers, drummers, quack professors, professional embalmers, or more properly speaking, embalming-fluid fiends, and the thousand and one other frauds that hang on to and suck the very life blood out of this profession."

The practice of "jobbing" lots of caskets to the funeral director, ostensibly to permit him to buy more economically in light of larger purchases, was an outgrowth of conditions in the casket manufacturing industry itself. In 1888, although there were about 700 coffin shops and casket manufacturing houses, fewer than 175 of these were companies of any considerable size, and perhaps some two dozen were what might be called large-scale producing units.

Moreover, fewer than half of those in existence could easily have supplied the nation's funeral directors with a sufficient number of good burial receptacles. Yet, with the field so crowded, it was almost inevitable that competition would produce less than the best product. Often, cheap, shoddy, competitively priced coffins and caskets were literally dumped upon the funeral director.

Curiously enough, because of the necessity of maintaining standards, the larger companies, despite their ability to mass-produce units, could not undersell and drive out the smaller, uneconomically organized coffin shops. The latter, through the "jobbing" system of sending out high pressure "drummers," could either cut prices to obtain an account, or would try to induce anyone with the desire to become an undertaker to lay in a stock of coffins "on consignment."

Thus, one of the most important *trade* problems of the funeral director of the late-19th century was protection against the kind of competition that would eventually ruin whatever community goodwill and social acceptance already had earned.

In 1888, even in the more densely populated areas, the ratio of single-purpose to combination establishments was scarcely better than one to five. Pennsylvania, for instance, had about 23% of its funeral directors operating independently of any other business; Georgia, 21%; Vermont, 24%; and Illinois, about 25%.

Of all the funeral directors in the country in 1888, about 23% held membership in the National Funeral Directors Association. Many in combination businesses did not belong to funeral director groups because, to them, the funeral portion of their work was only a sideline.

While many of these part-time operators were individuals of excellent business and personal character, and represented a transitional stage in the emergence of a trade into a profession, the degree of commercialization at which a few combination undertakers occasionally operated is illustrated by the advertisement reprinted from a country newspaper "in one of the Middle States" by *The Casket* in 1879:

DUTCH CHARLEY
MEANS BUSINESS.

IF YOU WANT TO STOP AT A GOOD HOTEL, go to the Bodman House, at Dutch Charley's.

IF YOU WANT A GOOD METALLIC COFFIN, go to Dutch Charley.

IF YOU WANT A WOODEN COFFIN, GO to Dutch Charley.

IF YOU WANT YOUR HOUSE INSURED, go to Dutch Charley.

IF YOU WANT A GOOD DRINK OF BOURban Whiskey, go to Dutch Charley.

IF YOU WANT A GOOD GLASS OF LAGER Beer, go to Dutch Charley.

IF YOU WANT TO BUY WESTERN LAND, go to Dutch Charley.

IF YOU WANT TO BUY A CHEAP TICKET to California, go to Dutch Charley.

IF YOU WANT TO BUY CHEAP FURNIture, go to Dutch Charley.

IF YOU WANT YOUR PICTURE FRAMED, go to Dutch Charley.

IF YOU WANT A JUSTICE OF THE PEACE, go to Dutch Charley.

Figure 33. The Many Businesses of Dutch Charley.

Another major factor motivating funeral directors to organize into an association was the desire on the part of certain outstanding and farsighted members to professionalize their occupation, thus gaining for it, and for themselves as well, a higher degree of social estimation.

During a period when sanitary reform and the general social movement embracing public health had gained widespread attention — and, with this interest reinforced by terrible epidemics and plagues — many funeral directors found it natural to associate their functions with those of the sanitarian. This concept seems to have been present at the very inception of the national association, at least among the acknowledged leaders of the group and, more or less, has been incorporated into the self-conceptions of funeral directors ever since.

Again, in arrogating to themselves the function of embalming, funeral directors were inevitably drawn into the company of the surgeon, the physician and the physiologist. At first, physicians were solely the ones to perform embalming. Later, as physicians and physiologists were drawn into closer association while funeral directors learned embalming skills and techniques, the practitioners of medical and biological science became the instructors, if not the founders, of schools of embalming. Thus, the association between the two continued.

Even today, due to the demands of modern schools of mortuary science for cadavers, the tendency continues for them to be located near medical centers. In many cases, physiologists, pathologists and other categories of medical scientists are brought into the schools as instructors.

It seems a fair statement, then, that the association of funeral directors with members of the medical profession, sanitarians and public-health officials tended to contribute toward the development of the self-image of the progressive funeral director of the late-19th century as a sanitarian. The funeral director's role as "sanitary embalmer," during a period when epidemics and plagues had the whole society fearful, conceivably enhanced the public estimation of this work and, consequently, that of practitioners.

This image, it should be remarked, like the image in other professional groups, was not equally appropriated to themselves by all funeral directors. As with other occupations, all funeral directors did not share an equal sense of the high social importance of the round of tasks, nor were they equally prepared to make the personal sacrifices needed to translate the high ideal into a daily way of working.

The terms "professional" and "profession" were seized upon at the first national association meeting and were used repeatedly. As will be pointed later, the leadership of the association during the period was highly dedicated to the proposition that a program of action was essential to bring professional status to funeral directors, and that words alone would not suffice.

Nowhere is this better shown, perhaps, than in the 1886 presidential address of Hudson Samson, one of the most influential and, incidentally, best educated of the leaders of the association. In blueprinting future policy, he noted the failures of the past before reiterating some suggestions that bore fruit in succeeding decades:

> We have to decide whether we will follow in the wake of the broom makers', box and basket-makers', bakers',... and butchers' associations. (They)... are intended to benefit men who work at manual labor; they resort to the boycott and the strike to carry their cause through, right or wrong. I will mention a few who take a different view of the realities of citizenship: the members of National, State, County, and City Medical Societies... the legal profession... clergymen... educators and Civil and Mining Engineers (have societies which)... assist one another across the hard places.
>
> I would advise (funeral directors)... to convince our state Board of Health of the necessity of having a law passed that will compel all who have not been a certain number of years serving as Funeral Directors to pass an examination, and to serve a given time as an apprentice. I would have a Board of Examination appointed by the Governor whose duty it shall be to determine the fitness of applicants for license to serve as Funeral Director: the Board should make such arrangements

with the County Boards of Health as will best serve the purpose of keeping a complete register of all Funeral Directors...

I would have a law regulating the care and burial of the dead the same as there is for the practice of medicine — the same as you will find in the several States to insure the better education of practitioners in dental surgery... I would advise an active step be taken in some State to have an act passed regulating the burial of the dead and we, as a National Association, to help, aid and assist in bringing about such legislation.

Do not think that we can get the public to RECEIVE US AS PROFESSIONAL MEN by simply meeting in convention and making constitutions and by-laws, by adopting a code of ethics, or getting our State Legislature to pass an act governing the burial of the dead, or by getting the National Burial Case Association to do what will be of as much advantage to themselves as to us, guarding against funeral reform, building crematories, or having a report on our trade journals, or providing a textbook that will assist you in beating the Egyptians.

All of these are means toward the desired end. One thing that will do more to bring about a professional feeling among the Funeral Directors is for us to act and talk as though our competitors were gentlemen; if we gain professional fame it will be by us as individuals leading pure, upright, professional lives.[25]

Characteristics of Early Leadership: Among the funeral directors of the latter part of the 19th century, leadership was in the hands of fairly well-to-do and fairly well-educated middle-class individuals who leaned in the direction of creating a profession out of their trade.

A check of the social characteristics of 42 better-known morticians of the day, whose biographies appeared in *The Casket* from 1876-1880 and who played an active leadership role in associations, reveals several interesting facts: most of these men were born in America, and a preponderant number resided and operated their establishments in the Middle Atlantic and New England states.

Investigation of the occupational backgrounds of the fathers of these men indicates that, with few exceptions, they were *not* sons of practicing undertakers. Of the 42, 14 had fathers who were farmers; six, professional men; four, manufacturers and executives; and the rest, with the exception of 4 undertakers (all operating combination shops), were engaged in small businesses, skilled and unskilled trades, or clerical and sales work.[26]

Given this, by no stretch of the imagination could funeral direction be conceived of as a "family" occupation during this period, as it justifiably could in the first quarter of the 20th century.

With respect to the occupational background of the 42 directors themselves, the pattern indicates that the majority entered the trade through some traditionally related occupation, such as cabinet- or furniture-making, or through the carriage or livery business. In other words, funeral directors of the period *worked* their way into the trade and did not merely succeed their fathers. Consequently they were less likely to be rigorously bound by occupational traditions than the sons who succeeded them.

Moreover, there were, at the time, few legal and quasi-legal restrictions regulating how they could operate. It is not surprising, then, that during the period under discussion, a high degree of independence and individualism became characteristic of the occupation and its practitioners. Some of this mood has persisted into modern times.

Code of Ethics: The drive toward professional status made by state, local and national associations during the late-19th century took the form of a series of efforts, some of which — such as getting railway agencies and baggage agents to recognize their embalming techniques as standard, professional operations, and the constant, eventually successful pressure applied to state legislatures to secure licensing legislation — have already been discussed.

Other efforts to achieve professional recognition were based on the recognition of the need to develop a sense of inner cohesion or colleagueship among funeral directors; to establish a sense of responsibility; to provide formal instruction in the special skills and techniques of the occupation, along with increased backgrounds in general education; to develop lines and media of disseminating information to funeral directors themselves, their business associates, and the public; and to indoctrinate all these groups with the new concepts.

Simply talking about professionalism, however, as Hudson Samson wisely pointed out to the infant national association, would lead nowhere.

A major early step toward developing honor and colleagueship among funeral directors was taken with the establishment of a code of ethics at the third meeting of the national association in Chicago, Illinois, on October 2, 1884. About 600 words in length and patterned after other professional codes of the times, this code alternated between general statements indicating the character and occupational morality aimed at and injunctions against specific kinds of actions.

Beginning, "A funeral director, on entering the profession..." it went on to posit the necessity of obeying the law and maintaining a high standard of conduct and propriety at all times. This was imperative because (it said):

> The nature of our calling takes us to the inner circle of the families that are afflicted. Secrecy and delicacy, when required by peculiar circumstances, should be strictly observed. The obligation of secrecy extends beyond the period of our professional services. None of the privacies of personal and domestic life should ever be divulged.[27]

Advertising was dealt with in a negative vein, and, among other things, advertising in the "daily prints" was prohibited. Proper procedure and protocol was indicated, in the case of two directors being called at the same time, for instance, as well as the injunction to the profession to carry on in times of epidemic and contagious diseases.

Also outlined in this code were the correct methods for dealing with shipping and removal cases. The first code of ethics closed with this statement:

> There is, perhaps, no profession, after that of the sacred ministry, in which a high-toned morality is more imperatively necessary than that of a funeral director's. High moral principles are his only safe guide.[28]

NFDA's ethical code appeared in the appendix of all of its subsequent printed proceedings, and was also broadcast among the various trade papers and journals.

The most controversial section, as it turned out, was that dealing with advertising. Undertakers had traditionally printed and distributed private cards, handbills and, in the daily papers, invited the attention of the public to their wares. (*See Chapter 6, Plates 25 & 27*.) Although the code was reaffirmed as "law" at the 1889 Toronto meeting, it was evident that the tradition of advertising had not been erased and that, instead, some concessions to the practice eventually might have to be made since, in cities, many, if not most, funeral directors were continuing to advertise.

A related problem, foreseeable in the not-too-distant future and more difficult to make rules for and to dispose of, was the mass-operation type of funeral home, whose business was based on a large volume of cases attracted by cut-throat advertising and other highly questionable promotion methods.

These developments did not come to a focus until shortly before World War I, however. As the 19th century closed, the code of ethics remained in precisely the same form as when created and adopted by the national association in 1884.

Communication Within the Trade: In a rapidly growing country such as America during the 19th century, the expansion and proliferation of industries and businesses posed many problems of organization, not the least of which was establishing an effective system of liaison and communication among and within related vocations and businesses, and between these and the public.

For funeral directors, their dispersion, their highly fluctuating number, and their diversification complicated this problem. Nearly four-fifths were operating their establishments in combination with other businesses, or practiced undertaking as a sideline to other services offered to the public.

One of the first agents of communication to directors was the casket salesman or "drummer." Casket salesmen and jobbers covered extensive territories, competed briskly, and were not without some self-consciousness as to the out-of-the-ordinary nature of the products they were distributing.

The itinerant nature of this occupation was put to verse by "Timber Awl," an anonymous individual who composed and submitted "The Song of the Coffin Drummer" to one of the trade papers:

> From Illinois, Iowa
> Nebraska and Dakota,
> To Michigan, Wisconsin too,
> And lovely Minnesota.
> From Lake Superior's Copper mines
> Through Hoosier Indiana,
> To Mississippi's cotton field,
> and Low Louisiana,
> I furnish wooden overcoats
> To many an Undertaker;
> For Banker, beggar, one and all,
> The Butcher and the baker —
> Baker —
> Butcher and the baker.[29]

These "commercial knights of the road" could be expected to bring with them news of the trade and interesting information concerning other funeral directors. Their importance in this respect declined somewhat with the appearance of trade papers and journals dedicated to different, and often many, sectors of the field of funeral service.

In 1871, Henry E. Taylor, a funeral-goods manufacturer of New York, published the first trade paper, which he chose to call *The Undertaker*. Subtitled "A Monthly Paper Dedicated to the Interests of the Undertaker and to the Discussion of Grave (*sic*) Matters," this subtitle possibly contained only an inadvertent play on words.

Regardless, this trade paper, as well as those that came after it — reflective apparently of the desire to dispel the dismal and gloomy public image traditionally held of undertakers and the trade — followed a definite policy of "spicing up the copy" with jokes, puns and anecdotes, some connected with the subject at hand and others drawn from various sources.

The Undertaker continued under its original title only until the following year, when it was changed to *Sunnyside*. Taylor continued to publish it until 1885, at which time it passed into the hands of independent publishers, although he continued to show his interest in the enterprise by bringing news and information to the trade through its columns.

In 1876, the most pretentious morticians' trade paper of the 19th century, *The Casket*, began publication in Rochester, New York. (Some 50 years later, its publisher was to buy *Sunnyside*; henceforth the journal appeared as *Casket and Sunnyside*.)

Subsidized heavily by the Stein Patent Burial Casket Works, and James Cunningham, Son & Co., hearse and carriage builders, and subtitled "A Monthly Journal devoted to and officially treating on all subjects of vital importance to UNDERTAKERS AND KINDRED PROFESSIONS," *The Casket* was sent *gratis* to funeral directors everywhere for the first year. After that, the subscription was $1 per year.

In the "Salutatory," the editors protested the need for such a journal, noting (with some historical inaccuracy concerning the sexton as the sole progenitor of the undertaker):

> Over six thousand men are rated at this date in this country "Undertakers." From the menial obscure church-yard sexton, there has within a quarter of a century been developed a recognized professional — represented by men of means, intelligence, taste and refinement; reading and thinking men, who have elevated their profession; therefore, why should they not be represented by a Journal and control an organ devoted solely to their interests; an official authority, in which they can interchange their professional views?[30]

Indeed, such views were expressed in its pages. Moreover, one of its most significant services to the field was the publication of a long series of articles by the celebrated embalmer Auguste Renouard on all aspects of the embalmer's work, the proper conduct of the funeral, and the necessary demeanor for those aspiring to be truly professional.

One of the less "professional" services of this journal during the following years, however, was its effort to clearly establish, by editorial comment, the fact that cloth-covered burial cases and caskets need not be cheap, shoddy imitations of wood or metal. These efforts indicated that the Stein Co. could be relied upon to produce an artistically conceived, aesthetically pleasing cloth casket suitable even for the president of the United States. (In point of fact, several Stein caskets were later so used.)

Following *The Casket* in 1879 came *The Western Undertaker* (which became *The American Funeral Director*), and, in 1880, *The Shroud*, a journal edited and published independently by Richard McGowan, a colorful figure among casket salesmen, that continued long enough to be accredited in 1884, along with *The Casket*, as one of the official journals of the American Funeral Directors' National Association. The journal expired shortly thereafter but others were not long in taking its place.

The decade 1885-1895 was prolific with trade papers and journals, which appeared, ran for a few issues and then passed out of existence. By 1894, not only had *The Shroud* ceased publication, but also *The Embalmer*; *Our Paper*; *Shadyside*; *Progression* (a competitor to *The Casket*); *The Canadian Casket*; and *The National Undertaker* had all become casualties to the rough road of early trade journalism. (***See Plates 66, 67, 68 & 69***.)

The Embalmers' Monthly was a notable exception. Launched auspiciously in Sioux City, Iowa, in April 1892, it appealed directly to the embalming side of funeral service and stayed strong through the years following.

Captain A.J. Millard, the first publisher, and W.W. Harris, editor, banked on an increasingly bright future for what they saw to be an important profession in the making. Their contribution to this development brought before the field the names and knowledge of early American leaders in embalming, such as Hohenschuh, Barnes, Carpenter, Worsham, Dhonau, Dodge, and others.

In 1903, the *American Undertaker* merged with *The Embalmers' Monthly* and, as a consequence, the range of subject matter covered by the journal increased. It remained in print until 1959, when it changed its title to *National Funeral Service Journal*, remaining in print until 1966.

These journals, whether designated "official" or not by NFDA, played an important, if not clearly assessable, role as media of communication in the field of funeral service, and as an instrumentality for placing before the public-at-large the claims of professionalism that funeral directors felt justifiably should be made.

Growth, Problems and Change: During the last two decades of the 19th century, associational activities on the part of funeral directors covered a broad range of interests and problems, some of which had been pressing since the Civil War, while others grew out of the changing times.

Although the following activities to some degree impinge upon one another and even intermingle, they will, in part, be discussed separately. These interests and problems include the relationships of funeral directors' associations with individual manufacturers and with manufacturers' associations; the general baggage agents of the nation's railways and health agencies in the matter of the transportation of the dead; and with public-health agencies generally.

Other matters of moment at this time include mortuary education and training, communication within the occupation itself, and professionalism.

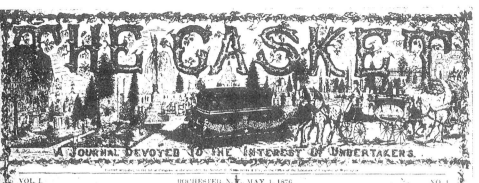

66. Front Cover of First Issue of *The Casket*, May 1876.

Some indication of the state of business affairs involving funeral directors and casket manufacturers was given earlier. The rapid growth in the number of casket manufacturers, the lack of organization and standardization of their business practices, and the free-wheeling sales activities of the casket jobbers and drummers left the average funeral director of the 1870s and '80s with little assurance that he was being dealt with fairly and would receive satisfactory funeral merchandise.

"The time is at hand," one irate undertaker wrote to the editor of *The Casket* in 1879, "when the undertakers must form a union to protect themselves and their trade on account of the many different frauds that are practiced by some of the wholesale coffin and casket as well as undertakers' hardware and trimming manufacturers."

In his presidential address of 1883, the first president of the national association, Charles L. Benjamin of Saginaw, Michigan, spoke directly to the funeral-goods manufacturers, calling for their cooperation, deploring the resolution passed in the association's first meeting asking for an exposition subsidized by them, and lecturing them to let the "Strife between them not be who shall sell the cheapest goods, but who shall sell the best finished and most desirable at the price."

In keeping with this conviction, expressed or implicit, that their association could address itself equally well to trade and professional problems, the membership called for rather stringently defined, restrictive trade practices. In terms of these, state or local associations would be party to an agreement with the manufacturers' association whereby members of the funeral directors' associations would trade *only* with recognized and accredited members of the manufacturers' association, the latter guaranteeing that its manufacturer-members would sell their funeral goods only to funeral director members in good standing with their respective associations.

This proposed relationship was generated at the local, or grassroots, level and found formal expression in the report of the first Committee on Resolutions during the second (1883) meeting of the national association:

> *Resolved*, That we request every manufacturer or jobber of funeral goods or supplies not to sell, six months after this date, any individual or firm wishing to establish a new business without a certificate of consent from the Executive Committee of the State or Local Association under whose jurisdiction they may be, or a committee appointed for the purpose of examining the field they propose to occupy, the probabilities for their success, the reputation for honesty and integrity, and the financial and professional ability of the new firm.
>
> *Resolved*, That we request all manufacturers and jobbers after this date not to sell or to supply goods to any person or persons, who shall be reported to the Secretary of the Manufacturers' Association by the proper authority of a local, district, or state association, for having violated the Constitution or By-Laws of the Association under whose jurisdiction they may be.
>
> *Resolved*, That we respectfully request the manufacturers not to supply any jobber who shall be complained of by the Secretary of the National Association as supplying any person or firm who may have been condemned by the Grievance Committee for violating the Constitution and By-Laws of any State Association.

PLATE 67

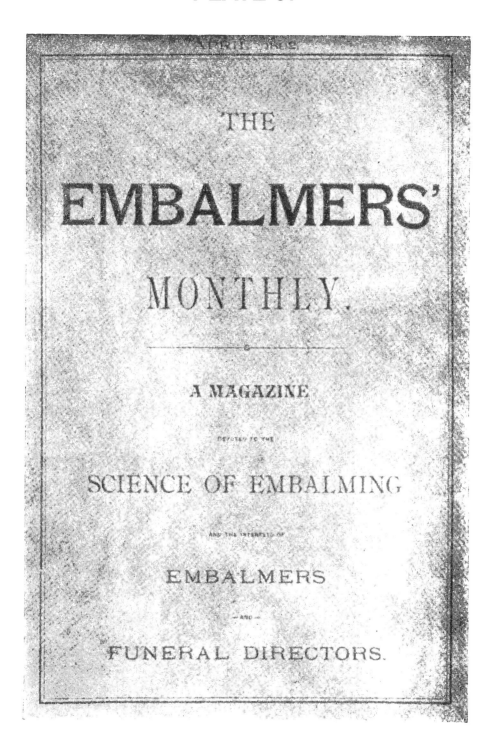

67. Front Cover of First Issue of *Embalmers' Monthly*, April 1892.

Resolved, That we, as funeral directors, condemn the manufacture of covered caskets at a less price than fifteen dollars for an adult size; and that we would be pleased to see the manufacturers of covered work form an association similar to that of the National Burial Case Association, and pledge ourselves to support them in a movement of this kind.

> Respectfully submitted,
> Chas. T. Whitsett, Indiana
> A.C. Burpee, Illinois
> L.A. Jeffreys, New York[31]

On the same day, a Committee on Manufacturers was appointed, which drafted a resolution calling for the creation of a standing committee to meet with a committee of the National Burial Case Association "for the purpose of considering any and all questions that may arise between manufacturers and dealers." This resolution was adopted, and a Committee on Manufacturers (at times slightly altered in title) continued to function throughout the remainder of the decade.

At the third annual meeting in 1884, the subject was brought up again by the secretary, Samuel Lippincott, who related the problem of non-compliance on the part of manufacturers, along with the burden of correspondence occasioned by members of state associations writing him to protest the sale of funeral goods by members of the National Burial Case Manufacturers' Association to non-members of funeral directors' associations.

President Robert R. Bringhust later submitted this report, in which the matter of restrictive agreements was proposed to be standardized for all funeral directors. The instrumentality would be a formal contract, or compact, signed by funeral director and funeral-goods manufacturer alike. It read as follows:

> This is to certify that I,_____, of the firm of _____, of the City of _____, do hereby covenant and agree, for said firm, that we will not sell, loan, advance or consign our goods to any undertaker or funeral director not a member of a local organization under state jurisdiction, when such local organization exists, pledging ourselves to the bearer thereof, to forfeit to him the sum of ten (10) dollars, if, by legal proof — proof sufficient to convict in law — we fail to carry out such compact; provided, that the holder thereof, _____, of the city, _____, State of _____, doing business as a funeral director therein, party of the second part, does in return, guarantee that he will not buy, receive on consignment or otherwise, for sale, any goods, directly or indirectly, from any firm or jobber of coffins and caskets known in the trade as wooden goods, or dealer therein, who is not a member or authorized jobber of the National Burial Case Association, does not further pledge himself yearly to submit his account and books to a member of the National Burial Case Association, for examination, and does further agree to freely testify, under oath, on demand, as to his business affairs, so far as this compact is concerned.[32]

When brought up for vote, this section of the report was tabled.

PLATE 68

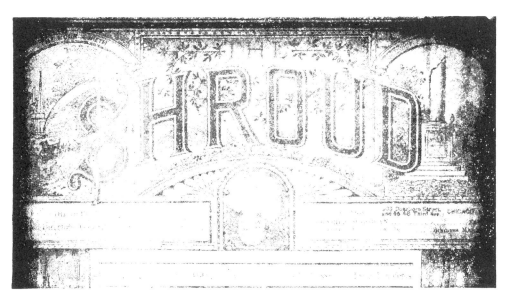

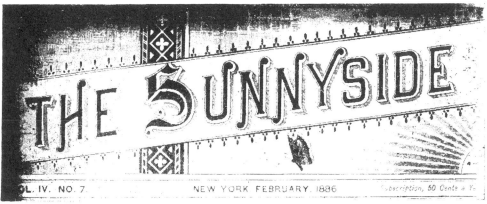

68. Portions of Front Covers of Early Undertaking Trade Journals.

There were two important reasons for this action: The first was that many funeral directors felt that the "combination" of manufacturers into what was popularly becoming known as the "coffin trust" had served only to increase prices without noticeably standardizing quality at a reasonable level. The second reason was that many "old line" undertakers were still in business, and some of these maintained their own cabinet and woodworking shops, while others were coffinshop proprietors. The objection of this group to such contracts is obvious.

Nevertheless, contracts between various burial-case manufacturers' associations (there were four by 1888) were entered into by members of state and local funeral directors' associations. (It should be pointed out that these agreements were *never* entered into at the national associational level.)

The results of these contractual agreements were so highly mixed that the eventual relations between funeral directors' and manufacturers' associations seldom proved satisfactory to either of the contracting parties. Regardless of their effectiveness, such agreements were nullified in 1890 when Congress passed the Sherman Anti-Trust Law, "An Act to Protect Trade and Commerce against Unlawful Restraints and Monopolies."

But while these contracts lasted, each side apparently was lax in enforcing its part. As a result, some members of the various funeral directors' associations bought indiscriminately from organized and unorganized case manufacturers alike, while certain members of the manufacturers' associations sold indiscriminately to funeral directors, without regard whether they were members of one of their associations.

In Canada, however, similar agreements made between the province associations and the Dominion Burial Case Association operated with singular effectiveness. Despite this, complaint was made to the national association that American casket manufacturers were shipping their merchandise into Canada, and, by so doing, were breaking down the structure of restrictive trade practices.[33]

In 1889, these agreements were mutually abrogated in consequence of legislation passed in Canada prohibiting written agreements between manufacturers and associations in restraint of trade.

Meanwhile, one year earlier, the Canadian Provincial Association was brought into the national association, with the result that the name of the latter was changed to the "International Funeral Directors Association." After several years, cooperation between the two groups began to decrease until, in 1893, the affiliation was discontinued and the American group adopted the title it still bears, "The National Funeral Directors Association of the United States."

As experiments in trade restriction and international organization failed, or proved less than entirely successful, other problems, many of them present in the background for decades, assumed new importance and claimed the attention of the funeral directors' association.

One of these was the matter of transporting the dead. As pointed out earlier — in default of any set of comprehensive federal regulations or a codification of rules and restrictions laid down by the several states, municipalities and other governmental agencies — funeral directors faced exasperating and time-consuming red tape and delays in their efforts to secure needed transport for the dead.

PLATE 69

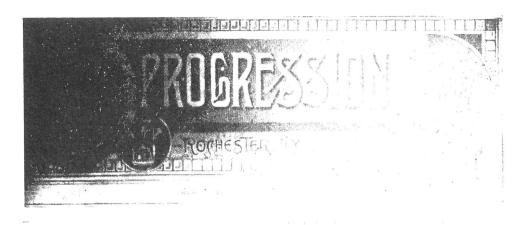

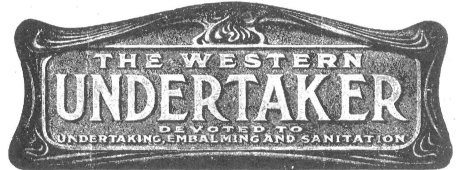

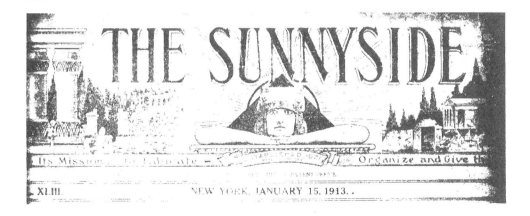

69. Additional Front Cover Titles of Early Undertaking Trade Journals.
(Note changed format on *The Sunnyside* vs. Plate 68.)

To further complicate this problem, there were no general rules governing the practices of railway baggage handlers in this matter. Under these conditions, it became apparent to funeral directors that collective action was necessary to provide solutions for these, and related, problems to be worked out cooperatively — not only with governmental agencies but also with other organizations concerned. The relationships with the railway baggage-handler's union were as wide as the group's jurisdiction among the railroads.

Because these problems were national in scope, their answers could not be local, state or even regional, but must be national and provide national answers. Therefore, an effective national association was essential.

Thus, the need for concerted action on the problem of railway transportation of bodies was first brought to the attention of the national association in 1888, when a special committee of the National Association of General Baggage Agents listed seven suggested rules. These rules included the recommendation that they be laid before the several state boards of health, the National Conference of State Boards of Health, and the National Association of "Undertakers," with a view toward "establishing some simple, effective rules which could be the guide for all Railroads, and other Transportation Companies in the United States and Canada."

The response of the national association was to send a committee to meet with the baggage handlers at their next regular meeting. The subsequent conference resulted in a list of rules adopted by the baggage agents' association and sent to the various boards of health, with the recommendation that they become universally adopted and put into effect.

In the majority of cases, the health boards were highly receptive to these recommendations and incorporated them into their own growing body of health and sanitation rules and regulations. Impetus was given to this reception by the decision of the Conference of Officers of the State Boards of Health at Nashville, Tennessee, in 1897 to accept, virtually unchanged, the suggested rules as they had been worked out by the railway baggage agents and the funeral directors.

The committee deliberations of the latter two groups lasted almost a decade and turned out to be well worth the time, inasmuch as the resulting joint decisions could be clearly, authoritatively and decisively stated at the Conference of State Health Officers, somewhat to the surprise of the "distinguished physicians present" who "conceded to the funeral directors who were present superior knowledge of the subject in hand."[34]

The rules, in brief, prohibited transportation of bodies dead of certain deadly and contagious diseases; permitted the transportation of others dead of less-virulent diseases only when thorough embalming and disinfecting had been completed; specified conditions under which bodies dead of non-contagious diseases might be transported; dealt with the problem of persons accompanying the dead body; and listed the steps in securing transit permits, applying pasters (labels), and the like. These rules, finally, were approved by the National Board of Health.

In light of this important development, funeral directors could henceforth look forward to increased standardization of public-health rules regarding transportation of the dead.

For the first time, they were also able to convince somewhat-skeptical baggage agents — who, after all, oversaw the handling of these dead in transport — and the even more-skeptical physicians and public-health officers, that embalming could render a corpse germ-free and innocuous to the living.

Finally, they gained *professional* recognition for their work in embalming; that is, the affidavit of a funeral director who embalmed a body was accepted at face value henceforth by baggage agents and public-health functionaries alike.

Little wonder that NFDA's meeting in 1897 was carried out in an atmosphere of jubilant excitement, and that, in addition to the formal report they received, the delegates insisted on informal recitations by all of the committee members of the inside story of the "victory at Nashville."

All problems of transportation were not solved by this one success, however. With the development of checking systems and the increase of transfer companies, new issues were brought before the association. Thus, the major point of discussion of the 1907 national convention centered around new transportation problems, as brought up in an address by Mr. A. Traynor, general baggage agent, Union Pacific Railway Co., on the subject of "The Silent Passenger."

Problems relating to health and sanitation, however, were not exhausted by the work accomplished by the funeral directors on rules and regulations for transportation of the dead. During the last quarter of the 19th century, the most important concern in this area — one that had involved both trade and professional aspects — centered on setting up licensing apparatus to regulate and control the practice of embalming, along with an extension of effort to bring about other health-related legislation in the mutual interests of both the public and of funeral directors.

As early as 1884, a Committee on Resolutions in the national association stressed the need for uniformity in death certificates in order that "a great many important facts might be obtained, and tables of vital statistics prepared that would be of use to our National Board of Health."[35]

In that same year, the evils of the quack professors of embalming were brought to the attention of the national association by the Association of Undertakers of the State of Illinois, who asked that it "recommend that the several State Associations in their respective States, charter such schools as would be above reproach; recommend a course of instruction, to embrace anatomy, chemistry and a thorough course on disinfectants, and to last at least three months."

In light of the fact that the so-called "schools" often were conducted for periods of three days to a week, this proposal sounded only slightly less than revolutionary.

Another delegate, a Mr. Russ of Chicago, hoped for a form of state or federal control of the occupation in such manner that any man who put up his name as an undertaker would be "compelled by the State, and indorsed by the United States, that he should be a man of good integrity, sober, industrious, and truthful in every respect."

Oscar N. Crane, second president of the national association, stressed the same point in his presidential address in 1885 when he remarked:

> It seems to me that the time is not far distant, if not already dawning on us, that there should be a legal standard; some qualifications; some governing laws; some moral fitness; necessary, which should be required and regulated by Statute both of State and Nation; a standard of ability, and morals which on strict examination, the applicant should be, must be, found to possess.
>
> And then, and not till then, will he be permitted to engage in a calling so solemn and at the same time, so full of professional responsibility.[36]

Later, during the same meeting, a resolution passed encouraging members and trade journals to urge legislatures to create state boards of health in order to further better sanitary measures, and to facilitate and expedite the transportation of bodies in and through their respective states.

Hudson Samson also pointed out during his 1886 presidential address that two universities — Michigan, at Ann Arbor, and Pennsylvania, at Philadelphia, as well as a medical college in Chicago — had already "manifested a willingness to provide a course of study that would be desired by a student preparing for the Funeral Directorship."[37]

During this speech (printed in part earlier in this chapter), Samson also stressed the need for legislation setting up training and education requirements for a license to enter into the profession of funeral directing, and regulatory requirements for remaining a funeral director.[38]

Samson also urged all members to join the American Public Health Association, which had, among its various committees, one on the burial of the dead; to participate in its activities; and to write and present papers on sanitation and the funeral director at its annual meetings.

Following his own advice, within the year, and with the aid of several of his outstanding colleagues, Samson prepared a model legislative act designed to ensure better education for funeral directors. This document was distributed to the executive committees of the various state associations. Titled "An Act Pertaining to the Care, Preparation and Disposition of the Dead, and to Insure the Better Education of the Funeral Directors," many of the features and provisions that went into the first licensing legislation of the states drew from this document.

State legislatures were not readily convinced, however, either of the public-welfare aspects of such legislation or of the quality of the practitioners who pressed for it. Despite the example of the province of Ontario in setting up a board of examiners in 1887, nearly eight years elapsed before the passage of a law by a U.S. state legislature regulating the practice of embalming.

In this case, Virginia led the way on March 5, 1894, when its governor signed the regulatory bill. The following year, Alabama, Missouri and Pennsylvania, passed similar legislation and set up a board of embalmers, or its equivalent, and laid down certain regulations concerning the educational and technical preparation necessary to enter and practice the art of embalming.

Before the turn of the century, the ranks of regulating states had swelled by 20 more names, making a total of 24 states having passed *some* sort of embalming legislation.[39]

The 1890s were a period in which the efforts of funeral directors to achieve occupational licensing — and thereby to underscore their claim to be practitioners in a profession rendering necessary and important personal services legitimated by the community — slowly began to bear fruit.

20th-century Traces of Professionalism: In spite of much spadework, it could be said that, at the dawn of the 20th century, funeral directing in America had managed to organize, establish and gain public recognition as a distinct occupation, but it still had a very long distance to go in becoming a full-fledged profession.

For one thing, even among its own practitioners, its aims and interests were by no means universally agreed upon. For another, the procedures or controls whereby any profession secures its aims and brings it members into conformity by social and legal pressures were only partially developed.

Many problems faced the aspiring profession of funeral directing as 1900 drew to a close. Some of these arose out of the processes, equipment and materials available for use in its practice. Embalming procedures, techniques and fluids (especially the latter) had, by no means, been perfected. Adequate controls over the quality of embalming fluids were lacking and, as a result and side by side with the standard brands produced by reputable companies, the market was flooded in the late 1870s to the end of the century with an incredible variety of untested and uncertain compounds, produced both by fluid houses and by individual compounders.[40]

Other problems arose from a lack of a firm, universal definition of what constituted proper training to enter the occupation. Most undertakers by 1900 felt that a diploma from some kind of embalming school was sufficient evidence of proficiency to qualify a candidate. As with medical schools of the day, however, there was no general agreement as to what should be the educational requirements for admission to the course, what the course content should be, how long the training should last, and what qualifications schools should meet in faculty and physical equipment.

Thus, a diploma from an embalming school might still mean anything from exposure to three days of demonstration made by an itinerant "professor" (whose purpose might be to sell a particular brand of embalming fluid) to graduation from a several-months' course offered by a well-established, formal school of embalming.

The lack of state laws for licensing constituted another problem to challenge the movement of the occupation toward a profession. While the states of Washington, Oregon, Nevada, Texas, California, Arizona, Arkansas, Louisiana, Mississippi, Wisconsin, Michigan, Ohio, Kentucky, Tennessee, North Carolina, Florida, Vermont, Maine, Massachusetts, Connecticut, New Jersey, Rhode Island, and Maryland, as well as American Indian territory, all had scattered bits of legislation regarding embalming and burial of the dead, each lacked formal licensing laws.

In addition, the viewpoint held by some members of state legislatures that funeral service legislation was passed only to secure the benefit of the funeral director — and, therefore, as wholly a favor to practitioners — constituted a serious impediment to the development of much-needed licensing and regulatory law.

Unsavory advertising and cut-throat competition had not yet reached its peak in 1900, but the lack of an unequivocal and general definition of what constituted legitimate promotional practice led later to grave abuses. This issue has by no means been successfully resolved.

Even though the term "public relations" was unfamiliar in 1900 (and the collectively felt need for such probably proved lower than today), then as now, good public relations constituted another problem for the profession. The successful efforts of funeral directors to reach an agreement with funeral-goods manufacturers, and the resultant practices in restraint of trade, did little to reassure the public of the service-basis of a funeral director's work.

If the medical profession looked askance at funeral directors, so too did the American press, which sustained the stereotype of the funeral director as the traditional undertaker — the "dismal trader" of doubtful character and indifferent feelings.

These and similar problems were not then, and are not now, unique to the occupation of funeral directing. They are the problems that, in a general sort of way, every profession met during its emergence and, from time to time, is called upon to solve again.

Perhaps the most difficult problem still facing the funeral director at the start of the 20th century was the all-encompassing question of professionalization itself. How far should the effort to professionalize the group be carried? By its very nature, the occupation could have swung sharply and far toward one or the other of opposites, or remained in some intermediate position. It faced the choice of becoming either an out-and-out trade or business, or a profession, or of compromising these extremes.

It merits repeating that the *personal service* elements in funeral directing have a natural "professional" orientation; the *impersonal service, or merchandising, elements* have a natural "trade" orientation.

Up until 1901, the great decision had been straddled, although the movement was toward professionalization. But it was apparent that, in order to create a cleavage in the public mind between the undertaker who furnished merchandise *and* rendered services, and all other undertakers, a strong element in the occupational group, using NFDA as its chief instrument, was successfully building a set of standards or measuring sticks that could be incorporated into a licensing procedure.

In order to eliminate the competition of merchants and others who sold caskets but did not furnish service, and later "facilities," both professional and trade-minded groups endeavored, by means of trade agreements with manufacturers and supply houses, to restrict opportunities for buying such merchandise.

Further, these groups attempted to penalize competing manufacturer-merchants by not buying from them, and by encouraging other funeral directors to buy only from recognized manufacturers who were not engaged in, or directly supporting, the service-end of the business.

In 1900, in the minds of most undertakers or funeral directors, both forms of conducting one's occupation, and thus serving self and mankind, merged into a vocational concept. In addition, like most of those occupations that, during the 19th century, had become self-conscious and sought to improve their economic and social status, funeral directing had achieved some kind of organization and internal order among its members but, by no means, had fully accomplished its aims.

Meanwhile, it was not considered necessary to make the choice of being either a professional or trade practitioner as the point of self-designation for funeral directors. The impulse to associate, however, provided the impelling motive for directing and molding the desires of those who would better the status of their occupation, and thereby elevate the condition of their work, their security and legitimate rewards, the good opinion in which they were held by other occupations and by the public at large, and finally, their own self-esteem.

CITATIONS AND REFERENCES FOR CHAPTER 11

1. *Occupational Licensing in the States* (Chicago: The Council of State Governments, 1952), pp. 16-17.

2. *Ibid.*

3. *Ibid.*, p. 18, quoting from A.M. Carr-Saunders and P.W. Wilson, "Professions," in the *Encyclopedia of Social Sciences*, vol. VI, p. 477.

4. *Ibid.*, p. 21, *passim*.

5. *Ibid.* Figures taken from Table A, p. 23.

6. See *ibid.*, p. 22.

7. James A. Tobey, *The National Government and Public Health* (Baltimore: The Johns Hopkins Press, 1926), pp. 21 ff.

8. James A. Tobey, *Riders of the Plague* (New York: Charles Scribner's Sons, 1930), p. 78.

9. For a more complete account of the activities of the "Sanitary Commission," see George W. Cooke, *Unitarianism in America* (Boston: American Unitarian Association, 1902), pp. 180-184.

10. Habenstein, "A Study of the Cremation Movement in the United States," *op. cit.*, p. 82.

11. Augustus Cobb, *Earth Burial and Cremation* (New York: Putnam, 1892), p. 136.

12. Adapted from the table on page 117 of John Storer Cobb's *A Quarter Century of Cremation in North America* (Boston: Knight and Millett, 1901).

13. O.B. Frothingham, *The Disposal of Our Dead* (New York: D.G. Francis, 1874).

14. *Proceedings of the First National Convention* (Detroit: Cremation Association of America, 1913), p. 4.

15. *The Keystone State Echo*, Golden Jubilee Number, June 1931, p. 97 ff.

16. Proceedings, National Funeral Directors Association (NFDA), 1909, p. 49.

17. *Ibid.*, p. 50.

18. *Ibid.*

19. *Ibid.*, p. 52.

20. *Ibid.*

21. *Ibid.*, pp. 56-57.

22. Proceedings, American Funeral Directors' National Association, 1882, p. 22.

23. *Ibid.*, 1884, p. 76.

24. Proceedings, International Funeral Directors' Association, 1888, p. 14, *passim*.

25. Proceedings, American Funeral Directors' National Association, 1886, pp. 5-10, *passim*.

26. Habenstein, "The American Funeral Director," *op. cit.*, p. 173 ff.

27. Proceedings, FDA, 1884, p. 11.

28. *Ibid.*, p. 12.

29. From *The Casket*, 1886, Archives of NFDA, Milwaukee, Wis., *op. cit.*, no month, n.p.

30. *The Casket*, May 1, 1876.

31. Proceedings, American Funeral Directors' National Association, 1883, pp. 31-32.

32. Proceedings, *op. cit.*, 1884, p. 53.

33. Proceedings, *op. cit.*, 1888, p. 29 ff.

34. "Rules Governing Transportation of Dead Bodies, Adopted by the National Board of Health" in Proceedings, NFDA, 1897, *op. cit.*, pp. 147-149.

35. Proceedings, *op. cit.*, 1884, p. 75 ff.

36. Proceedings, American Funeral Directors' National Association, 1885, pp. 14-15.

37. Proceedings, *op. cit.*, 1886, p. 7.

38. *Ibid.*, pp. 7-8.

39. Proceedings, NFDA, 1900, p. 53.

40. For example, in *The Casket* between 1876 (when the journal started) and 1880, at least a dozen different brands of preservatives and body disinfectants were advertised. A few examples: John Gallagher's (patented 1873) "American Segestor — Great Preservative and Disinfectant. Removes mortification in the worst cases in 2-3 hours"; and the much-touted George M. Rhodes "Electric Balm — Discoloring, Deodorizing, Disinfection, and Embalming the Dead on Sea or Land. Warranted the Best and the Cheapest (Considering what it will accomplish.) A Poison and Contagion Preventative for Sick Rooms or on Shipboard."

Interestingly, the renowned Champion Embalming Fluid, which first advertised in *The Casket* in the September 1880 issue, was preceded by some eight or nine other brands in earlier issues. Also, during this half-decade, at least four or five brands of embalming kits were on sale with pump, syringes and several tubes at about $15 to $20 per set. (Personal communication from Melissa Johnson Boffey, Chicago, Illinois, 1976.)

PART THREE:
Organization of Modern Funeral Service

Chapter 12

Institutional Growth and Modern Associational Developments

In the conditions of their emergence and change, occupations differ considerably. Some grow slowly, adding new workers and, possibly, new functions to the basic work or service performed. Others, especially in modern times, appear almost overnight, born of technical innovations and inventions. Yet, no matter what the specific conditions of emergence, all occupations face a general problem of institutionalization — that is, of putting order, harmony and certainty in the minds of those who work in them. One of the major functions of an occupational association is to create a definite and positive image of that livelihood in the minds of those who engage in it, and to impress this image as the true representation of the occupation in the view of the public.

Therefore, this chapter describes some of the historical developments in funeral directing as they reflect the problems and actions of persons trying to introduce order, harmony and certainty of mind into a rapidly changing field. The path is not entirely new since Chapter 11, dealing with the associational impulse, has in many ways already cast light on the organizing activities to build an orderly vocation. In dealing with recent institutional growth and associational developments in funeral directing, we will consider five related matters: mortuary (funeral service) education; developments in mortuary law; multiplication of associations; economic growth and expansion; and, finally, evidences of integration and stabilization.

Mortuary (Funeral Service) Education: In the process of becoming instituted as one of the more important sectors of present-day funeral service, mortuary education has developed into four divisions: 1) the schools of mortuary science, as they have come to be known; 2) the agencies controlling the activities of these schools, as they have come to be known; 3) the committees that represent the various interests in the general field of mortuary education, and which advise and recommend action to the agencies; and 4) the body of legislative actions and the rules and usages laid down by the boards of the states and the federal government. Although these divisions overlap somewhat, they will be taken up in the order listed.

(1) *Schools*. As we know from brief references in Chapter 8, which dealt with embalming, schools of mortuary science before 1900 were more notable for the men who conducted them and the products they used and supported than for the quality and thoroughness of the instruction they provided and the range of subject matter their courses covered.

Included in this group are such individuals as Dr. Auguste Renouard, who, as early as 1874, independently instructed a small number of undertakers in the back room of a furniture store in Denver, and whose *Undertaker's Manual*, written in 1876 and published in 1878, marked a first; his son, Charles A. Renouard, one of the first to establish an independent, non-commercial-house-connected school of embalming in 1884; W.P. Hohenschuh, later to become an authority in the field of funeral service generally; that showman Dr. Carl Lewis Barnes, founder of many schools of embalming and compounder of several varieties of fluids; C.B. Dolge, founder of the United States School of Embalming in 1887, and president of the Brooklyn Embalming Fluid Co.; Felix A. Sullivan, itinerant teacher of embalming and founder of schools, whose embalming of well-known persons led to his moniker as "the dean of embalmers of the English-speaking peoples"; Joseph H. Clarke and A. Johnson Dodge, described earlier; and the scholarly physician, text-writer and embalming-school pedagogue Dr. William S. Carpenter. These make up only a partial list of the pioneers in the field of mortuary education.[1]

"In the beginning," remarks Charles O. Dhonau, an early funeral service educator, "the training of individuals to be practical operators was largely promoted by those who were either associated then, or later, with concerns whose business it was, or is, to produce and to distribute embalmers' supplies."[2] Yet, the commercial support of these early schools was not an unmixed evil since there was probably no other way at the time by which the practice of embalming, crude as it might be, could be diffused so rapidly through the field. To this point, Dhonau states:

> In all fairness to commercially operated "schools" of that early period, they were quite successful in enrolling students from existing "undertaking establishments," "livery stables," "furniture stores," and "cabinet makers," as well as from the ranks of that one-out-of-ten-thousand individuals who had a natural bent toward rendering what was then the service of an "undertaker." Many of the leading members of our profession "graduated" from these commercially motivated schools… Their "professional education" did not end with their short school term, but they improved themselves, their knowledge, their conduct, their personalities, through that agency we may call the "university of hard knocks," to the point where their success was unbounded.[3]

Non-commercial schools of embalming before 1900 were rare mainly for two reasons: the limited demand for embalmers, as contrasted with the demand for physicians or dentists, and the relatively high cost of instruction. In addition to the Renouard's school (both father and son operated it until 1912), there were the Cincinnati School of Embalming, established in 1882 by Joseph H. Clarke and now functioning as the Cincinnati College of Mortuary Science; the Illinois School of Embalming, opened in Chicago in 1884 under the sponsorship of the Chicago Association of Undertakers; and the Iowa School of Embalming, founded about 1890. These were four of the more lasting "independents" before 1900.

A feature of many of the other early embalming schools was their itinerancy. It was customary for a team of demonstrators to travel from city to city, holding sessions that each lasted from three or four days to a week. School diplomas were granted at the end of each session. Occasionally, examinations would be given.

After 1894, with the introduction of embalming legislation in several states, these schools were forced to perform an added function: the preparation of the student who expected to take the examination prepared by the state board of embalming.

Other innovations at the turn of the century were the "quiz compend" (a list of questions commonly used by the state boards, together with the correct answers to be memorized), and the mortuary correspondence schools. At this time, the course prepared by H.S. Eckels was perhaps the most popular. Again, the emphasis was upon preparation for the state board examination.

Instruction in all the "formal" schools was limited primarily to lectures and demonstrations in anatomy, bacteriology, practical embalming, disinfectants, and contagious diseases. Memorization, again, was one of the ends of instruction and demonstration. By 1900, courses at the more reputable schools (there were no formal standards or grading systems at the time) lasted about three weeks.

Literature on the subject was scanty, and often the founder of the school would find it necessary to prepare his own texts, as well as to lecture and handle administrative matters. Between 1874 and 1893, only seven texts dealing directly with embalming were written in America, according to a list drawn up by Charles O. Dhonau. In the next two decades, the figure tripled. In comparison with the amount of literature being produced in the last few decades, the period of 1895-1914 may be looked upon as prolific from the standpoint of works in the field of embalming. Many of the basic texts and reference works written during this period were substantial products written by men trained in anatomy, physiology and chemistry, whose theoretical knowledge was amplified by practical experience in the field.

The quarter century of growth in embalming schools after 1900 produced some rather striking developments, most notable of which, perhaps, were the rise of the proprietary school with the beginnings of a standardized curriculum, and the lengthening of the term of instruction. If, for example, one wished to study embalming in Chicago at the Barnes School of Anatomy, Sanitary Science, and Embalming around 1905, he would have no trouble enrolling any day of the year — Sundays included.[4]

In 1910, the average length of courses in embalming schools was about six weeks; in 1925, it was eight weeks; in 1928, three months; in 1930, six months; and in 1934, the nine-month course was originated at Eckels College of Mortuary Science.[5] The American Board of Funeral Service Education now requires each of its accredited schools to offer an associate-degree program or its equivalent.

At least 12 schools of mortuary education were founded between 1900 and 1920: The Simmons School of Embalming in 1902; the American College of Embalming in 1903; the Indiana School of Embalming in 1905; the University of Minnesota Course for Embalmers, the Cleveland College of Embalming, and the Boston School of Anatomy and Embalming, all in 1909; the Worsham College of Embalming in 1911; the Los Angeles College of Anatomy, Embalming and Sanitation in 1918; and the Gupton-Jones School of Embalming in 1920. With the exception of the University of Minnesota, these schools were proprietary in the sense that they represented private ownership of an educational enterprise by an individual or individuals. Although the tendency was to operate these schools without outside help from the embalming fluid and other morticians' goods companies — the reorganized Cincinnati School of Embalming was an outstanding example in this case — such was not always possible.

The next phase in the development of schools of mortuary education took place in the late 1920s and early '30s, after many pioneer founders retired or died, and the institutions were faced with the problem of survival without the personal guidance, inspiration and, often, the unstinted time of their founders. In numerous cases, these schools, never more than 25 at one time, faced crucial problems of reorganization. One solution was to reincorporate along non-profit lines, with the faculty assuming responsibility for administration of the school itself.

The current phase of these schools started with the establishment of the Wisconsin Institute of Mortuary Science in 1936. This is the first instance in which the term "mortuary science" appeared in the title of a school of mortuary education. By 1962, most of the old schools, and practically all of the newly established ones, had adopted this term.

Many of the present schools of mortuary science came into existence through mergers and combinations, and it was often the case that at one of these junctures, a change in title would occur that would reflect the changing emphasis in mortuary education. For example, the Hohenschuh-Carpenter College of Embalming was organized in Des Moines, Iowa, in 1900, and shortly thereafter absorbed the Western College of Embalming. In 1930, it moved to St. Louis, Missouri, and merged with the American College of Embalming, founded in 1903 by another "pioneer," M.H. Alexander. In 1943, it merged with the Williams Institute of Mortuary Science to become the College of Mortuary Science, St. Louis, organized as a non-proprietary institution. Likewise, the Los Angeles College of Anatomy, Embalming and Sanitation, founded in 1918, simplified its name to the California College of Mortuary Science. It was eventually absorbed by Cypress County Community College as part of the state of California university system.

Thus, the mortuary schools in their changing structure have tended, on the whole, to follow the pattern set by other professional schools. The final stage seems to be incorporation into the organization of large universities and colleges. As far back as 1908, the University of Minnesota, for example, offered a regular course in applied mortuary science.

There are currently 59 accredited funeral service programs in the United States, of which 13 are offered at private schools. The majority of the remaining schools with accredited programs are community colleges that confer associate degrees. The 59 institutions offer a total of 55 associate degrees, eight baccalaureate degrees, and five certificates and/or diplomas. The development of mortuary schools reflects the important influence exerted through associational committees, licensing boards, legislative acts, and the collective endeavors of other relevant and interested groups.

For most of its history, American funeral service has been a male-dominated, family heritage profession. Since 2000, however, the number of female enrollees has been greater than the number of males. In program year 2013, for example, approximately 61% of new enrollees, and 56% of graduates, were female. In addition, the average age of new students has increased since the early 1990s: today, 52.5% of new enrollees are over 25 years of age. Other changes include increasing minority student enrollments.[5]

(2) *Agencies, Conferences and Councils.* One of the most significant steps taken to raise examination standards, and to otherwise improve the service of the state boards of examiners to the profession and public, took place with the organization of the Joint Conference of Embalmers Examining Boards and State Boards of Health in 1904, under the guiding genius of J.H. McCully of Idaville, Indiana.[6] The first meetings of this conference were held in conjunction with the annual convention of the National Funeral Directors Association (NFDA) at St. Louis that year.

The project had been talked about for some time before actual organization began; the first stirrings had come in 1900 at the Denver meetings of NFDA with an informal conference of the members of the various boards for licensing embalmers. J. Newton Nind, editor of *The Embalmers' Monthly*, attended and, about three years later, he and McCully joined forces to bring about the St. Louis meeting.

In a circular letter written to the field at large, the hope expressed by these two, and seconded formally by H.M. Kilpatrick, secretary of NFDA, was that "such a conference might result in unifying the regulation of embalming in the several states, in the interchange of recognition of licenses issued by the different Boards, and expedite the adoption of the new transportation rules." Meanwhile, a Committee on Education of NFDA, with McCully as chairman, had brought under scrutiny the problem of providing some uniform system of requirements, both in the receiving of applicants for examination before licenses were granted, and in examining them. The work of this committee was incorporated into the deliberations of the newly formed Joint Conference of Embalmers Examining Boards and State Boards of Health.

One of the first issues taken up by the latter was reciprocity with regard to licenses. Although it became increasingly apparent that the problems of the examining boards were more specific than the state boards of health would care to discuss, an effort was made to keep the two groups together. In 1906, at the Chicago meeting, the organization changed its name to The Association of State and Provincial Boards of Health and Embalmers' Examining Boards of North America. A prominent figure in public health, Dr. H.M. Bracken of St. Paul, secretary and executive officer for the Minnesota State Board of Health, was elected president, but the combination survived only for a year.

In 1907, the Conference of State and Provincial Boards of Health of North America again returned to its unaffiliated status, and the Conference of Embalmers Examining Boards of North America, with a slate of officers drawn from its own functionaries, was organized as a more limited-interest group dedicated to problems more specifically relating to embalming and funeral directing. Some of these were matters of concern to the entire field of funeral service, such as transportation of the dead; the quality, efficacy and reliability of embalming fluids; the relations of funeral directors with casket manufacturers; and self-improvement in the service of the state boards.

Several developments, not necessarily representing direct actions of the conference, need mentioning. In 1907, McCully was able to secure from the attorney general of Indiana an opinion that the burial associations operating in that state were violating the insurance law. In the same year, the Conference of State and Provincial Boards of Health endorsed a particular embalming fluid.

In 1913, again due mainly to the persistence of McCully acting in the capacity of a representative of the NFDA, the conference, as one of its first important actions, adopted a set of rules pertaining to the transportation of the dead.

Meanwhile, the Conference of Examining Boards of North America revised its name in 1914 and became the North American Conference of Embalmers Examining Boards. For the next several years, it devoted itself to pressing for adoption, by individual legislatures and state boards, of the transportation rules it had set in 1913. The difficulty of welding together such a conference, representing about half of the state boards of health and embalmers' examining boards (with membership in these boards often a matter of political appointment and, in each state, the result of a different legislative act) can well be imagined.

Charles O. Dhonau, reminiscing over the early years of the conference, underscores the differences that prevailed:

> As I remember, particularly in the Conference meetings of and since 1914 at New Orleans, there were usually committees reporting on the possibilities of different kinds of uniformities. From the beginning, nearly every state delegate opined that his license law was superior in some provisions. Practically everyone thought his own law as a suitable pattern for all and was willing to try for uniformity provided his own law was the pattern. In 1914 much was talked about concerning license reciprocity between states and for a few years there was more actual reciprocity than in later years, when many board members began to believe that there must be something iniquitous about a licensed individual changing his state of residence.[7]

After World War I and during the early 1920s, the conference displayed a growing interest in the curricula of the schools. Under the inspiration of Dhonau, it strove to convince state board examiners that the responsibility for a student passing or failing an examination should, in part, be shared by the school that provided him with his training. Consequently, it was incumbent upon the several boards to learn more about the actual character and operation of embalming school programs.

Among education-minded funeral directors, it has become traditional to look upon the year 1927 as marking the turning point for the conference. In that year at its Cincinnati meeting, a decision was reached to adopt a topical curriculum for a six-month course — then the longest being given. The length of this term merits passing attention. As early as 1913, the Cincinnati School had offered a six-month course but other institutions in the field of mortuary training had by and large not followed this advance, so that, 14 years later, the average course still was of less than three month's duration, although a few schools had converted to a six-month basis. After the passage of the 1927 resolution, most of the schools that had been offering shorter courses voluntarily lengthened their programs.

A second step toward raising standards was taken in 1927 when the conference decided to take positive action toward placing embalming college training on some basis of national accreditation. Its initial move was to adopt as standard one of the six-month curricula in use in 1927. It also set four years of high school as an entrance requirement — which prerequisite had already been demanded by at least one existing college of embalming.[8]

To finish setting up an accreditation system, the conference adopted a plan for the grading of colleges of embalming according to revised standards, as partly listed above. A three-man accreditation committee was appointed to oversee this function. Although schools had already begun to revise their own programs, it was not until 1928 that the first grading system, consisting of the grades "A," "B" or "C," was worked out to the satisfaction of the conference itself, and of the 11 schools that were represented at its Kansas City meeting. Later, the system was changed to "A," "AA" and "B."

In 1934, the "grading committee" became the National Conference Board Committee of Embalming Examiners, later to become the Examination and National Board Committee, operating under the authority of the board of directors of the conference. Its functions were, and are, to develop examinations to be used by the state boards; to distribute and, when directed, to grade these examinations for a stipulated charge; and to carry out continuous evaluation of its own efforts in the examination program with a view to constant improvement.

In 1938, the graded schools were encouraged to change their legal names from schools and colleges of "embalming" to schools and colleges of "mortuary science." In 1940, the conference became the Council of Funeral Service Examining Boards, Inc., and later substituted the term "Conference" for "Council." In 1999, its name was changed to the present form: the International Conference of Funeral Service Examining Boards (ICFSEB).

Since 1948, the conference has served graduates of accredited schools of mortuary science by making available to them national board examinations. A certificate is granted to the successful applicant, and a certification notice is sent to the state board(s) of the applicant's choice.

Another mortuary education agency, which eventually came to represent embalming schools and colleges, was founded in 1942. Originally formed as the Mortuary Education Council, its corporate name was registered later as the National Council on Mortuary Education. The purposes of the council were primarily educational and its operations non-profit. It sought to formulate the proper educational, scientific and professional principles and standards to be used in placing schools and colleges of mortuary science on an approved list. Acting as an agency independent of any one interest group — although trying to represent all impartially — it conceived its function as to accredit and approve the programs of mortuary education and training being offered in the schools. It set up and carried out this function at the request of those schools that elected to join the council.

Although the original intent of this council was to include within its membership representatives from all of the mortuary education interest groups, the Conference of Funeral Service Examining Boards elected not to participate because its members, for the most part, felt that a duplication of the accreditation function would result. In some degree this feeling was also present among NFDA members, and although representatives of the latter did participate for several years, the council ceased to function by 1948, although its legal dissolution was not completed until 1953.

While this agency was short-lived, it nevertheless brought under its influence most of the major schools and colleges of mortuary science, many of which revised upward their standards, facilities and operations, and, apparently, benefited by the accreditation they received.

(3) *Interest Group Committees.* Turning for the moment to the various committees and groups that represented the different interest groups — other than those of the colleges and state examining boards — our attention is first drawn to the committees on education of NFDA, which were first appointed in 1903 and whose initial reports in 1904 coincided both in time and in point of view with the first meeting of the Conference of Embalmers Examining Boards.

Proposed and adopted at this time was the creation of a three-man educational committee, whose members would be elected for periods of one to three years, and whose function would be to prepare a workable plan whereby "this association may pass intelligent judgment upon the quality of professional attainment offered by any educational institution catering to the ranks of our profession."[9]

In some detail, the committee was also charged with the function of "working as far as possible in conjunction with the State Associations and State Embalmers' Licensing Boards." This committee was to "arrange and prescribe and present to this association for approval a detailed schedule of instruction which shall represent a standard that is in keeping with the dignity of our profession." Having determined upon such schedule, this committee was further to "arrange with standard educational institutions for giving the necessary instruction to meet the requirements of such schedule."[10]

In the succeeding years, this committee and its various elected members worked in close cooperation with the newly formed Conference of Embalmers Examining Boards. The meetings of this conference were usually held just prior to those of the national association and in the same city. Occasionally, a member of the conference would also be a member of NFDA's Educational Committee.

While this committee received many recommendations designed to better mortuary education, and recommended for adoption a considerable number of them, actual progress was not always as rapid as enthusiastic committee reports would seem to indicate. It was not until the 1920s, when the number of licensed embalmers in the field had soared above 35,000, that the committee's repeated pleas for increased requirements and higher standards of educational and technical instruction began to receive serious notice. By 1924, an overture from the Conference of Embalmers Examining Boards, made to NFDA through the Committee on Legislation, suggested the formation of a new joint committee consisting of three members from the conference, three from NFDA, and three from the National Selected Morticians. This joint committee would be set up to "coordinate activities looking toward the enactment of more uniform laws in the various states requiring higher standards of entrance into the profession."[11]

In the same year, the Committee on Education recommended establishment of the American Institute of Funeral Directors.

> 1. The affairs of the Institute shall be in charge of a commission of five funeral directors who have state licenses... The purpose and duties of this Commission shall be: To endeavor to establish uniform preliminary requirements in all states willing to cooperate.
>
> 2. Said Commission shall be ready to furnish, under seal, original examination questions and answers for the use of those State Boards, which may desire this service.

3. To provide increased opportunities for self-development for individual licensed funeral directors and embalmers by providing for the conducting of a course (or Institute) in funeral directing, embalming, cost accounting and other business methods for funeral directors and embalmers.[12]

Only NFDA members in good standing were permitted to become students in the institutes, which were to begin as soon as the commissioners felt conditions warranted. In 1926, plans to hold a two-week institute at the University of Chicago failed when an insufficient number of members enrolled.

In 1927, the two days prior to the annual meeting of NFDA in Cincinnati were given over to a highly successful institute, presided over by "Dean" Harry G. Samson, son of Hudson Samson, who was one of the outstanding 19th-century Pittsburgh funeral directors, past president of NFDA in 1885 and 1886, and resolute champion of increased educational standards and professionalism among his colleagues. Lectures by well-known experts in the field covered a variety of topics, ranging from anatomical and physiological subject matter to discussions of modes of pricing funeral services. Attendance was excellent, and it was generally agreed that such institutes should become permanent adjuncts to annual NFDA meetings.

1928 saw this conviction fulfilled, and "Dean" Samson again presided over another two-day session. At this second meeting, 14 speakers were present, each presenting a paper and leading discussions afterward.

These two meetings marked the high point of the NFDA pre-convention institutes. Although they were held regularly until 1932, and through the years 1937-1939, both the length and educational quality of the sessions diminished perceptibly until, at the end, they offered little more than an address or two, generally on trade matters.

Like many other similar ventures in occupational self-education, this one became a casualty of the Depression of the 1930s. It was reported by a representative of the burial goods industry, who was the main speaker at the 1932 institute, that between 1929 and 1932, funeral directing had dropped $100 million in volume of business.[13] During these difficult times, in which shrinkage characterized all phases of professional and economic life, many funeral directors faced the all-absorbing question of survival, to the exclusion of less-urgent matters. The fact that a number went out of business is in itself eloquent of the crisis the group was facing.

With the return of moderately prosperous times, mortuary education for funeral directors already established in the field assumed a somewhat different character. Two additions had been incorporated. One was a tendency to view business and marketing-research problems as not only highly important, but also as belonging to any program of education by "institutes," "forums," "in-service courses" or "lectures." The other was the tendency to accept the growing field of "public relations" as a likewise important part of any program of mortuary education.

Among funeral directors, academic and technical subjects were gradually relegated to the formal schools of mortuary education. When directors or their representatives demanded additional training for admission to such schools, their requests were less likely for specific course content as they were to be for an increased number of years of formal schooling; that is, for more general education.

The conception of public relations received concrete expression in 1930 with the establishment, within NFDA, of the Institute of Mortuary Research. The function of the institute staff was to disseminate information about the various media of communication (radio, newspapers, journals, spokesmen and the like) and to "troubleshoot" points of hostility and attacks on the occupation.[14] It was also to serve as an information center for all persons, whether connected with funeral service or not, who sought answers to questions in any way related to the funeral field. It likewise published *The Director*, the trade organ of NFDA. The institute operated enterprisingly through 1939. After that year, the newly created office of executive secretary of the association absorbed most of its functions.

More specifically concerned with mortuary education, but conceived in the narrower sense of the training and indoctrination of new personnel in the field, were the Joint Conference Committee and the Joint Education Committee, both closely related although separated in time. These joint committees represented the various interest groups and agencies in the field of funeral service and licensing and examining boards. In 1924, the National Funeral Directors Association and the National Selected Morticians each appointed three representatives to form a "Committee of Nine" with the Conference of Embalmers Examining Boards. This group, known within NFDA as the "Joint Conference Committee," issued its first report in 1924, which stated its "readiness to function any time on matters pertaining to the Three Nationals," and indicated its liaison activities in its support of the American Institute of Funeral Directors.

Substantively, along the lines of educative advancement, the license board of each state was urged to "step up its requirements of the applicant, and to make the examination, both oral and written, of a still higher standard." However, the committee felt that, because such harmony prevailed among the major organizations, it had no further usefulness, and, despite its continued existence on paper, no meetings were held for the next several years due to the difficulty of assembling the members from the different organizations at one place.

The 1929 committee report to NFDA called for a cut in representation to one from that group, but little more was heard from the committee during the next several years.

In 1933, the NFDA Education Committee proposed during the national meeting that a somewhat familiar sounding "committee of three be appointed to meet with the like committee from the Conference of Embalmers Examining Boards and the National Association of Embalming Colleges, to be known as a Joint Educational Council... to consider any and all questions referred to it by its constituent bodies, and to make such recommendations as may be advisable."[15] This group, known within NFDA as the "Joint Committee on Education" (with slight variations in its title) found sufficient common interests and problems to hold together as a coordinating agency from its 1933 inception at Rochester, New York, until its change in name to the Education Issues Task Force.

In 1956, NFDA's Commission on Mortuary Education, a panel of distinguished educators, set about to examine the work of the funeral director and programs of mortuary education. A year later, the panel's report, *The Future of Funeral Service Education*, based on a national survey, concluded with 58 recommendations for revision and upgrading of mortuary education and funeral service. Highlighting these were the proposal for a single license for the all-around "funeral service practitioner"; a basic three-year program for mortuary education emphasizing liberal arts pre-professional courses; and, significantly, a change in name and expanded functions for the current Joint Committee on Mortuary Education.

Although the commission's report remained, for the most part, a blueprint for the future, the joint committee was renamed the American Board of Funeral Service Education (ABFSE) in 1959, and incorporated two years later. From 1960 until 1972, the board was active in seeking recognition from the U.S. Office of Education as the official accrediting agency for mortuary science schools. This recognition was first sought by the conference in 1956. When it was refused such recognition, ABFSE began a restructuring process in cooperation with the U.S. Office of Education, which culminated in success on March 16, 1972. This, perhaps, is signally the most important milestone in institutional growth in the history of funeral service/mortuary science education. Today, the U.S. Department of Education and the Council on Higher Education Accreditation recognize the board as the sole accrediting agency for academic programs that prepare funeral service professionals.

ABFSE members include representatives from the accredited institutions, the National Funeral Directors Association, the National Funeral Directors & Morticians Association, the International Conference of Funeral Service Examining Boards, and the International Cemetery, Cremation & Funeral Association, as well as representatives from the public. The ABFSE meets annually; most of its work is carried out through various standing committees.

The expanded purposes of the board, outlined in its Articles of Incorporation, are "To further education in the field of funeral service and in the fields necessary thereto or allied therewith, and further to formulate standards of funeral service education and to give accreditation to proper colleges of Mortuary Sciences, and to do all things necessary to the foregoing."

Today, subject areas comprising the funeral service education curriculum established by the board include the sciences, business, social sciences, and law and ethics. An associate degree or its credit-hour equivalent is required (a minimum of 60 semester hours of academic course work, of which 25% must be general non-technical education courses). Most state programs additionally require the successful completion of a practicum with a funeral home. Specifics in each state differ.

(4) *Licensing Laws.* One of the highest hurdles facing all agencies, councils and committees concerned with the betterment of mortuary education has been the structure of state licensing laws. Although this matter has been referred to above, especially in the context of early associational developments, and will again be commented upon later in this chapter, its relevance at this point merits brief mention.

The crux of the situation seems to be that in the haphazard growth of state licensing legislation, few if any of the states have identical or corresponding rules that pertain to the organization, curriculum, programming and operation of schools and colleges of mortuary science. Licensing, as a state function in the realm of embalming and funeral directing, has carried with it an inclination on the part of the several legislatures to spell out in some detail the substance, structure and function of mortuary education within their respective states. The difficulties of achieving such standardization are succinctly reviewed by Dr. Robert McFate, professor of pathology:

> Some 20 or 25 years ago, the scope of funeral service had grown so wide that our modern funeral director began to appear. With many demands made upon him, he realized the value of a more complete educational background. As a result, state legislatures passed new laws requiring a high school diploma for entrance into a college of embalming or mortuary science.
>
> At this time, however, a major mistake was made. State laws were passed prescribing complete college curricula for the courses in embalming and funeral directing, so many hours of this subject, so many hours of that, and with no flexibility allowed. Furthermore, the requirements of one state would generally vary markedly from the requirements in a neighboring state. These requirements were not determined by a conference between the colleges and the members of the profession, but usually were based on the ideas of just one or two persons, often individuals not too well informed.
>
> For the past 25 years then, the colleges of embalming and mortuary science have been faced with the problem of meeting the requirements set up by state laws with no opportunity to change their curricula to meet the advances in funeral service. In fact most state laws, as they refer to education in this field, are completely impracticable and impossible.[16]

Developments in Mortuary Law:[17] Although the framework of legal controls over sepulture in England was set in ecclesiastical law — which, in turn was compounded out of earlier Church or canon law, generously mixed with components of civil, common and statute law — in America, the tendency has been to ground these controls in common law, and to look for precedents no further back than 1607, the year of the founding of Jamestown, the first English settlement.

The common law of England, founded on a concept of property rights, had little to offer the colonists in matters pertaining to the burial of the dead that was applicable to the New World situation. As a result, through the ensuing centuries, Americans have evolved mortuary laws of their own.

These are no less mixed and complex than those evolved by the English, however, in spite of the fact that, with temporal courts in complete charge of matters pertaining to the dead, it might have been expected that an integrated, organized body of principle and precedent would have developed. Such has not been the case; and to repeat for emphasis: in America, traditional ecclesiastical usage has been mixed with common law, *ad hoc* decisions of the courts, statutes enacted by the several legislatures, and municipal ordinances, until the sum total has almost defied reason, much less codification.[18]

In the evolution of traditional usage, along with items of sumptuary legislation, now long in disuse, and scattered court decisions — there were only about 20 of any significance between 1821 and 1900 covering all aspects of sepulture[19] — there were few regulatory laws governing the actions of the embalmer and funeral director. Most do not appear until the 20th century. Those of most significance were the first state licensing laws, mentioned earlier, beginning with Virginia in 1894, and, in the next several decades, encompassing a majority of the states. These, however, were statutes primarily dealing with the licensing and control of embalmers, and the impulse to license funeral directors or bring them under the control of state laws was a later development.

Nevertheless, a few states had such laws before 1900: Pennsylvania in 1895; Virginia, 1897; and New York, 1898. By 1910, the total had increased to 12, and by 1930, to 19. Today, the District of Columbia and all states, except Colorado, license embalmers and/or funeral directors. That these laws have been enacted for the purpose of protecting the public interest has been sustained as valid and constitutional, without exception, whenever any attack has been made upon them.[20]

There has been some difference of opinion as to whether the funeral director and the embalmer should have separate licenses, whether each should be compelled to have both licenses, or whether there should be a combination license. There have been decisions that have held it is improper to compel a funeral director to have an embalmer's license and vice versa,[21] and there has been at least one decision that has upheld the provision that each should have both licenses, or that both should have the combination funeral director-embalmer license.[22] The majority of court decisions have leaned toward the doctrine that the two callings differ so clearly that to compel one to take an examination for the license of the other is interfering with one's constitutional rights.

From the very beginning, the laws regulating both embalmers and funeral directors were held to be right, proper and legal, and were regarded as a reasonable exercise of the police powers inherent in the state. Both legislatures and courts felt that the enactment of such laws was in the interest of public health and welfare. Embalming, although not compulsory by federal law, has been regarded as a valid preservative and sanitary measure, and therefore as having implications for public health.

Since the 1970s, however, there have been a growing number of challenges to the public-health value of embalming; today, the claim of many years that embalming is essential to public health is seldom, if ever, made. Embalming is required by law in some states where death occurs due to certain infectious diseases, and/or when the body must be transported by common carrier, and/or when final disposition of the body does not take place within a specified number of hours. A caveat to these requirements is that they may be limited by certain religious beliefs and the mandates inherent in them.

Also, since the late 1970s, many funeral director/embalmer/mortuary science laws have been reviewed through "sunset" and other procedures. Only in Colorado has there been the abolishment of a mortuary science (funeral service) license law and licensing board. Despite this, the Mortuary Science Code of the Colorado Revised Statutes, effective 2011, does prohibit individuals from advertising, representing or holding themselves out as, or using the title of, funeral director or embalmer without evidence that minimum education and internship requirements have been met. The Colorado Funeral Service Board offers voluntary certification programs administered by the Colorado Funeral Directors Association. Because licensing changes might be enacted in states at any time, practitioners must always be aware of current rules and regulations that govern licensure.

There have been other indications of statutory recognition of the economic hazards flowing from the very nature of the functions of the funeral director. In setting priorities in estates, the statutes of a majority of the states have placed payment of funeral expenses only after the costs of administration and taxes. This preference is based on awareness that the funeral director must perform his or her services before the estate of the deceased is inventoried and declared.

A number of court decisions have underscored the liability of the funeral director for his or her own or an employee's negligence with respect to funeral procession accidents.[23] But, the funeral director is not liable for accidents due solely to the negligence of others. A few cases supply some precedent governing the action of the funeral directors themselves. The courts have decided, for instance, that a funeral director cannot hold a body as security for a debt,[24] nor can the funeral director delay a funeral against the wishes of the next of kin.[25] If this occurs, he or she is subject to legal penalty in the way of damages; likewise, he or she is liable if it is proved that an embalmer, while in his or her employ, improperly embalmed a body.[26]

The practice of zoning a particular municipality into various districts, such as residential, commercial and industrial, began about 1900 and, in the past 25 years, has become widespread. The purpose is to maintain property values and to limit the use of land for the public welfare. The establishment of zones is a legislative function, and before the courts will declare a zoning ordinance invalid, it must clearly appear that the ordinance is discriminatory or unreasonable in its operations, or has no substantial relation to the public health, safety or morals or to the general welfare.[27]

While a funeral home has generally been held not to constitute a nuisance as such, or as legally stated "per se,"[28] nevertheless the general rule is to the effect that, in the absence of zoning ordinance, the operation of a funeral home in a strictly residential neighborhood does, by its very nature, constitute a nuisance. The reason behind these cases is the theory that the hearse, the ambulance and the procession of mourners are reminders of the presence of death and can bring depression and discomfort to the normal person unused to such conditions.[29]

Where a funeral home is operated in an area permitted by existing local zoning ordinances, the courts will not interfere with the use of the home because it is not a nuisance "per se"; however, should the funeral home be so operated as to constitute a nuisance by the failure to observe such rules and regulations pertaining to the use of proper equipment for preservation of public health, a court may well grant injunctive relief to persons in the neighborhood who are suffering, or who may suffer, by the careless operation of a funeral home.

Shortly after 1950, a number of "preneed" (meaning prearranged and prefunded funeral and cemetery plans) appeared around the country. These promotional plans were created and operated by persons outside the funeral directing profession. The basic danger in these plans was that they lacked adequate safeguards for the public. There were no assurances that the contracted funeral merchandise, or funeral or cemetery services, would be available when needed.

Through actions of the state and national associations, statutes or regulations have been enacted by all states specifically designed to control these operations. Such preneed statutes, which vary among the states, are framed in the interests of both the funeral directing profession and the public. In general, when a preneed contract is entered into, certain protections are afforded in the contract to the consumer through specified contract disclosures and requirements. The licensing requirements of preneed sellers and agents, if state law permits an individual to arrange or sell preneed funeral services without holding a funeral director's license, are also addressed, as well as issues such as the solicitation of preneed consumers, and the cancellation, revocation, transfer, ownership, portability and other requirements of preneed contracts and funding. Some state statutes establish a preneed guarantee fund to make restitution to any preneed contract purchaser when the seller or other provider defaults on its obligations under the preneed contract. Laws governing how cemeteries may or may not offer preneed contracts or sell caskets or other funeral merchandise vary by state.

In the execution of duties, the funeral director is enjoined to respect the sentiments and feelings of the bereaved, but such is the nature of this work that obligations to a client can never be explicitly or totally defined by contract. There remains always a residue of things to be done and said appropriate to the circumstances of particular situations as they arise in the course of the care for the funeralization of the dead. While it is more or less universally accepted that this vocation is carried out within a context of individual enterprise, and for remuneration adequate to support a member of the community, it does not carry with it a sanction for dealing with the dead as merchandise, nor with the bereaved as merely customers seeking to maximize the value of their purchases.

In the course of the last century, in caring for the dead and serving those who survive, the funeral director has come to recognize that the legal and cultural sanctions for this vocation place it somewhat beyond general business practices in light of the special care and judgment that must be used. In other words, the customs and usages of our time make it so that the funeral director cannot seek to operate within the confines of our present legal and cultural definitions of judicious handling of the bereaved with a "let the buyer beware" attitude. All of the funeral director's obligations cannot be covered by the instrumentality of the contract.

Multiplication of Associations: During the 19th century, the associational impulse found concrete expression in the founding of a number of municipal and state associations, and two national associations — the National Funeral Directors Association, and the American Cemetery Association. This impulse to organize along occupational lines has continued, evidenced by the further development of local and state associations, and by the appearance of several new national organizations. A brief outline of the organizational characteristics of the primary national groups follows.[30]

AMERICAN MONUMENT ASSOCIATION

The American Monument Association (AMA) is a group of American memorial manufacturing companies that joined forces to promote the use of American-manufactured memorials. Incorporated in 1925 and originally named the American Granite Association, AMA members have been the leading quarries and manufacturers of monumental stone products in America.

Its offices are in Saint Cloud, Minnesota. Website: www.americanmonumentassociation.com.

CATHOLIC CEMETERY CONFERENCE

The National Catholic Cemetery Conference was founded in 1949 and is the largest and oldest Catholic cemetery association serving Catholic cemeterians nationally and internationally. In 2006, the conference was renamed the Catholic Cemetery Conference (CCC) in recognition of its international constituency. A guiding principle of the CCC is that burial of the dead is one of the corporal works of mercy. CCC is committed to cemetery advocacy and education, and to:

- providing a forum for discussion and dissemination of information concerning all phases of Catholic cemetery development, operation and maintenance.
- assisting Catholic cemetery personnel in the understanding and solution of their cemetery problems by assembling accurate information with reference thereto.
- assisting Catholic cemetery personnel in the continuous improvement of cemetery services in the archdioceses and dioceses they serve.
- fostering and promoting the religious, charitable and educational interests of Catholic cemeteries and their beneficiaries in cemetery service.

CCC meets these objectives by sponsoring educational programs, referral of products and services, providing information necessary for the successful operation of Catholic cemeteries, an in-house library file for idea exchange, and by providing members with legislative information.

CCC publishes a monthly magazine, *Catholic Cemetery*, a yearly *Membership & Resource Directory*, and various reports and forms. It holds an annual convention and tradeshow, as well as regional seminars.

The association offers the Certified Catholic Cemetery Executive professional designation. Membership is open to all Catholic cemeterians and suppliers providing goods and services to Catholic cemeteries.

Its offices are in Hillside, Illinois. Website: www.catholiccemeteryconference.org.

CASKET & FUNERAL SUPPLY ASSOCIATION OF AMERICA

Originally founded as the Casket Manufacturers' Association of America in 1913, the Casket & Funeral Supply Association of America (CFSA) represents the interests of suppliers to licensed funeral homes and funeral directors. Its members manufacture or distribute virtually every type of product used by funeral directors. CFSA's objective is to provide useful information and perspectives on the funeral industry and the funeral supply industry to support manufacturers and suppliers of funeral goods and/or services.

The association offers the following services to its members: education and networking opportunities through seminars and an annual conference and trade show; government and industry representation and liaison; industry credit services; targeted supplier lists; a monthly newsletter and website; and extensive research and statistical data, including trend analyses, market projections, and a proprietary sales-statistics program for members.

Its offices are in Lake Bluff, Illinois. Website: www.cfsaa.org.

CREMATION ASSOCIATION OF NORTH AMERICA

The Cremation Association of North American (CANA) was founded in 1913. Today, it is an international trade association of more than 3,300 members, comprising cremationists, funeral directors, funeral home operators and owners, cemeteries, industrial suppliers, and consultants who believe that cremation is preparation for memorialization. CANA originally was formed to promote cremation as the "safe and hygienic way" of dealing with a dead human body at a time when cremation was simply a form of disposition. CANA is now concerned with the proper treatment and respect for those who have chosen cremation. All CANA members must sign the "Code of Cremation Practice," which upholds the highest standards of ethics, education and consumer information.

CANA is a recognized national authority for information, education, products, services and support for cremation. Its annual statistics report includes cremation projections for North America at the state, province and national levels, as well as international cremation statistics. CANA publishes a quarterly magazine, *The Cremationist*, and also publishes a consumer brochure and information on its website. Member benefits include educational, networking, public relations, directory, certification and seminar offerings, in addition to the annual CANA convention.

Its offices are in Wheeling, Illinois. Website: www.cremationassociation.org.

FUNERAL SERVICE BUREAU OF AMERICA (1927-1935)

Of the several attempts made in the 20th century to develop more sound and workable business relations between funeral directors and casket manufacturers, and among funeral directors themselves, the movement to introduce cost accounting into the funeral service field deserves paramount attention. Although the need to know such an elemental fact as the funeral director's business cost has been recognized by many funeral directors, it was sharply underscored at the Public Relations Conference called by the Casket Manufacturers' Association in May 1923. Here it was discovered that, without this datum, it was impossible to organize an intelligent discussion of the business relations of the funeral directors and manufacturers.

Subsequently, in 1925, NFDA and NSM jointly sponsored a uniform cost-accounting study. Although participation was less than expected, records were secured from a sufficient number of funeral directors from different sections of the country that indicated most of them were operating without any certainty as to the soundness, from a business standpoint, of their practice.

The lessons of cost accounting were apparently so imperative to several of the officers and leaders of both the major associations that they were willing to put this subject above all other associational considerations. When their own enthusiasm failed to elicit the desired response, they formed the Funeral Service Bureau of America (FSBA) on October 8, 1927. Although the new group was independent of both NFDA and NSM, some of the groundwork had been laid in the former organization's Cost Accounting Committee, which had been in existence for several years prior to 1927.

Although the aims of the FSBA ranged widely, it can be fairly stated that its basic purpose was to promote the study and use of cost-accounting methods to foster the business interests of its members and to help dispel the aura of mystery that was felt to exist in the public mind regarding the business of funeral directing.

Seventy-six representatives of the better-established funeral homes formed the nucleus of the organization. This number was broadened later to include nearly 200 members. Ample funds were pledged to support the organization and ensure the prosecution of its major aims. Not only were cost-accounting procedures introduced to these members, but actual observation over periods ranging up to a year were also included by the agency that formulated them. Additionally, advertising problems were studied, and the organization also submitted the elements of a standard funeral service to the Federal Trade Commission for its consideration.

After a period of several years of rather intense activity, these organizational projects tapered off and little was heard of the activities of the bureau during the early years of the Depression. However, the principle of cost accounting was given impetus through the work of the organization, and cost accounting became an established practice in many, if not most, of the better-run funeral homes.

A brief renaissance of the fortunes of the bureau took place in 1933 when it joined with other groups representing the funeral service field, and with federal officials, to work out a code for funeral directors in conjunction with the National Recovery Act, which had been put into operation the previous year. At this time, FSBA, NFDA, NSM and other associational representatives worked together and, while not always in complete accord, set up a Code Authority comprised of a committee representing 12 major geographical regions, with three at-large members.

This group managed to work out a code for the field, but the brief life of the National Recovery Act provided funeral directors with only a short period to bring a widely scattered field of practitioners under a specific code of operations. Two important results may be noted, however. First, in light of the deference shown by federal officials to the FSBA for its claims to have a vast body of information and data on the activities of funeral directors everywhere, it became clear that associations that claimed to be representative of the field, or a segment thereof, would henceforth have to build up bodies of reliable knowledge concerning the actual practices of their members. Second, in a figurative sense, notice was served that funeral directors could no longer remain aloof of all that transpired outside the province of their immediate scope of operations — in other words, that occupational organization had become a necessity for all who wished to practice their vocation.

Shortly after the demise of the National Recovery Act, the FSBA slipped out of public notice and, by 1935, had passed out of existence. Much of the data gathered, and the experiences gained by its members, were passed on to the major associations in funeral service and allied fields. Some of their materials went to NFDA, but the lion's share was passed on to the NSM and to the Casket Manufacturers Association — known now as the Casket & Funeral Supply Association of America, referred to previously.

THE FUNERAL SERVICE FOUNDATION

In 1932, a group of funeral service leaders recognized the need for a national organization dedicated to improving mortuary management through education. This vision was realized in 1945 when Wilber M. Krieger and other visionaries established the National Foundation of Funeral Service (NFFS) as an educational trust in Evanston, Illinois.

The National Research Information Center, a division of NFFS, produced two landmark studies for the times: "Attitudes toward Death and Funerals," conducted by Northwestern University; and "Project Understanding," conducted by Notre Dame University. Since then, the foundation has evolved and adapted into the Funeral Service Foundation (FSF), the philanthropic voice for the profession.

The Funeral Service Foundation became the charitable arm of the National Funeral Directors Association (NFDA) in 1997 when the NFFS Board of Trustees transferred the foundation's assets, as a separate entity, to NFDA. This strategic decision gave the foundation more administrative power as part of the world's largest funeral service organization. The asset transfer included educational resources and the foundation's Beryl L. Boyer Library, now the primary collection within NFDA's Howard C. Raether Library, which is housed at NFDA's headquarters in Brookfield, Wisconsin.

Dedicated in perpetuity via establishment of its Hand-in-Hand Endowment in 2002, the Funeral Service Foundation receives operational support from NFDA and donors across the profession that help advance its mission to support funeral service in building meaningful relationships with the families and the communities it serves. The foundation fuels the careers of funeral service professionals through scholarships and professional-development opportunities, and funds and promotes initiatives and outreach that make a measurable impact on funeral service.

FSF's office is located in Brookfield, Wisconsin. Website: www.funeralservicefoundation.org.

INTERNATIONAL CEMETERY, CREMATION & FUNERAL ASSOCIATION

The International Cemetery, Cremation & Funeral Association (ICCFA) was founded in 1887 as the American Cemetery Association. At first, the association only served cemetery owners; this was later changed to include members from the cremation field. Today, the association has expanded to include cemetery, cremation, funeral, memorial industry members, students and industry suppliers to serve as a national problem-solving forum for managers and employees working in all aspects of the funeral service industry. ICCFA has international members, as well.

It offers seminars and conferences, such as its annual training conference designed to groom current and prospective managers for leadership positions in the cemetery and funeral service industry; an annual sales management and marketing conference for cemetery, funeral home and insurance preneed sales managers; and cemetery operations and management programs.

ICCFA holds an annual conference and expo, and publishes *ICCFA Magazine* 10 times per year. The association provides consumer information on its website.

Its offices are in Sterling, Virginia. Website: www.iccfa.com.

THE INTERNATIONAL CONFERENCE OF FUNERAL SERVICE EXAMINING BOARDS

The mission of the International Conference of Funeral Service Examining Boards (ICFSEB), a not-for-profit voluntary association, is to provide examination services, information and regulatory support to funeral service licensing boards and educators, governmental bodies, and other regulatory agencies. The organization was started during the 1903 NFDA convention in St. Louis, Missouri, when a group of state licensing boards came together to discuss common problems in transporting bodies across state lines. The name "The Joint Conference of Embalmers Examining Boards and State Boards of Health" was adopted in 1904. In 1928, the organization established a system to grade schools of mortuary science and education.

By 1934, 27 states required that applicants for licensure had to be graduates of conference-approved schools. The first National Board Examination was established in 1930 and sent directly to state boards for grading. By 1932, a committee was established to grade exams and report on the results to state boards. The organization's name was changed in 1940 to "The Conference of Funeral Service Examining Boards of the United States, Inc." "International" was added to the name in 1997 to reflect Canadian membership. Currently, all states, with the exception of California and the District of Columbia, accept the results of the National Board Examination as an assessment of content knowledge needed to practice as a licensed funeral director or embalmer.

ICFSEB provides consulting services, seminars and presentations for its constituent state regulatory boards at their request, as well as seminars for mortuary colleges. ICFSEB publishes and archives comparative statistics of examination results, holds an annual conference, continually monitors the regulatory environment, and provides other services to meet membership needs.

Its office is located in Fayetteville, Arkansas. Website: www.theconferenceonline.org.

THE INTERNATIONAL ORDER OF THE GOLDEN RULE

The International Order of the Golden Rule (OGR) traces its roots to the Hahn Rodenburg Advertising Agency of Springfield, Illinois. Beginning in 1919, the agency developed a variety of advertising programs that were widely used by area funeral directors. In 1927, an executive of the firm, S.P. Wright, began discussing the idea of grouping the agency's funeral director clients together in an association for the purpose of serving their common interests. In May 1928, the "Order of the Golden Rule" was officially formed, with its activities controlled by the advertising agency during the organization's early years.

By the mid-1950s, the need was recognized for more emphasis on the group's potential as a professional association. Numerous services and products other than advertising were now available through the "Order," and a plan was developed for reorganization to help members make good use of business and promotional services that were not provided by other funeral service organizations.

In 1956, a not-for-profit corporation was organized under the laws of Illinois for purposes of carrying on the activities of the association. Goods and services were provided through a separate for-profit organization, which was then privately owned.

By 1970, membership had grown to more than 1,000 funeral homes, and there was a general consensus that the association should control its own destiny in terms of providing goods and services to its members. In 1971, an executive director was employed for the first time who was charged with the responsibility of working directly with both the not-for-profit corporation and the supporting, privately held service organization.

The "OGR Service Corporation" was created in 1974 to consolidate the newly formed for-profit organization into the existing membership-owned corporation. In 1975, the new service corporation, owned by the members of the International Order of the Golden Rule, commenced operations to provide professional consultation on general business practices, products and services, and cooperative support to members of the association. A 1980 reorganization resulted in a unified management of both the association and service corporation. From 1983 through 1994, OGR facilitated the necessary changes to help members adapt to an evolving regulatory environment.

Today, OGR is an organization of independently owned and operated funeral homes worldwide, retaining its commitment to outstanding service, care and compassion to families in need, and to high ethical standards through educational seminars, conferences, publications, a resource guide, and cooperative buying opportunities, among other services. Members adhere to a basic set of principles that guide their practices with "service measured not by gold, but by the Golden Rule." OGR publishes *The Independent*, a quarterly publication for the benefit of its members.

Its offices are in Austin, Texas. Website: www.ogr.org.

MONUMENT BUILDERS OF NORTH AMERICA

Monument Builders of North America (MBNA) was incorporated in Chicago, Illinois, in 1906 as the National Retail Monument Dealers Association. For its first 15 years, the association functioned with no paid staff. Then, a series of executives were employed to provide leadership and relieve the volunteer officers of staff functions.

Among the programs was an early trial of a national advertising program, and efforts to persuade Congress to authorize a cash allowance in lieu of a marker or headstone for veterans, which is now in place. A monthly pocket-sized magazine called the *Monument Builder News* became a reality during World War II.

The following is a synopsis of the historical developments of the MBNA:

• 1950s: Creation of the Monument Institute of America; development of regular educational sessions.

• 1960s: Cemetery Assistance Program co-sponsored by the American Monument Association and the Monument Builders of America; Canadian Granite and Marble Dealers merge with Monument Builders of America to form MBNA; Monument Industry Educational Foundation created.

• 1970s-1980s: Association support of litigation resulted in landmark decisions with tremendous impact on the rights of monument retailers to do business in cemeteries, resulting in the 1986 development of the "Recommended Installation Guidelines" approved by both MBNA and the American Cemetery Association; scope shifted to industry-wide organization to include monument manufacturers, wholesalers, bronze manufacturers and suppliers to the trade; attained congressional approval for cash allowance to veterans families; was instrumental in organization of International Monument Federation; introduced certification program for memorialists.

• 1990s: "Mausoleum Study Report" published, an exhaustive research project examining challenges and solutions in the erection and maintenance of private family mausoleums; Consumer-advocacy program established to assist members and consumers regarding regulatory and legislative issues, as well as proper memorialization of loved ones.

• 2000-2012: Member benefits expanded; MBNA University (learning center) established in 2006. Three key areas of focus identified: education, legislative/regulatory affairs; branding of memorialization and the independent monument retailer. Bylaws changed, reducing districts from 20 to 10. MBFilms introduced.

The MBNA offices are in Dayton, Ohio. Website: www.monumentbuilders.org.

NATIONAL CONCRETE BURIAL VAULT ASSOCIATION

The National Concrete Burial Vault Association (NCBVA) was chartered in 1930 as a voluntary nonprofit organization of concrete burial vault manufacturers throughout the United States and Canada. Its membership includes independently owned and operated concrete burial vault companies. The purpose of the organization is to provide a unified voice for the concrete burial vault industry regardless of product affiliation, brand recognition or location. Every major brand affiliation of concrete vault manufacturer is represented as a member of the organization. NCBVA represents groups that provide in excess of 70 percent of all outer burial receptacles interred within the boundaries of its membership.

The association takes a leadership role to continually research and develop, specify and promote minimum-performance standards for the burial vault industry in specifications that serve as the standards whereby burial vault producers, customers and all interested parties may judge the structural integrity of outer burial receptacles brought to the marketplace. Procedures outlined by NCBVA are designed to demonstrate performance under the wide variety of soil and vehicle loads that the typical concrete burial vault and graveliner must withstand. The NCBVA intends to establish testing procedures to demonstrate whether manufactured units meet minimum performance specifications and criteria. NCBVA holds an annual convention.

Its offices are in Dayton, Ohio. Website: www.ncbva.org.

NATIONAL FUNERAL DIRECTORS ASSOCIATION

On January 14, 1880, a group of 26 Michigan undertakers held the first meeting of what would later be established (in 1882) as the National Funeral Directors Association (NFDA). Today, NFDA is the oldest and largest national funeral service organization in the world. From its national headquarters in Brookfield, Wisconsin, NFDA's membership spans the globe.

The National Funeral Directors Association is the worldwide source of expertise and professional resources for all facets of funeral service. Through information, education and advocacy, NFDA is dedicated to supporting members in their mission to provide families with meaningful end-of-life services at the highest levels of excellence and integrity. Funeral firms, licensed funeral directors/embalmers, retired funeral service professionals, mortuary science students, interns and apprentices in the United States and its territories are eligible for membership. International membership is open to funeral firms, individual funeral service practitioners and students across the globe.

NFDA's governing structure includes a nine-member board of directors, and a policy board consisting of representatives from every state and the District of Columbia. NFDA's Bylaws comprise the association's primary governing document. Upon joining NFDA, members agree to abide by NFDA's enforceable "Code of Professional Conduct," which addresses funeral directors' obligations to the families and the decedents they serve, as well as to the public, the government and to NFDA. The code assures consumers of the high ethical standards upheld by NFDA and its members.

Members have the opportunity to showcase their commitment to service through NFDA's Pursuit of Excellence program. This awards program, established more than 35 years ago, honors funeral homes that exceed customer service expectations and serve families with distinction.

NFDA's International Convention & Expo is the world's largest annual event of its kind and features speakers, workshops and a trade show. In addition to this event, NFDA delivers other annual programs, including advocacy, leadership, women's, mentoring programs, and more. It also offers more than 80 live and distance-learning continuing-education options for U.S. and international members and non-members; awards various performance certificates to member funeral homes; delivers exclusive professional certification programs; and offers comprehensive cremation resources.

NFDA conducts and funds research in areas of health, safety, the environment, and consumer and member interests to help funeral professionals meet changing needs. Through these endeavors, the association tracks comprehensive information, vital statistics and trends concerning its members, the funeral profession, and the funeral industry. NFDA houses the Howard C. Raether Library, a unique collection of books, periodicals, proceedings and other materials dealing specifically with funeral service through the ages, which is open by appointment. NFDA's in-house publications include *The Director* magazine, with a larger total circulation than any other funeral service magazine; the *NFDA Bulletin*, a biweekly electronic newsletter for members; the *Memorial Business Journal*; and the *Director.edu* for mortuary students. NFDA also publishes consumer brochures, offers online consumer information and resources, and operates a consumer-assistance helpline.

Its national headquarters are located in Brookfield, Wisconsin; NFDA also maintains an office in Washington, D.C. Website: www.nfda.org.

NATIONAL FUNERAL DIRECTORS & MORTICIANS ASSOCIATION

The Independent National Funeral Directors Association was organized in 1924, under the leadership of R.R. Reed, by a group of licensed funeral directors seeking to maintain high professional standards for the benefit of the public and their own business community. The funeral directors had been meeting with the National Business League, but there was a feeling that the funeral directors were not able to develop their full potential in the league because it was made up of general business groups. The first official president of the national association was G. William Saffell Jr. of Shelbyville, Kentucky.

In 1926, the association's name was changed to the Progressive National Funeral Directors Association. In 1940, a merger of the National Colored Undertakers Association and those members still a part of the Independent National Funeral Directors Association took place to form the National Negro Funeral Directors Association. In 1949, Robert "Bob" Miller, a Chicago funeral home owner, was elected the first general secretary of the association and, in 1957, the association's present name was adopted, the National Funeral Directors & Morticians Association (NFD&MA).

NFD&MA members include professional funeral directors and embalmers, and its members and members-at-large also belong to state funeral service associations dedicated to promoting common professional and business interests of members. The objectives of NFD&MA are to foster research; conduct workshops and seminars; investigate funeral practices; develop and maintain standards of conduct designed to improve the business condition of its members, and to maintain high standards of service for the benefit of the public; provide a continuing program of service and to develop and disseminate information beneficial to members and the public at large; represent the common professional and business interests of its members before various federal, state and local legislative, administrative and judicial bodies; and to engage in any other activities consistent with its purposes and objectives.

African-American funeral directors have had vast involvement with many historical events. During the yellow fever epidemic in the 1880s, the Free African Society furnished volunteers. In 1978, African-American funeral directors traveled to Dover Air Force Base in Delaware to recover victims of the Rev. Jim Jones mass-casualty from Guyana. Member and past national treasurer Andrew W. Nix Jr. was in charge of handling the human remains from this tragedy. NFD&MA members were also of instrumental service in the Albany, Georgia, flooding of 1994; the Oklahoma City bombing in 1995; and the Croatian air crash that took the lives of U.S. Commerce Secretary Ron Brown and other members of his party.

A number of organizations are part of NFD&MA, including the Epsilon Nu Delta Mortuary Fraternity, Inc., founded in 1944 in Chicago; the National Ladies Auxiliary, founded in 1952; the Birdies; and 100 Black Women in Funeral Service, founded in 1993. NFD&MA is comprised of chapters throughout the United States, the Caribbean, and South Africa. NFD&MA publishes *The Scope* magazine quarterly.

Its national office is in Decatur, Georgia. Website: www.nfdma.com.

SELECTED INDEPENDENT FUNERAL HOMES

Formerly the National Selected Morticians, Selected Independent Funeral Homes (SIFH) is a nonprofit, limited-membership organization of independent, locally owned funeral service firms founded in 1917. The association actively monitors its members to help ensure that consumers receive the best care available when they work with an SIFH-member funeral home.

The mission of this association is to study, develop and establish the highest standards of service for the benefit of consumers; to provide a continuing forum for the exchange, development and dissemination of knowledge and information beneficial to members and the public; to furnish information to members and the public regarding all aspects of funeral service; and to cooperate with communities and other organizations, public and private, to achieve its purposes and objectives. Membership is worldwide.

Selected Independent Funeral Homes holds annual and group meetings for its members and for special member constituencies; offers professional- and public-education programs; community involvement and veterans memorial programs; news and information; a management assistance program and other resources; and customized materials and programs for its members based on its standards of excellence in service embodied in the SIFH "Code of Funeral Service Practice."

Its offices are in Deerfield, Illinois. Website: www.selectedfuneralhomes.org.

Economic Growth and Developments: From 1850 on, innovations in the manufacture of coffins, burial cases and caskets, the spread of embalming as a sanitary and preservative measure, the rise of associations, and the changing popular taste in funerals all combined to mark the great social and economic developments in funeral service in the 19th century.

The task remains to point out some of the changing economics of modern funeral service — seen as a process of development in which the *organization* of economic relations has become something more than a promise, but less than a complete reality.

So closely are funeral directors and manufacturers of funeral goods related in the total complex of funeral service that the economic features of one group can hardly be discussed without describing, in the same breath, the like features of the other. In this respect, it has already been pointed out previously that one of the first concerns of the associations of funeral directors was with casket manufacturers, and, until the passage of the Sherman Anti-Trust Act in 1890, vain efforts were made by the two groups to protect each others' business interests through compacts in restraint of trade.

In 1899, there were 189 manufacturers of funeral goods (emphasizing casket manufacture) of sufficient size to fall outside the United States Census designation of "hand shop." The latter (and there were hundreds of them) consisted of small shops in which coffins and caskets were occasionally made by craftsmen, usually along with cabinet-making, furniture-making, rough carpentry, and the like.

By 1925, the total figure for both small- and large-scale manufacturers (again excluding "hand shops") had risen to 326 and, by 1947, to 568. The total volume of business of these establishments had increased likewise from a little better than $12 million in 1889 to almost $190 million in 1947.

With this almost sixteen-fold increase of dollar volume, there was, for the most part, little increase in the size of these industries, as the average number of employees per establishment grew only slightly during this period — from about 30 in 1889 to just under 40 in 1947, with less than one-fifth of all establishments having more than 50 workers each that year.

Casket manufacturing remained a diverse industry, with very large and very small companies, but the industry experienced rapid change during the last 60+ years. In 1950, it is estimated there were more than 700 casket manufacturers in the U.S., employing more than 20,000 workers. U.S. Census Bureau data from 2012 shows only 98 casket manufacturers employing approximately 3,800 (down from 161 manufacturers listed in 1997).

These changes resulted from the declining market for caskets due to the rise in cremation, as well as other reasons, including foreign manufacturers entering the marketplace, consumer preference for less-expensive burial options, industry consolidation, etc. Today, an estimated three companies produce more than 70% of all caskets sold annually in the United States. Total shipment value in 1997 was $1.3 billion; $817 million in 2007; $734 million in 2010; and $731 million in 2012.[31]

Behind the scenes, the relationship of the manufacturers to funeral directors through the early part of the 20th century continued to prove unsettled and unorganized. In 1920, the wholesale mortuary and merchandising business evolved into five central elements: large manufacturers; small manufacturers; large-scale funeral directors; small-scale funeral directors; and, finally, traveling salesmen and "jobbers." Jobbers represented many types of businesses: some manufactured certain products and jobbed others; some jobbed only one line; others jobbed several; and some salesmen sold practically anything and then shopped for it, and, thus, in a sense, became jobbers, as well.

The circumstances of casket manufacturers were such that small concerns could vary standards of quality, workmanship and materials to the extent that it was possible for them to cut wholesale prices and undersell the larger establishments, whose products had long since been standardized in quality, as well as price. Those funeral directors that operated, or tried to operate, on a large-scale basis would often try "price pressure" tactics on casket salesmen, attempting to get special discounts for large orders. Salesmen of quality-line products were often distressed by what they considered a misplaced emphasis on the price over the quality of the merchandise.

As a result, old-line casket accounts were lost when salesmen refused to cut prices, and smaller manufacturers found that by offering special and unscheduled discounts, it was possible to capture new orders at the expense of the larger concerns. Volume-buying funeral directors were not above entering the casket manufacturing field themselves, thus increasing the total number of establishments in an already crowded field.

In retaliation for competition — in the form of funeral director-encouraged, or funeral director-operated, small-scale casket manufacture — the larger and better-established houses encouraged new talent to enter the field of funeral service and made introduction easier by setting up showrooms (display rooms to which the funeral director could take a client for purposes of casket selection, the price to be set by the funeral director); by the cheap rental of equipment; and through the use of quite-liberal credit. During the 1920s, it was not uncommon for a casket house to have more than a quarter of its assets tied up in accounts receivable from its funeral director customers.

Casket manufacturers were also in the habit of extending long-term credit to competing funeral directors. For those who paid promptly, this created a hardship because their money actually permitted the manufacturers to build working funds upon which they based such credit operations. On the other hand, the manufacturers extending the normal trade discounts had a proper complaint against funeral directors who were paying in advance and financing competitive manufacturing concerns.

Still another intrusive factor (that of increasingly rapid style changes in caskets) made itself felt through the first quarter of the 20th century. A funeral director who would buy 100 caskets in 1910 would hesitate to stock a quarter of that perhaps 10 years later; five years later, a funeral director might consider 10 caskets in any one style a precarious inventory. As the factor of taste in caskets gained strength, manufacturers found the battleground of competition for style-acceptance had widened its lines. The impulse to standardize a product for large-scale distribution conflicted with consumer desire for a *variety* of styles. Often, the funeral director would seek some kind of individual expression, demanding certain markings or refinements on all the caskets purchased. The upshot was an opportunity for other manufacturers, often quite small, to enter into and remain in competition.

A funeral industry development of the 1980s and '90s was the growth of large consolidation companies. By 2009, three publicly traded companies accounted for an estimated 10% of available U.S. market share (Service Corporation International/SCI, Stewart Enterprises, Inc., and Carriage Services, Inc.). Today, the major market share company is SCI, which acquired Stewart Enterprises in 2013; SCI accounts for approximately 16.5% of the U.S. market. Carriage and StoneMor Partners LP are the other two prominent industry operators with a national presence, with a combined estimated market share of nearly 6% in 2017.[32]

Another industry development in the 1980s and '90s was the proliferation of "preneed" funding instruments for prepurchasing funeral goods and services. In the 1800s, religious groups first established "death insurance" (now called life insurance) to help survivors defray funeral expenses. In the 1930s, burial-certificate plans, mostly in the South, were followed by the development of funeral insurance, payable in cash toward funeral/burial expenses. Prepayment became prominent in the Midwest shortly after World War II. Today, every state regulates preneed practices. In 2012, it was estimated that nearly 12% of total funeral home revenues derive from preneed.[33]

Along with consolidation and preneed, increases in the U.S. cremation rate have had an effect on industry economic growth and development, since cremation tends to generate lower funeral home revenues. According to NFDA's latest published figures, the U.S. national cremation rate exceeded the burial rate for the first time in 2015 — just over 47.9%, from only 17% in 1990. By 2035, NFDA predicts the U.S. cremation rate will grow to 78.8% of all deaths.[34]

To return to our historical perspective, between 1900 and 1935, "curbstone" operators flourished with little investment as ventures offered the rental of their equipment and funeral paraphernalia, including a hearse, funeral coach, chapel or parlor, and possibly the services of an embalmer. In the 21st century, not unlike these "curbstoners" of decades past, casket stores, third-party sellers, funeral "event planners," and other sellers of funeral-related products or services increasingly operate outside of traditional funeral home establishments.

Integration and Stabilization: The stabilization of the number of practitioners in any field where there is a limited demand for services is an essential of any occupation. To entrust the problem of achieving such stabilization simply to the operations of competition and the fluctuation of the business cycle has apparently not sufficed for the funeral directors of the past century. It should be noted that there are proportionately fewer business failures among funeral directors than among many other types of businesses — even those with expanding markets.

Licensing legislation, as noted before, has had the effect of setting up standards of competence and performance necessary to the public health and welfare of the community, as well as for the funeral directing profession itself. Matters of reciprocity, renewal and assignability of licenses and other items pertaining to the circumstances of practicing these vocations likewise are almost universally covered in state licensing acts.

As is the case with other licensed groups, the responsibilities of the licensing agency in a few states are assigned to special agencies, such as the state board of health. In other states, the responsibility is assigned to a centralized department or agency that supervises all professional licensing within that state. And, in most states, enforcement of laws and regulations is dependent on the office of the attorney general or other legal officer.

A vast majority of states have a separate board that controls the issuing of licensees, which is involved in the enforcement of laws and regulations within its jurisdiction. Some such boards consist solely of funeral service licensees, while a number of state boards also have public members from outside funeral service. Some licensing boards, through both public and private representation, have become agencies for the control of personnel in the field, and thus have exercised some small influence in the restriction of competition for the market.

The burden of legislation goes beyond the stipulation of basic requirements for licensure. A sometimes ill-formed, but nevertheless recognizable, image of the practitioner and the service he or she performs orients this legislation; that is the image of the skilled practitioner dedicating all of his or her professional efforts to the task of serving the community on a full-time basis.

Although imperfectly realized, perhaps, by the lawmakers themselves and the funeral directors who have pressed for such legislation, there is, it seems, an implicit recognition of the need to keep the care of the dead from becoming perfunctory, impersonal and commercial, and from being brought into the workings of highly bureaucratized business organizations.

In *Funeral Customs the World Over*, Gordon Bigelow, past executive director of the American Board of Funeral Service Education, writes the following on licensure:

Most states issue what are called "combination licenses." This form of licensure authorizes the individual to perform both funeral directing as well as embalming functions. There are, however, a few states in which funeral directing and embalming licenses are separate and an individual can be both or either, depending on their background, education and training. The majority of persons licensed in funeral service hold both a funeral directors as well as an embalmer's license. There are still a few states in which the only license granted is for embalmer, while in a few other states, to become a funeral director the embalmer's license is prerequisite. Every state but one requires persons to be licensed before practicing embalming. Most states recognize the National Board Examination given by the Conference of Funeral Service Examining Boards.

A majority of state licensing laws specify the physical equipment of the funeral home/mortuary, such as a sanitary preparation room in compliance with safety standards. Some states license the funeral establishment. Typically, such licensure results in issuing a "permit" for the firm to hold itself out as a place in which funeral service is practiced. Such a "permit" is placed in jeopardy by the illegal acts of a licensee, or any other person associated with, acting on behalf of, or for the benefit of the firm.

Funeral directors, as well as most people in occupations that directly serve human beings, have developed or sought to develop a set of inner controls, or moral restraints, by creating through their associations codes of professional practice, professional ethics, credos, and pledges to each other and to the public they serve. While these might often serve as goals or ideals of conduct, their appearance marks the recognition by those who created them that their conduct must be subject to something other than simple, concrete rules of practice.

In the funeral home, the framed code of ethics complements the publicly displayed license to practice. Each deals with a form of control over vocational behavior, and while neither of these symbols absolutely guarantees orderly ethical, competent and professional behavior, their presence nevertheless expresses a form of occupational and quasi-public consensus concerning the need for and value of organization in the field of funeral directing.

CITATIONS AND REFERENCES FOR CHAPTER 12

1. The authors are indebted to the late Helene Carpenter Craig for putting unpublished materials dealing with early mortuary education at their disposal.

2. Charles O. Dhonau, "Influence Back of Mortuary Education," unpublished document, written at request of authors.

3. *Ibid.*

4. Advertised in the trade journals of the period.

5. American Board of Funeral Service Education: "Fact Sheet: 1975-2005," 2009 Administration Reports; "2014 ABFSE Directory"; ABFSE Annual Report, Program Year 2013.

6. See Proceedings, NFDA, 1904; also revealing: Correspondence of J.H. McCully, 1904-1917, NFDA Howard C. Raether Library.

7. Charles O. Dhonau, *op. cit.*

8. *Ibid.*

9. Proceedings, NFDA, 1904, *op. cit.*, pp. 60-61.

10. *Ibid.*

11. Proceedings, NFDA, 1924, *op. cit.*, p. 60.

12. *Ibid.*, p. 74.

13. Proceedings, NFDA, 1932, *op. cit.*, p. 147.

14. See the scattered reports of the Director of the Institute of Mortuary Research in Proceedings, NFDA, 1930-1939.

15. Proceedings, NFDA, 1933, p. 55

16. Proceedings, NFDA 1947, p. 33.

17. The authors are indebted to Thomas H. Clark and T. Scott Gilligan for their considerable help in preparing this section on the development of mortuary law as it affects funeral directing.

18. Jackson, *The Law of Cadavers*, *op. cit.*, pp. lxxv-lxxvii.

19. Thomas F.H. Stueve, *Mortuary Law*. (Cincinnati, Ohio: The Cincinnati College of Embalming). See "Table of Cases."

20. *Prata Undertaking Co. vs. State Board of Embalming and Funeral Directing*, 182 Ati. 808; *Nugent Funeral Home Inc. vs. Beamish*, 173 Atl. 177; *People vs. Ringe*, 197 N.Y. 143; *Keller vs. State*, 90 Atl. 603.

21. *Wyeth vs. Board of Health*, 200 Mass. 474; *People vs. Ringe, Supra*; *State ex rel Kemplinger vs. Whyte*, 188 NW 607.

22. *State Board of Funeral Directors and Embalmers vs. Cooksey*, 147 Fla. 337.

23. *Grothmann vs. Herman*, 241 SW 461; *Greenberg Bond Co. vs. Yarbrough*, 106 SE 642.

24. *Gadbury vs. Bleitz*, 133 Wash. 134.

25. Mass. 1932 Ch. 272, Sec. 42; N.Y. Penal Code, Sec. 2220; Okla. Tit., 21, sec. 1166; S.D. Sec. 13.1421; Wash. Sec. 2492.

26. Jackson, *The Law of Cadavers*, *op. cit.*, p. 462.

27. *Pritz vs. Messer*, 112 O.S. 628; *Euclid vs. Ambler Realty Co.*, 272 U.S. 365.

28. *Jordan vs. Wesmith*, 269 Pac. 1096; *Meldahl vs. Halberg*, 214 NW 902.

29. *White vs. Luquire*, 129 Southern 84; *Leland vs. Turner*, 230 Pac. 1061.

30. Information primarily based on March 2014 website self-descriptions of each organization.

31. U.S. Census Bureau, 2012 Economic Census.

32. Kelsey Oliver, IBISWorld Industry Report 81222, "Cemetery Services in the US." February 2017.

33. Caitlin Moldvay, IBISWorld Industry Report 81221, "Funeral Homes in the US." June 2012.

34. *The 2017 NFDA Cremation and Burial Report: Research, Statistics and Projections*. July 2017.

Chapter 13

The Panorama of Modern Funeral Practice

Even to the most superficial observer, it must seem apparent that significant changes have taken place in the American mode of life. Among these changes is a general rise in the standard of living; a continuing exodus from rural to metropolitan areas, with a resultant urbanization of a much larger segment of the population; increasing mobility; growing centralization of government, with the role of government impacting the lives of people; the decline of illiteracy and the rise in general education; increasing demographic diversity; the penetration of computers, the Internet, and social media into the workplace, home and other areas of life; changes in family dynamics; and, less tangible but no less real, changing patterns in religious beliefs and thoughts concerning human relationships — among them the meaning of death.

In light of these and other changes, we must ask what changes have taken place in American attitudes toward dying and death, and in the immediate and extended post-death activities.

In the sections that follow, two complementary lenses will be used to focus on the modern panorama: first, the funeral patterns of modern America; and, second, the work patterns common to the majority of American funeral directors today. In dealing with funeral patterns, comparisons will be made whenever expedient with American funeral practices of nearly a century ago, as described in Chapter 10; in dealing with the practices of funeral directors, contrast will be sought with former occupational usages.

THE FUNERAL PATTERN IN MODERN AMERICA

Responses to Death: In any society, death stops the orderly processes of daily life and necessitates the mending of broken personal and social attachments. Societies differ, however, as to the way their members act in bereavement and the manner in which they dispose of their dead. Historically, the pattern of mortuary behavior in any society is subject to change, although basic death beliefs remain fundamentally unchanged.

It bears repeating that the roots of American funeral behavior extend to the nature of God, man and the hereafter, and that, in turn, these beliefs and practices were influenced to some extent by even older beliefs and practices. Despite the antiquity of these roots, their importance in respect to the treatment of the dead in American society cannot be overemphasized. Nor can changes in practices to meet the needs or wants of those who survive a death be disregarded. For most Americans in the 21st century, there still is a reverence for the dead, with the concept prevailing that decent and respectful care and disposition be made of the remains. But changes initiated in the 1960s and '70s provide some incidental, and even inherent, differences in attitudes of the past 150 years and the practices predicated on them. In other words, there are some now who feel it makes no difference what is done with a dead body.

Because American funeral beliefs have undergone some changes, we will examine pre- and post-death customs and usages as they reflect changing social conditions, along with marked shifts in the very foundations of our funeral beliefs. Two of the more significant social conditions or social processes important in this connection are the growth of an urban mass society, and the changing form and functions of the American family, including the mobility of its members.

Along with industrial progress and business expansion have come the growth of cities and the concentration of the American people in urban centers. Of the host of social consequences that followed, one of the more important, especially from the standpoint of this study, has been the decline of communal or "folk" ways of living. Students of modern society have noted the manner in which groups of people, held together by ties of blood, religion and ethnic background, have become dispersed and scattered throughout cities and across the country. Although these groups still hold together with sufficient strength to keep many customs intact, and still might demand and support their own institutions (including funeral service), the broader picture over time is one of a weakening of the influence of traditional community ties, and the appearance of masses of individuals more aware of their individuality and self-interest, and more responsive to the inducements of fashion, popular taste and the currents of popular opinion.

A closely related development — the changing form and functions of the American family — has held the attention of many social scientists, government agencies, religious leaders and others. As the economic, protective, recreational, religious and formal educational functions formerly fulfilled by the family have tended to be given over to outside institutional agencies, the family has become a unity of persons thrown together in more intimate association, with a higher degree of personal involvement and an intensification of emotional relationships. Because of smaller family size, problems and crises that produce stress on individuals tend to be distributed among proportionately fewer family members — much more so than was the case in the 19th century, when families were larger and the sense of family ties extended to more-distant relatives who still closely involved themselves in the affairs of any family.

Thus, in a family circle today, death can produce the kind of crisis with which few members are ready and able to cope. Aside from the shock of loss, often overwhelming even among those who have expected the death, and the confusion that is magnified by the natural upsurge of grief, complicated questions develop to which the average person does not have certain and ready answers. How does one deal appropriately with an object both profane and sacred, i.e., the body? In what forms do the bereaved acceptably express mourning? What legal regulations bear on the subject of final disposition of the body?

These only sample a multitude of questions and problems that confront men and women at a trying time in their lives. And even without such disturbed conditions, there is a whole area of professional information and skill that, in a society operating with a high division of labor and resultant specialization of competence, has been assigned to the funeral director.

Contrast this modern response to Americans living in 1880, particularly in less-advanced rural areas, when there still existed customary modes of response to death that, although perhaps not too well attuned to the tenor of the times, were generally known well enough by the bereaved to enable them, if they so desired, to see themselves through the trying situation produced by death. Moreover, enough defined roles clearly remained so that not only family members, but also other relatives and, often, many community members, might be able to participate usefully in the care of the dead.

In 1880, the role of the undertaker in rural areas was minimal. In the cities, this work revolved around the deceased's home, the church of the family's choice, and the cemetery. The assumption of the direction of funeral proceedings was as yet a new role — somewhat imperfectly, if not less sincerely, conceived, perhaps — and certainly not as important or as central to funeral matters as it is these days.

Americans today, in addition to natural confusion and disorientation to death (except for those who have experienced a recent death in their family or who have arranged the details of a funeral service), are somewhat at a loss for knowledge of what is appropriate behavior toward the dead. From one's religious and cultural background may be drawn important cues as to what should be done, and the ecclesiastical rules and social norms that must be observed.

Yet, with the general decline of birth and death rates — which means smaller families and therefore fewer deaths within them — one is less likely to have experienced a funeral in the family, and only a minority have actually taken charge in matters of death. Missing today, for the most part, are the friends and neighbors who laid out the dead as a simple matter of community duty. Also missing in the culture of each family are the family traditions and remembrances of all the actions necessary after the death of one of its members.

While the burden of responsibility for immediate and subsequent action taken as to the deceased is still, for the most part, assigned to the funeral service licensee, there have been shifts in attitudes and action toward the emotional needs of those who survive the death. Some people, for example, want nothing to do with a dead body except to dispose of it.

The Funeral Director — Death Call to Disposition of the Body: In 1880, when the undertaker received a call to come to a home and help prepare the body for burial, one of the major concerns was to arrive as quickly as possible in order to begin preservation procedures. Until it was properly "laid out" and ready for funeral and burial ceremonies, the body would most likely not leave the home. Today, the funeral director and/or his or her assistants make the first death call primarily to remove the body to the funeral home.

The general inclination in American society to avoid considering death realistically and as a fact of everyday life often leads to confusion in the minds of those experiencing the death of someone close. The death of a loved one is one of the most distressing events to befall any person. Funeral directors today are expected to deal not only with the dead body but also with the state of mind of the survivors.

The varieties, alternatives and options of the survivors in respect to modes of caring for the disposing of the dead now make it necessary for funeral service personnel to be able to perform manifold funeral tasks and services. With few exceptions, a funeral service licensee is prepared and willing to do as little as arrange for a direct disposition of the body — without viewing or attendant rites or ceremonies — or as much as provide a united, personalized/customized service with a clergy person, if desired, during a one- to three-day period of the funeral.

Howard C. Raether, executive director of the National Funeral Directors Association from 1948-83, summarized the primary tasks and services of the licensed funeral director and embalmer as follows. The summary has been updated and expanded where necessary.

Today, most deaths do not occur at home as they once did. Per the most recent National Center for Health Statistics data, approximately 29% of deaths now occur in hospitals, down from 43% in 2007. Hospice growth may be one factor in fewer hospital deaths. From 1989 to 2010, deaths at home grew from 16% to 27%.[1]

The telephone call to the funeral home telling of a death and requesting the services of the funeral director is generally made by someone other than the next of kin, and is sometimes received by someone in the funeral firm other than the individual who will personally serve the family.

The first face-to-face meeting the funeral director has with a member or members of the family following the telephone call announcing a death is most important. If death occurred at a residence, this usually is a traumatic experience. If the family knows the funeral director, this will often result in a visible expression of grief. Sometimes a clergy person will be present and the funeral director and clergy person will begin to offer their coordinated services.

The funeral director must secure various details from the family for the purposes of completing the death certificate, newspaper notices, and for other purposes. If information is not readily available, the family is told they can furnish it later, such as bringing it with them when the detailed arrangements are made for the funeral.

Some people may be in the room where death occurred while the body is placed on the removal cot. This is especially true where there has been hospice care. When death occurs at a medical institution, or is the subject of a medical examiner or coroner's investigation, the body is usually in a morgue at the hospital or at some public facility, from where it is removed by the funeral firm. Seldom does the funeral director see the family at the medical institution or morgue, and then, hardly ever in the presence of the body. When the funeral director has not seen the family at their home or at the hospital or morgue shortly after death, generally the first meeting is at the funeral home.

Before any funeral arrangements are made, the funeral director asks to know who is the spiritual leader (if there is one) of the deceased and/or of the family. The funeral director ascertains if such clergy person has been notified of the death. If this has not been done the funeral director suggests it be done and offers to do it for the family.

During the arrangement conference, the funeral director will request the following types of information:

- Vital statistics regarding the decedent and the decedent's family
- Service in the Armed Forces, if any
- Educational background
- Occupations and employment
- Religious affiliation, if any
- Membership in organizations
- Awards received
- Whether there had been a funeral or alternative prearranged/pre-financed
- Form of body disposition desired
- Ownership of cemetery plot, mausoleum space or cremation niche
- Selection of funeral/burial/cremation merchandise
- Visitation with open or closed casket
- Clothing for deceased
- Type of service: public, private, none
- Personalization/customized funeral requests
- Flowers and other remembrances
- Casket bearers
- Donation of body preference, if any.

The preparation of the body for funeralization is undertaken by a licensed embalmer. To temporary preservation and sanitation, the major purposes of embalming in the late-19th century, has been added the function of restoration (restorative art). Using skills akin to those of the sculptor, artist and plastic surgeon, the embalmer (working, if possible, from a photograph of the deceased) restores the facial features to the appearance of the person prior to a devastating illness or accident.

Most decisions regarding a funeral, an option within it, or an alternative to it include some type of merchandise — generally a casket or an urn. Today, there are many casket, outer burial container, and other merchandise display options for the funeral home, from the traditional full-casket display room to closed quarter-casket display systems to virtual selection rooms. The accelerating move from the full-casket selection room of the past in part results from the discomfort and sense of intimidation that many people experience when they enter this type of selection room. Many have never seen a display of burial merchandise before; some experience distressing reactions, perhaps predicated on a subconscious picturing of the deceased in the casket. The array of caskets might be uncomfortable reminders of mortality that some might wish to deny. Some funeral directors enter the selection room with the family to explain the merchandise and to answer questions, and stay with the family until a selection is made. Others leave families to explore the selection room on their own, after some explanatory remarks, and might rejoin them there at their request to answer questions, or meet with them after they have made their decision as to the kind of casket and other funeral merchandise they want. Many funeral homes today have multi-purpose merchandise display rooms including a range of cremation and memorialization items, sometimes including monument selection options.

Prior to the Federal Trade Commission (FTC) Rule for Funeral Industry Practices (Funeral Rule), the price of the funeral was directly related to the casket selection, using one of the following methods of pricing/quoting a funeral. When a family decided on the kind of service and merchandise desired, the funeral director provided a memorandum or agreement for the family to approve or sign.

• In the *single unit* method, the price on the casket or associated with it included the casket, services, and facilities of the funeral establishment.

• In the *bi-unit* method, there was a charge for services and facilities and a separate charge for the casket.

• In the *tri-unit* method, there were charges for (1) the services, (2) the facilities, and (3) the casket.

• In the *multi-unit* method, there was a separate charge for each major component of the funeral and also for items within one or more of the components.

With the implementation of the mandatory FTC Funeral Rule on April 30, 1984, following 12 years of meetings and public hearings, some of which were attempts to establish voluntary guidelines instead of a mandatory rule, the way that funerals are priced was radically changed. The purpose of the Funeral Rule is to enable consumers to obtain complete information about funeral arrangements so they can make informed decisions, paying only for the goods and services they want or need. The Funeral Rule requires funeral homes to provide written price lists of the goods and services available, including the prices for all available caskets and outer burial containers, with the intent of ensuring that funeral homes do not misrepresent state, local, or crematory or cemetery, requirements.

The current amended rule went into effect on July 19, 1994. The basic provisions of the amended rule, in addition to prohibiting misrepresentations and requiring numerous disclosures, require:

• A printed or typewritten General Price List (GPL) must be physically given for retention to anyone inquiring in person about goods and services, prices or the overall type of funeral to be arranged (at-need and preneed).

• A printed or typewritten Casket Price List must be offered to anyone inquiring in person about casket offerings or prices before showing the caskets. It can be printed or contained in other formats and must contain at least retail prices for merchandise that does not require special ordering.

• A printed or typewritten Outer Burial Container Price List must also be offered and must contain at least retail prices for merchandise that does not require special ordering.

• A Statement of Funeral Goods and Services Selected must be given to the client family at the conclusion of the arrangement in accordance with FTC requirements.

The amended rule prohibits charging the family any type of "casket handling fee" when the casket is not purchased from the firm conducting the service.

Before the Funeral Rule, most firms offered complete funeral packages based on the casket price, from which credit would be given for declinations of some components. Under the rule, itemization allows for the selection of components of the funeral or alternatives to "build" what is desired. Packages can be offered but they must be on the General Price List, along with the itemized prices of services and use of facilities, as stated previously. Funeral home practices to comply with the rule are subject to the interpretation of the FTC and court decisions (case law).

Some rite or ceremony that incorporates the embalmed body or the cremated remains follows a significant majority of deaths. If the body is placed in state, relatives and friends may call during the "visitation," "wake" or "calling hours." In most instances this is done in the afternoon and evening prior to the funeral service, and in most areas, viewing is limited to specific visiting hours.

Sometimes the visitation and funeral are held on the same morning, afternoon or evening of the funeral service. However, in some sections of the country, especially in the East, Midwest, and South, this period may be extended to several days. In "paying their last respects" to the dead, many of the friends of the deceased establish their only social contact with the immediately bereaved, since more persons in most sections of the country view the body or visit the family in its presence than attend the funeral services and burial. The viewing is controlled in some parts of the country by the funeral director to the extent that certain visiting hours are established. The custom of all-night wakes and sitting up with the deceased has all but disappeared; yet it is not entirely out of keeping with the routine of modern funeral home operations.

On the second or third day following death, the actual funeral service ceremony often takes place. Custom today sanctions for most the use of either a funeral home, place of worship or both. For Catholics in regular practice of their faith, for example, a church ceremony is required, except in the case of infants; Protestants and those of the Jewish faith may or may not bury their dead from their place of worship.

The funeral service ceremony is perhaps the most important facet of the modern funeral. Mourners gather along certain lines of protocol, and are seated in the main room of the funeral home or place of worship, while the family and immediate relatives often are withdrawn in another location that affords privacy in almost direct contrast to the older custom of putting the family on display. In the 1970s, there was a trend to return to the older custom of having the family sit with the rest of the mourners in the front of the room, as during a church funeral where family members will most likely occupy the front seats, nearest the casket.

If the funeral service is a religious rite, the wishes of the clergy prevail, subordinate only to those of the family in those areas where choices are available. When it is a religious rite, the viewing is usually completed before the service begins, with the casket closed for the service and from that point on. Whatever the situation, the family usually wants to have an opportunity to see the body of the deceased for the last time. Sometimes they will want their "leave taking" in private.

Until Vatican II (1962-65) the funeral rite of the Roman Catholic Church was rigid. It centered on death and its religious aspect; the liturgy did not include reference to those who survived with the exception of a statement that could be used at the committal. Vestments were black and cremation was prohibited in most parishes. After Vatican II, there have been slow but steady changes to post-death rituals. Survivors can now participate in the wake and funeral mass with readings or eulogies; vestments are white and the paschal candle is lit during the funeral service; and cremation is generally permitted.

The general pattern of the Protestant funeral service comprises four segments: the ritual, consisting of the reading of scripture and prayers; the funeral sermon; music; and the committal service. Participation in the service by family and other mourners is encouraged by some clergy members. Prayers for the most part are intercessory to bring comfort, consolation and strength to the bereaved. Many religious services have become more adaptive, and contemporary music may be used along with or in lieu of traditional hymns.

Jewish funeral ceremonies are traditionally kept very simple, with interment taking place as soon as possible after death. Cremation is not allowed in Jewish law. Typically, in Jewish communities of faith, a group of volunteers aid the bereaved and ensure that appropriate practices are followed. In some communities this is carried out by local cemetery societies or by funeral homes that observe Jewish customs and traditions.

Like other religions, Islam has laws and customs regarding the preparation of the body and funeral rituals. It is important that burial takes place as soon as possible after death, within 24 hours. Cremation is not practiced. Types of customary funeral practices may differ by Islamic community or national heritage.

A growing segment of the U.S. adult population is not affiliated with any particular religion. According to the 2015 Pew Forum on Religion & Public Life report, nearly 23% identify themselves as unaffiliated — an increase from just over 15% in 2007. Fewer Americans report belonging to various forms of Christianity: 70% in 2014, from 78% in 2007. Six percent report belonging to Jewish, Muslim, Buddhist, and Hindu faiths.[2]

When death is not followed by a rite or ceremony with the body present, there are alternatives to this practice, such as, but not limited to: (1) a memorial service without the body present; (2) a direct disposition as soon after death as the law would allow with no viewing or attendant rites or ceremonies; (3) the donation of the body to medical science with the possibility of a service with the body present prior to delivery to the medical institution; (4) a memorial service after delivery of the body; or (5) a committal service after delivery of the body by the institution. The method of final disposition also is a variable, with earth burial remaining the most common choice in the U.S.

Following services, or following the committal, a funeral gathering generally awaits mourners. The gathering might include a meal, whether at the place of worship where the service was held, the home of a family member or friend, a restaurant, or perhaps the funeral home (if state law allows food service in funeral home establishments).

There usually is a public committal at the cemetery, mausoleum or crematory. A funeral procession to the place of final disposition remains traditional in many parts of the country today. However, due to safety concerns, the practice has become less frequent or has been eliminated in a number of jurisdictions.

In place of the long drawn-out array of vehicles (carriages before 1910, and afterwards motor cars whose number often was interpreted as indicating the respect and popularity with which the deceased was held), the average funeral procession of today contains fewer persons, most of whom ride in privately owned automobiles. For many years, the funeral procession consisted of a funeral casket coach or hearse, and a seven- or nine-passenger limousine, as well as mourners' private automobiles. It would journey through sometimes heavily trafficked city streets to the place for the committal service and the final disposition of the body. Sometimes, the procession would go past the workplace or home of the deceased. However, increased costs and regulations have caused a cutback in the use of traditional vehicles today, and as we have seen, due to traffic-safety concerns, funeral processions are no longer allowed in many jurisdictions except for certain special circumstances — for example, funerals for dignitaries or civil servants, such as police officers and firefighters.

The committal service is performed at the site where the deceased will be interred. While some physical elements involved with the setting have changed in modern times (the use of artificial turf, chairs, tents), the purpose of the service has not. Members of the community gather to commit their loved one and friend, to pray, and to comfort one another. Depending on the tradition, those gathered may leave prior to the casket being lowered into the ground. For others, assuming an active role in the burial process by placing dirt onto the casket that has been lowered into the ground is symbolic of their farewell. In the Jewish tradition, the act of covering the grave is seen as the final "mitzvah" (good deed) that those present can perform for the deceased. All of these practices are meaningful because, as Paul Irion writes:

> The committal service provides, as nothing else... does so graphically, a symbolic demonstration that the kind of relationship which has existed between the mourner and the deceased is now at an end.[3]

The end of the committal service marks the end of the period of the funeral, although not necessarily the end of the relation of the funeral director to the bereaved. The funeral director finds there are many tasks to complete after the funeral is over, including insurance paperwork, obtaining certified copies of the death certificate, preparing Social Security forms, veteran requests, reviewing other funding, such as union death funds, and other tasks. The amount to be done depends on the benefits available to the deceased or the surviving family, the circumstances of the death, and the extent to which a family needs assistance.

Funeral directors may render many other post-funeral services, usually referred to as "aftercare" services. Funeral home aftercare may be defined as organized, often individualized, ways to provide and maintain services, support and education to families and the community, based on the unique nature of the funeral home and its personnel and the type of community in which it does business.

There are many levels of aftercare service, depending on the funeral home, its staff, budget and other considerations. At the least, funeral homes may offer an informal program based on active listening and the compassionate services of all staff members. A comprehensive, formal aftercare program might include facilitating self-help grief support groups, presenting grief education programs in the community, becoming an aftercare resource, and making informed referrals to licensed counselors, such as those specializing in grief counseling.

Since lawsuits can be brought against non-professional counselors alleging malpractice, funeral directors make it a practice to avoid misrepresenting their expertise or skills, so that they remain held only to the standard of aftercare expected of a funeral director, not a licensed counselor or therapist. Other ethical issues extend to a funeral home's aftercare operations: funeral homes should establish a formal aftercare code of professional conduct and expect strict compliance by staff, according to guidelines that delineate and separate aftercare job functions. To avoid even unintentionally misleading the public, funeral homes do not refer to aftercare services as "counseling" or "therapy."[4]

OPERATING THE MODERN FUNERAL HOME

The Contemporary Funeral Establishment: In physical appearance, the well-equipped funeral home of the modern period bears only a passing resemblance to the funeral establishment of the 1800s. Whereas modern establishments are, for the most part, constructed around the chapel or service room, the earlier types — which were not usually built as funeral homes but as private residences or stores and later converted into undertaking establishments — centered their emphasis around the "parlor(s)." Today, funeral homes are not located by chance or haphazardly, and their location and construction are governed by rules and regulations, including building codes and zoning laws.

Air-conditioning, comfortable furniture, easy access from the street, ample parking, the elimination of stairs, wall-to-wall carpeting, soft lighting, drinking fountains, and many other amenities reflect the goal of making mourners comfortable. In point of fact, after accessibility, for many years, beauty undoubtedly became the foremost consideration in setting the motif of the funeral homes of the 1950s and 1960s since they were either newly built, or in the process of rebuilding or redecoration.

A prime concern today is to make new or remodeled facilities multi-functional. Increases in building, renovating and utility costs, and the need for adaptability of portions of the building, depending on need, make this necessary.

While some ethnic, religious and other groups have had their own funeral directors skilled in their respective special services and customs, fewer funeral directors today count on a single ethnic or religious group for their clientele, although there are some Hispanic or Asian American funeral homes, for example, that specialize in serving those communities, usually in large urban centers. African-American funeral homes still predominantly serve African-American families.

Factors other than the traditional accessibility to, and services for, specific population groups are considered important when determining the location for a new funeral home today. It is critical to identify, for example, how many effectively competitive funeral homes already exist in the market area; how much investment is required to successfully compete with other establishments and to meet current and potential population needs; how accessible is the location; what are the demographic characteristics or changes operating in the area; or if there any environmental issues. When considering the purchase of an established funeral business, questions about its reputation, existing clientele, profitability and future market opportunities must also be answered. Of course, any new building or acquisition planning requires a formal business plan.

It has been noted before, but bears repeating, that it is characteristic of the business of funeral directing to persist under the same family name or operation, and to remain in the same area or site for several generations. While there are advantages to such permanence of site, the development of metropolitan areas nearly always brings with it an intensification of the problem of parking and, to a lesser extent, managing the traffic of funeral processions to existing or new cemeteries. The two related factors (increasing city size and density) have made permanency of site for funeral establishments somewhat less desirable than it was in the past. Today, a funeral home might move to a new location to follow its clientele or to relocate to a more desirable physical location with a population more apt to choose that funeral home.

It is sometimes difficult for the larger "volume" and chain mortuaries to anchor themselves into a community by any means other than a market relationship. The trend in the 1990s was for a multi-unit operation to acquire funeral homes, cemeteries and crematories in an area (*see Chapter 12*). The so-called "cluster" principle allowed for other than a strict market principle. Many of the firms acquired then continued their community roots as they competed with "independent" enterprises of one or more establishments, and with other national and international corporate operations.

Because of the nature of the work performed, all funeral homes have a basic physical and operational similarity. Since people die at all hours, and as funeral directors are expected to answer calls immediately, most mortuaries have a 24-hour availability.

The exteriors of most funeral homes are such that they add to the beauty of the neighborhood. Well-landscaped grounds, rock gardens, flowerbeds, evergreen plantings, etc., are all designed to create favorable public sentiment. Facilities are constructed in many architectural styles, from Colonial and other traditional styles to severely functional "contemporary." The "showcase" aspect of the funeral home adds to the funeral director's image in the community as a businessperson practicing in surroundings that are scrupulously clean and ordered, sanitary, dignified and even beautiful.

These standards make for important and costly problems in maintenance. For example, long before motor equipment wears out, it is felt to be obsolete, and long before funeral homes actually begin to look shabby, many funeral directors feel the urge to redecorate. Both the outside and inside of an establishment need constant maintenance and repair. Windows must be washed; lawns mowed; shrubs clipped; motor equipment washed and polished; walks swept;

floors waxed; furniture, caskets, and other merchandise dusted; and equipment and preparatory locations inspected and kept in good working order, as well as in compliance with all local, state and federal regulations and laws.

Funeral homes compete in many ways in a market area, including their standards and array of services, facilities and equipment. In fact, competition is not only with the firms in the market area, but also with funeral homes previously visited by their clientele. People make comparisons based on what they have seen or liked somewhere else.

Funeral home design-layouts today generally include an entrance hall or foyer, arrangement room(s), casket/vault/urn selection room(s), visitation rooms, a funeral service room or chapel, a preparation room, clergy room, reception or community room, offices, and receiving and storage areas. Room sizes and numbers, as well as the overall interior and exterior design schemes, reflect specific funeral home functions and community needs.

While funeral establishments do not exhibit the extreme variation in the number of workers found in commercial or industrial concerns, there is a significant difference between small and large funeral establishments. The range is between a small, family owned business (sometimes called a "mom and pop" operation) to an enterprise comprising multiple locations or a corporate enterprise comprising hundreds. On any scale, funeral homes today increasingly provide a combination of related services (when allowed by state and local regulations) that might include a cemetery, crematory, florist, monument company, trust and/or insurance preneed programs, or community meeting facilities for other rituals, such as weddings, graduations and retirements. These services might also reach beyond the local community to serve whole metropolitan districts or even larger geographical regions.

The nature of the relationships among funeral-establishment personnel depends mainly on the firm's size and its cultural and business perspective. In larger funeral homes with attendant specialization, there is considerable division of labor, and it is convenient to classify occupational personnel into three groups: (1) policy making — this group includes owners, proprietors, partners and active officers of the corporation, if there is one, and sometimes stockholders; (2) management, including those who function within the establishment — this classification includes managers, funeral directors, embalmers, receptionists, comptrollers, personnel managers and office staff; and (3) other staff, consisting of attendants, chauffeurs, garage mechanics, maintenance workers, etc.

This classification is by no means universally valid for all larger establishments and would be misleading if applied to smaller firms. The marginal or "gray areas" of the classification are made up of embalmer and attendant groups.

To some extent, the orientation of these groups depends upon how higher levels of management of a particular business look upon their personnel. For example, in establishments where embalmers assist in arranging and/or conducting funerals, classifying them as "labor" is unrealistic. Yet, embalmers as such have come to be regarded by many funeral directors, and by the courts, as performing a technical specialty today. Their training and functions cannot be placed at the same personal-service level as that of a funeral director unless they function within what is called the whole-man concept:

> The whole-man – total-funeral concept makes one person licensed to practice funeral service responsible to a family to try to meet all their needs in relation to the total funeral. While there undoubtedly will be some delegation of duty and authority, the person "waiting on" the family is responsible for the funeral of the one they loved. And if the funeral home owner is not the one, he will at some time or times check with the licensee responsible and the family to see how things are coming...
>
> *On the other hand...* the owner-manager-technician concept consists of... persons who do the arranging... others who are with the family for the casket selection... those who only embalm, and there might be some who just direct the actual funeral service. Most times these individual functionaries report to a central office or person. Sometimes that person to whom they are responsible is not a funeral service licensee...[5]

There are those who argue that this tiered concept is more efficient, less expensive and can affect economies of scale. Others maintain this concept could result in depersonalization because:

> The departmentalized or specialized services of the funeral home bring no single staff member in constant communication with the family so as to allow them a total picture of what is happening and what is needed. Also, because the family sees and makes various arrangements with two or three people, they are less likely to get sufficiently close to one of them to make some requests they might have, or to "unload" some of their feelings...[6]

Regardless, a funeral home's size or volume does not necessarily indicate depersonalization or less service. Many firms with hundreds of calls each year provide exceptional service that is just as personalized as that delivered by other firms performing fewer funerals.

In a few areas in the U.S., funeral personnel are unionized — usually embalmers or chauffeurs and drivers. In some locations, other non-licensed employees are also unionized, including pallbearers and cemetery workers. In larger operations, union organization is more likely as the inevitable association of employees along lines of mutual interest. There are no industry-wide, collective-bargaining patterns in the field of funeral service. "Trade embalmers" are self-employed, independent contractors who embalm for various funeral establishments and are not likely to participate in unions. Within smaller funeral homes, the funeral director, who also is a licensed embalmer, usually does embalming.

Traditionally, owners are apt to groom an employee as an eventual successor — a son or daughter, a relative or connection by marriage, or an employee whose performance and potential have impressed the owner. If interested in a career in funeral service, this person must naturally meet state-licensure requirements. Following a period of dedicated training and practice in performing the necessary skills of funeral directing and funeral home management, he or she may take over. Beginning in the 1990s, ABFSE graduation statistics show that significantly fewer individuals from funeral service families are receiving degrees than in previous decades: in 2014, 85% of graduates were from *non-funeral service families*. A growing number of attendees are non-traditional students with prior experience in different careers.

No reference to funeral home or mortuary personnel would be complete without pointing out the growing impact of young funeral directors. As we have seen, a higher percentage of newly licensed personnel are in no way related to someone already in funeral service. This "frees" them from having to do things "the way Dad wants it"; rather, they might tend to bring in new perspectives and innovation to the business.

THE FUNERAL: OPTIONS & ALTERNATIVE SELECTIONS

The Changing Scene: Some people who arrange a funeral, whether at-need or in advance, have an idea of what they want and what they are willing to pay. Others do not know what they want but think they know what they *don't* want. Much of what they learn about the funeral they get from the media, and the information is often negative, especially regarding costs.

What should constitute a reasonable funeral expense is not a simple matter, since there are many grounds for reasonableness. Empirical evidence reveals a decided lack of knowledge of funeral prices by most people, and even probate courts disagree on a standard for reasonable cost. Municipal, county, state and federal agencies have different ideas, and social reformers still other ideas.

The experience among funeral directors during the last century is that racial, religious, ethnic and social-class factors influence spending, but less than previously has been the case. A display of grief, flowers and open mourning are sometimes frowned upon as ostentatious and unnecessary by some groups; others might see a direct correlation between the amount of money spent on a funeral and the degree of respect for the deceased.

The cultural diversity brought about by increasing immigration of Asians and Hispanics beginning in the 1980s and '90s has raised the sensitivity of funeral directors to cultural differences and variations in funeral customs, many of which involve post-death activities with the body present. U.S. census information shows that the Hispanic population, for instance, is a large, growing and diverse population with geographical concentrations that vary by region, state and city.

In addition to cultural factors that influence funeral arrangements and help set prices and standards of quality in funeral service, there are several controls that, more or less, perfectly act to determine the business conduct of a funeral director. One of these is that the funeral director does not want to be in the position of selling an expensive funeral service for which a family cannot or will not later pay. Most funeral directors are aware that exorbitant funerals are bad investments for the consumer and can saddle the provider with the reputation of being high-priced, which ultimately results in less business.

Other important controls over the business practices of the funeral director are community perception, practices, expectations and opinion. These factors strongly affect the firm's service, facility and merchandise costs. There is the further control of local, state and federal laws, and the mandatory requirements of the FTC Funeral Rule. Among other things, state laws prohibit funeral directors from soliciting, taking advantage of a family, misrepresenting merchandise and services, and false advertising.

In concluding arrangements with a family or anyone else responsible for the post-death activities, and in all contacts with the bereaved, the funeral director must use his or her discretion as to what is appropriate to the particular circumstances. He or she needs to be in command of the social skills necessary to successfully deal with individuals who often feel uncomfortable and susceptible to increased distress. The funeral director must be sincerely empathetic to the suffering of others, and in a manner above and beyond mere commercial considerations.

Death benefits and burial allowances of the Social Security Administration, the Armed Forces, the U.S. Department of Veterans Affairs and other government agencies can be secured only by completing proper forms within a prescribed period. The funeral director performs this, or helps to get it done, by assisting the beneficiaries in completing the necessary paperwork to obtain insurance, lodge benefits and compensation awards, for example. It has been said previously that funeral directors serve the living while caring for the dead. Many times — days or weeks after a service has been conducted — the funeral director will be communicating with survivors.

RECENT DEVELOPMENTS: FUNERAL OPTIONS OR ALTERNATIVES

In the 21st Century: The "funeral," as used in this work, is defined by psychiatrist William M. Lamers Jr. as an organized, purposeful, time-limited, flexible, group-centered response to death. It traditionally involves personalized rites and/or ceremonies with the body present to commemorate that a death has occurred and that a life has been lived.

Although the majority of deaths today are followed by post-death activities with the body present, as described previously, the steadily increasing rate of cremation and the choice of personalized funerals or memorials by a growing number of individuals and families have changed the approach of many funeral directors. It can no longer be assumed that the next funeral a family arranges with the funeral home will be anything like the previous one that same family arranged.

Thus, today's funeral homes offer a variety of options: a visitation service that might or might not be followed by cremation; a religious service; a procession; a service offered solely at graveside; or other alternatives, such as the following, if arrangers do not want a viewing:

- A memorial service following the disposition of the body, usually via cremation.
- Direct cremation or immediate burial with no attendant rites or ceremonies.
- The donation of the body to a medical institution, if needed and medically acceptable. (State anatomical-gift acts were enacted starting in 1968.) Some institutions permit a service with the body present before delivery to the institution. Some have a committal service for the residue of the remains.

In the early 1960s, the vast majority of funerals included a religious rite and symbols. In the past 60 years or so, there have been many more humanist and other types of services without any rites or ceremonies.

Publicity regarding memorial societies, which began in the 1960s, has subsided, but some of the effects of these programs to ensure "dignity and economy in funeral arrangements through advance planning" remain. These societies continue to seek arrangements with funeral directors to provide particular services at specific prices and to publicize the arrangements they have made. The Continental Association of Funeral and Memorial Societies, now the Funeral Consumers Alliance, seeks to "protect consumer rights to choose meaningful, dignified, and affordable funerals." This group, located in Vermont, has existed since 1963.

The increase in cremation has changed the merchandise funeral homes offer. In addition to the standard items, such as caskets, vaults and clothing, there are additional options for families that choose cremation, including the availability of "rental caskets" used for a viewing only. (A removable receptacle containing the body is used for final disposition of the body). There are additional merchandise lines of caskets manufactured for cremation only, as well as the manufacture of many different kinds and styles of urns, in which the cremated remains are placed for memorialization.

Recently, in response to increasing consumer concerns about environmental issues — such as conserving energy, preserving natural resources, and choosing sustainable, biodegradable products — some funeral homes have begun to offer "green" funeral options. Basically, a "green funeral" does not include embalming or, alternatively, might include embalming with formaldehyde-free products; and it incorporates "eco-friendly" merchandise options, such as a biodegradable casket or urn, to meet the needs of the family requesting this type of funeral.

The expense of providing the services, facilities and merchandise by the funeral home has resulted in re-evaluating the cost-effectiveness of offerings, especially regarding those things not inherent in the value of the funeral, as perceived by the consumer. A 1962 study by sociologist Robert Fulton confirmed that the greater the education a person has, the greater the earnings, the less the religiosity, and the greater the doubt about the usefulness of funerals.

Today's research remains consistent with these findings, and Fulton's profile fits many of today's baby boomers. But funeral homes need to be profitable to continue to operate as a successful business enterprise. Hence, there will continue to be new approaches to delivering excellence in service, including the merging, acquiring and coalescing of firms, and the pooling of manpower, facilities and equipment to benefit from economies of scale.

RECENT DEVELOPMENTS: REGULATIONS AND ENTITLEMENTS

Federal: Myriad federal programs affect the day-to-day business operations of a funeral home. Funeral-specific regulations dealing with veteran and Armed Forces entitlements have affected operations since 1926. Government regulations, including those promulgated by the Department of Labor, the Environmental Protection Agency, the Transportation Security Administration, and others, as well as the Health Insurance Portability and Accountability Act, also affect funeral homes as business entities. As noted earlier, on April 30, 1984, the Federal Trade Commission (FTC) Funeral Industry Practices Rule went into effect, and it has had a major impact on the operation of funeral homes in the U.S.

In 1970, Congress passed the Occupational Safety and Health Act (OSHA), which, at that time, impacted funeral homes and funeral directors very little. However, many OSHA standards now directly impact the operation of the funeral home. In 1988, OSHA's Formaldehyde Standard, and its Hazard Communication Standard, became law; in 1992, the Bloodborne Pathogens Standard became law, mandating the use of universal precautions. More than 20 states now have state OSHA-approved safety and health plans that apply to private-sector employers. Those in the balance of the states comply with the federal OSHA regulations.

On January 26, 1992, the public-accommodations section of the Americans with Disabilities Act (ADA) took effect, prohibiting any public establishment, such as a funeral home, from maintaining policies, practices or procedures that deny persons with disabilities equal participation in, or access to, goods or services offered by a business. In July 1992, the ADA prohibited discrimination against disabled employees and job applicants by employers with 25 or more employees. In 1994, these employment-related provisions of the ADA were imposed on employers with 15 or more employees.

In 1981, Congress restricted eligibility for veteran burial and subsequent plot allowances. However, eligibility for burial or inurnment in national or state veteran military cemeteries, gravemarkers, headstones, presentation of the American flag and of a presidential memorial certificate remain. The federal government provides for the care and disposition of the remains of members of the Armed Forces, active and reserve, who die while in active-duty status. Military authorities will, in most instances, assist with the arrangements for these services within amounts allowed by the government, or the next of kin may make their own arrangements, if desired, and claim reimbursement in the amounts allowed.

The purpose of the lump sum death payment (LSDP) in the 1935 Social Security Act to guarantee a return of contributions was highly criticized. Congress enacted a small LSDP to become a benefit for every insured worker to help meet the expenses of death. In 1954, a ceiling of $255 was placed on the LSDP. In 1981, the payment was limited to certain members of the deceased's family.

Irrevocable funding of a preneed funeral contract constitutes "excludable assets" within certain state-defined limits under Supplemental Security Income (SSI) and Medicaid laws. SSI is a federal program that assures a minimum level of income to certain individuals with limited income and resources; Medicaid is a health insurance program, jointly funded by states and the federal government, for certain low-income and needy individuals. This asset "spend-down" to fund a funeral in advance does not affect the individual's eligibility for the programs.

State: For many years, most state laws affecting those in funeral service were associated with professional licensing. Over time, other laws were passed that dealt primarily with employee protection, such as various wage and hour laws. Currently, most state laws also control certain funeral business-related practices, including cemeteries, cremation, crematory operations, and preneed. In accordance with the FTC Funeral Rule, some states are allowed to administer and enforce state requirements that are more stringent than the rule. Entitlements, such as funds to pay or help pay for the funeral and final disposition of indigents, might be regulated at state, county or municipality levels.

RECENT DEVELOPMENTS: MANDATORY AND VOLUNTARY CONTINUING EDUCATION
Currently, 41 states and the District of Columbia require post-licensure continuing education for license renewal, varying from three to 12 credit hours per year. Continuing-education providers must meet state licensing board requirements. The Academy of Professional Funeral Service Practice (APFSP), founded in 1975, grants national accreditation to more than 50 qualifying course providers; a number of states automatically accept APFSP-approved courses for continuing-education credit.

Since the late 1970s, U.S. public and private schools have increasingly offered death education at elementary through post-secondary levels. In 1976, the Association for Death Education and Counseling was founded; as the oldest interdisciplinary organization in the field of death education, it works to promote and share research, theories and practice.

THE FUTURE: AN OVERVIEW

• The U.S. Centers for Disease Control and Prevention, using preliminary data, reports the 2011 death rate (annual deaths per 1,000 population) as 7.4, a record low. The 2000 rate was 8.72. The decline of the death rate to a record low value and an increase in life expectancy to a record high value are consistent with long-term trends. As the U.S. population progressively ages, the death rate is projected to increase to 10.0 by 2045-2050, and to 10.3 by 2050-2055.[7]

• Cremation rates, and a focus on memorialization options for families that choose cremation, will continue to increase.

• In 2016, it was estimated that 13.7% of total funeral home revenues derived from preneed, automobile parking services, and additional customized services.[8]

• The display and incorporation of memorabilia into the funeral — including personal items, photographs, and video and digital representations of aspects of the life of the deceased — will continue as part of the focus on personalizing funerals.

• Mourners and funeral directors alike will continue to decreasingly use the traditional color of black in their dress, ceremony and automotive equipment.

• Possible new EPA and OSHA regulations might limit the use and exposure limits for formaldehyde based on new scientific studies, which might have a significant effect on traditional U.S. funeral home embalming practices.

• The impact of the Internet on consumer behavior continues to grow. The proliferation of technologies — such as smartphones, online social networking, and user-review portals, for example — has facilitated a dynamic, multidirectional information flow that will continue to affect how consumers make choices and form opinions about businesses and services, including funeral homes and funerals.

• Future funeral home design, construction and renovations will continue to be influenced by innovative technologies, such as advanced computer-controlled audiovisual systems and the "green" movement, which is driven by growing consumer concern about environmental issues.

• As consumer beliefs change about what constitutes a "traditional" funeral, socially acceptable options or alternatives to the funeral will modify existing social norms and establish new ones.

In an address before the 1990 convention of the Association of Death Education and Counseling, Paul Irion observed that attitudes of various cultures toward death and mourning were being reshaped:

> Changes in our understanding of death and grief in the past few decades have produced corresponding changes in funerals — the ritual response to death. Protestant, Catholic and Jewish communities have developed new funeral services. Six common trends reflect a growing intentional awareness of the psychological and sociological insights into the mourning process. They are: 1. New funeral orders manifest an integrated, more comprehensive understanding of the function of ritual. 2. Emerging new orders see the funeral as a community function, not a private exercise. 3. New funeral services show awareness of the importance of facing the reality of death. 4. The funeral is set within the context of the mourning process. 5. New funeral orders are responsive to the religious pluralism we find in our society. 6. New funeral orders recognize that there are ministries to the bereaved for lay persons as well as for clergy.

The hallmark for American funeral service and its survival in the 21st century is to care for the dead and the living in a way that enhances the dignity of humankind. This must be done by meeting the needs of the deceased and of those who mourn before death, at the time of death, and for an extended period thereafter.

CITATIONS AND REFERENCES FOR CHAPTER 13

1. CDC/NCHS, National Vital Statistics System, "Health, United States, 2010 Chartbook"; National Center for Health Statistics, 2013.

2. *America's Changing Religious Landscape*, Pew Research Center, The Pew Forum on Religion & Public Life. May 5, 2015, 2012.

3. Paul E. Irion, *The Funeral and the Mourners* (Abingdon Press, New York), p. 110-111.

4. Howard C. Raether, "Person to Person Professional Service." *Successful Funeral Service Practice*. (Prentice-Hall, Englewood Cliffs, New Jersey, 1971), pp. 114-116.

5. *Ibid.*, "The Whole-Man Total Funeral Concept," p. 20.

6. *Ibid.*, p. 21.

7. "The 2017 NFDA Cremation and Burial Report: Research, Statistics and Projections." July 2017

8. "Funeral Homes in the U.S.: 812221," IBIS World Industry Report, October 2016, p. 13.

INDEX

A

Academy of Professional Funeral Service Practice 400
Acts of the Apostles 63, 75
Adams, J.F.A. 113
Adams, John 318
accreditation of embalming schools
.... 355, 356, 358, 359, 363
advertisements 162, 166, 167, 171, 173, 174, 175
advertising 325, 333, 334, 347
After-Life in Roman Paganism 73
Aiken, Alexander 164
"airtight" receptacle
.... 185, 186, 201, 221, 222, 224, 229, 252
Alexander, M.H. 356
Alexander V., Pope 109, 116
alienation of the dead 46, 144
Allen, F.D. 312
Allen, O.M., Sr. 242
"Alone in His Glory" 252
American Board of Funeral Service Education
.... 355, 363, 380, 381
American College of Embalming 355
American Encyclopedia of Etiquette and Culture 312
"American Funeral Director, The" 74, 159
American Funeral Director, The 252
American Language, The 137
American Monument Association 367
American Undertaker 336
anatomist, and embalming 108-110
Andrews, Charles M. 144, 152-159
Andrus Corpse Cooler 224
Andrus, R.C. 224
Angles and Saxons 72
    burial 79
    widow 87
Annals of the Barber Surgeons of London 121, 136
Anne of Austria 89
anointing the corpse 54, 60, 61, 63
Antigone 39
An Apologie or Defense of Brownists 142
Appian Way 64
arca 92
Ardron, Thomas 289, 307
Army and Navy Journal 252
Art of Embalming 26-27, 50, 116
Arts and Crafts in New York 178
Ashton, John C. 124, 137
Assoc. for Death Education and Counseling 400, 401
associations, development of 367-377
Aristides 59
Atherton, Lewis 283, 295, 312
Atkins, Robert F. 240, 242, 326
Attila 77

B

Babylonian Captivity 54

Bachtel, William H. 198, 212
Baddeley 115
Baillie, Matthew 119
Baker, A.A. 246
Baker, Lafayette C. 235, 253
Baker, Scipio 214
Baldwin, Mrs. A. 281, 312
Ball, James M. 184, 218
Baltimore, city directory 11, 164, 166, 182, 259
barbe 100
barber-surgeons 108, 120-122, 127, 128, 130, 136
Barber-Surgeons of London 121, 122, 130, 136
Barnes, Carl L. 354
Barnes School of Embalming 250, 355
Barron, Oswald 123, 137
Barstow, A.C. 186, 190
basketry coffin 202
"bearers" 256
"Beecher Flowers" 301, 312
Beecher, Henry Ward 301
Bellows, Henry 319
Bendann, Effie 74
Benjamin, Charles, L. 325, 338
Bennett, James Gordon 194, 196
Berner 83
Bigelow, Gordon 380
Bigelow, Jacob 303
bills, late-18th and 19th century 165, 170, 177, 183
Birch, Mrs. Benjamin 162
"Black Book" 322, 333
Black Plague 83
Blair, Robert 132, 138
Blair, Sherman 164
Blanton, H.J. 287, 295, 312
Bleak Age, The 137
Bleigh, Samuel 166, 259
Blind, Karl 70, 75
Blood, Thomas 327
body donation 387, 390, 397
body-lifting device 225
bone burial 89, 106
Bonnot, M. Raoul 266
Book of Common Prayer 94
Book of New England, A 158
Booth, Charles 135, 138
Boston, city directory 11, 12, 172, 190
Boston Evening Post 146
Boston Gazette 182
Boston School of Anatomy and Embalming 355
Bothick, Thomas W. 242
Boyce, William 127, 129
Boyd, George W. 209, 212, 214, 246
Boyer, Beryl L. (Library) 371
Bracken, H.M. 357
Bradford, Charles A.
.... 104, 105, 107, 115, 116, 120-121, 123, 137

Breasted, James H. 27, 50
Brewster, Ethel H. 52
Bridenbaugh, Carl 154, 156, 158, 159, 178
................................180, 181, 217, 218, 258, 259, 278
Bridgman's Patent Wrought Iron Coffin.........................184
Bringhust, Robert H. 340
broadside, Colonial 145, 147, 149, 151
Brooklyn Embalming Fluid Co. 250, 354
Brooks, Henry M. 155, 159
Brown and Alexander 233, 239
Brown, Isaac...174
Brownell's Hearse Repository.......................................260
Brownlow, W.R. 75
Bruce, Philip A. 152, 159
Brunetti, L. 238
Bryson, Charles, L. 312
Buckhout, Oskar K. 248
Buckley, Anthony 230, 239
Budge, E.A. Wallis................................... 28, 31, 50, 51
Buechel, W.P..57, 74
buffoon, Roman 48, 49
Bunnel, William 233, 253
Burch, George 230, 239
Burchard of Worms..88
Burial:
  cases 179-218
  cases, cloth covered 194, 196-197
  clubs 68, 96, 133-134
  dress, medieval 78-79
  extramural 64, 83, 303
  fees, medieval English...99
  immediate burial 142, 397
  in churches 69, 80, 82
  in cities 80, 82, 303-305
  "In Woolen Act" 96, 98
  mounds 70, 92
  of poor 46, 49, 50, 54, 56, 59
  ....68, 82, 94, 98, 106, 112, 174, 220
  practices, Egyptian... 28-36
  practices, Greek 39-44
  practices, Roman 45-48
  practices, Hebrew 53-56
  practices, early Christian 57-58, 59-66
  practices, medieval 79-95
  practices, Colonial 144-154
  practices, 19th-century American 279-313
  practices, 20th-century American 386-391
  receptacles, 19th-century "also-rans"
  ....197-198, 200-202
  safe...208-209
  and sanitary reform..133-136, 319
  vaults and outside boxes......................................208-217
Burial Reform Association of New York.......................321
Burpee, A.C. 340
Burr, Richard 235-236, 253

C
Cabinet-maker Undertaker 126, 162-164, 180
California College of Mortuary Science........................356
Calhoun, John C. 186-187
calling cards...297
Calvary Cemetery 304
Cambridge (Massachusetts), city directory 260
Camp, William J. 324
Canadian Casket 336
canon law... 59, 75, 156, 364
canopic chest 32
canopic jars 28, 29, 34
Canute the Dane 72, 107
Cardinal Bourbon...82
Carpenter, William S. 336, 354
carpenter 126, 127, 134, 135, 148, 164, 176, 180, 187
Carpi 118
Carr-Saunders, A.M. 349
carriages and hacks 166
Carriage Builders National Association.........................327
cartonnage 31, 33
Casket, The 231, 234, 250, 252, 253, 297, 312, 324
.... 325, 326, 327, 330, 332, 335, 336, 337, 338, 350
Casket and Sunnyside 51, 312, 335
Casket and Funeral Supply Association of America........368
Casket Directory of Manufacturers and
  Jobbers of Funeral Supplies 217, 254
casket hardware..215, 217, 328
caskets 179-218
  cement 185, 197, 198
  cruciform 202
  papier-mâché.. 185, 201
  rental 398
  sheet metal 193, 210
  straight sided 190
Casket Manufacturing 312
casket stores..380
Castiglioni 78, 113, 116
casting of earth 49, 100, 113, 295
catacombs 64-65, 75, 78
Catholic Times...300
Cattell, Henry, D. 233
cement-filled coffin 227
cement mold burial case 208
cemeteries:
  central 302, 303, 304, 305
  early Christian 63-66
  open air 66
  19th-century American.......................................302-305
  cerecloth 35, 98, 105, 107, 108, 148, 180
certification, Colorado 365
Chadwick, Edwin 133-134, 138
Chaffin, Hollis 175
Chamberlain, C.B. 235, 253
Champion College of Embalming 248
Champion Chemical Company 212, 214, 246, 250

INDEX

Chappel, Chase, Maxwell & Company 286, 327
charges 243
Charlemagne 80, 106
Charlestown (Massachusetts), city directory 175
Chaucer, Geoffrey 122
Chicago and its Makers 312
Chicago Association of Undertakers 354
Chicago Funeral Directors Association 327
"Christian Burial — What It Means" 74
Christian death beliefs and customs 57-69
Chrysostom, St. John 61, 63, 74
Church of England 100, 112, 142, 156, 258
churchyard 80, 82, 83, 84, 91, 99, 101, 102
.... 132, 134, 143, 152, 172, 174, 258, 303, 305
Ciba Symposia 50, 136
"Cincinnati Expert" 260, 262
Cincinnati School of Embalming 248, 354, 355, 358
Cities in the Wilderness 158, 278
Clark, Thomas H. 382
Clarke Chemical Works 242
Clarke, Joseph H. 246, 248, 250, 253, 254, 354
Clauderus 118, 119
clergy 66, 68, 99, 100, 101, 120
.... 132, 142, 178, 293, 295, 386, 389, 390
Cleveland College of Embalming 355
Clinical Topics 312
cloth burial cases 194, 196-197
cloth-covered bronzed cases 194, 196-197
Clover Coffin Torpedo Manufacturing Co. 204
Cobb, Augustus 320, 349
Cobb, John S. 321, 349
Code of Ethics 317, 332, 333, 334, 381
Coffin Manufacturers Association 327
coffin:
 and the aesthetic movement in funerals 183-185
 basketry 202
 celluloid 185, 201
 Egyptian 31, 34
 glass 92, 185, 192, 194, 200-201, 211
 Greek 42, 44
 iron 184-185
 lead 92, 107, 121, 184
 log 92
 stone 92, 185
 terra cotta 190, 198
 wood 94, 182
 protection against grave robbery 184
 and status indication 183
 in 17th- and 18th-century America 179-182
 variation in early function and type 183-185
coffin bill 183
coffined burial 92-95, 180-182
coffin furniture, Colonial 181-182
coffin pall 93
coffin shop 163, 182, 183, 187, 188, 329
coffin warehouses 172, 176, 182, 183, 308

cold air ice casket 244
College of Mortuary Science, St. Louis 356
Colonial Craftsman, The 217, 218, 278
Colonial Folkways 158
Colonial funeral behavior 141-159
Colonial hearse 258-260
Colonial undertaker 259
columbarium 46, 47
"combination" establishment 167, 169, 330
Commission on Mortuary Education 362
committal service, late-19th century 295
Committees on Education, NFDA 360-363
"Committee of Nine" 362-363
Concerning the Evolution of Styles in Hearses 278
Conclamatio 47, 49, 62, 202
Conil, P. 252
Conference of Funeral Service Examining Boards
.... 359, 363, 372, 381
Consolations of Death in Ancient Greek Literature 51
Constantine the Great 49, 58, 66, 68, 80
Constantinople 63, 77, 80, 90
Contagion, and the plaques 84, 90-91
Cooke, George W. 349
Cooley, William 172, 190
cooling boards 222-224, 244, 284
Coon, Carleton S. 75
Coover, Jacob 212
Corinthians 57, 73, 95
Cornelius, W.R. 233-234
"corpse bearer" 40, 93
corpse cooler 222-225
Cotton, Z. 168
couch casket 300
Council of Auxerre 59
Council of Funeral Service Examining Boards 357-359
Counter-Reformation 112
Course of American Democratic Thought 251
Cox, Charles 114
Craig, Helene Carpenter 381
Crane and Breed Mfg. Co. 187, 189, 193, 263, 270, 276
Crane, E. 238, 242
Crane, M.H. 187
Crane, Oscar N. 345
"Crane's Electro Dynamic Mummifier" 242
"Crane's Excelsior Preservation" 242
Creighton, Charles 50, 84, 98, 113, 114, 115
cremation 51, 113, 369, 371, 375
.... 378, 379, 382, 387, 390, 397, 398, 399, 400, 401
 among Germans and Scandinavians 69-72
 among Greeks and Romans 38, 42, 45, 49
 among Hebrews 56
 and the resurrection of the body 57-58
 as a protection from the dead 69-72
 as a transforming force 70
 movement in America 319-322
Cremation Association of North America 321-322, 369

cultural diversity 396
Cunningham, James and Son Co.
.... 260, 263, 270, 276, 327, 335
Cumont, Franz 57, 73
"curbstone" undertaker 380
customs, local medieval 100-101

D

Dana, Marvin 312
"dance of death" 102, 103
Danish invasions 72
d'Argellata, Pietro 108, 109, 111, 116, 118
da Vinci 118, 120
Davey, Richard
  .... 79, 85, 89, 94, 101, 108, 113, 114, 115, 116
Davis, M.L. 320, 321
Davis, W.C., and Co 186
Dawn of Conscience, The 37
Days of the Spinning Wheel 159
Death and Burial in Christian Antiquity 50
"death as sleep" 58
death beliefs:
  Egyptian 26-27
  Greek 38-39
  Roman 44-45
  Hebrew 53-54
  early Christian 57-58
  Scandinavian 69-72
  medieval 78-79
  Protestant 110, 112-113
  Colonial 144-146
  late-19th-century American 280-283
  modern American 383-386
death crier 85, 87
death dance 102, 103
death watch 85, 123
decanii 68
De Corpora Humani Fabrica 109
De Graff 118
De Moribus Artificum 113
Denis the Carthusian 101
de Palm, Baron 320
designator 48, 68
Deusterberg, H.B. 163
Devore, E.L. 176, 178
Dhonau, Charles 336, 354, 355, 358, 381, 382
Dictionary of Greek and Roman Antiquities 52
Dillon, John 182-183
Director, The 253, 362, 375
Directory for the Publick Worship Of God 142
Disbrow, W.B. 174
Disposal and contagion in the Middle Ages 84-85
Dionysius 39
Diodorus 28, 35, 36
Disposal of the Dead, The 114
"Disposal of Our Dead, The" 321, 349
Diuguid, W.D. 164
division of labor, mid-20th-century mortuary 394-395
Dobbin, John 168
Dodge, A. Johnson 250, 336, 354
Dodge, Arnold, J. 254
Dodge School of Embalming 250
Doge, Dandolo 84
Dolge, C.B. 354
door crepe 284, 296
Downey, Fairfax 158
"drummer" 329, 334, 338
dry burial 28
Duffy, John 251
Durfee, Allen 325, 326
"Dutch Charley" 330

E

Eames, C.J. 238
Earle, A.M. 145, 146, 148, 157, 158, 159, 180, 217
early Christian burial 63-66
Earth Burial and Cremation 349
*Ecclesiastical Sepulture in the
  New Code of Canon Law* 75
Eckels College of Mortuary Science 355
Eckels, H.S. 355
Economic and Social History of New England 158
education, continuing 375, 400
Edwin Chadwick and the public-health movement
  .... 133-134, 138
Egypt, Egyptian 25-38
  coffins 31-34
  death beliefs 26-27
  embalming 28, 30-31
  influence of death customs 36, 38
  undertaking specialists 34-35
Egyptian Chemical Co. 250
Egyptian coffin portrait 31, 33
Egyptian Embalmer Co. 250
Egyptian gold mask 33
Egyptian outer coffin 32, 33
Eighty-Fourth Homily on St. John 74
Eisenbrandt, Christian 202, 203, 204
elastic body shipping receptacle 226, 227
electroplating the corpse 226
Eliot, Charles, W. 321
Elliott, James S. 45, 52
Ellis, Hilda 69, 70, 75
Ellsworth, Elmer E. 230
"Embalmer" 122
Embalmers' Monthly 178, 336, 339, 357
Embalmers Supply Company 246
embalming:
  American, and the plague 226
  American innovators 226-241
  And the barber-surgeon 120-122
  Charge for late-19th century 241, 243, 283

INDEX

and the Civil War 229-236
   humanitarianism as a motive for................................246
   in America... 219-254
   in late-19th-century funerals..........................282-285
   medical... 117-120
   medieval... 106-110
   resistance to chemical preservatives..........................241
   Romans...46
   "schools" of...246, 248, 250-251
   with metallic salts...252
embalming fluid advertisement.......................245, 247, 249
Embalming Fluids................................... 116, 136, 254
embalming fluid patents 238
embalming literature before 1900 355
Encyclopedia Americana...115
Encyclopedia Britannica 114, 115
Encyclopedia of Religion and Ethics 50
Encyclopedia of Social Sciences 349
"end sealer" casket 191
"end sealer" grave vault..214
English Villagers of the Thirteenth Century 123, 137
Ensign, William..174
Epicureans 45
Epicurus..45, 73
Epidemics in Colonial America 251
Epitome of Medicine 109
Epitome of the History of Medicine 104
Epply, Charles M..248
Epply, J.P. 238, 240, 248
Erichsen, Hugo..321-322
Ethical codes 317, 332, 333, 334, 381
"Etiquette of Undertakers" 324
Etudes Historique et Comparatives
   sur les Embaumements 252
Euripides..39
Eustachius..118
Evarts, Jefferson...201
evolution of the modern casket 189-193
Everyman 101, 102, 115, 306
extramural burial...64, 83

F

"Facts About Casket Textiles".....................................312
Falconry, Dr..119
Fathers of the Church...78
Fearnaught, Albert.. 204, 206
Federal Gazette..162
Federal Trade Comm. Funeral Rule........388-389, 396, 399
female "layers out of the dead" 170, 172
feudal funeral..................... 123-124, 133, 135, 146, 295
Finer, Samuel 133-134, 138
Fire Burial Among Our Germanic Forefathers 75
"First Embalmer" 239, 252
First Fifty Years Were the Hardest, The 218
first responses to death...................................280-281
Fisk, Almond D...186-187

Fisk metallic burial case 186-187, 210, 218, 222
Fisk metallic coffin 186-187
Fisk mummy case 188
Flavius, Josephus 54
flower car..276
flowers 40, 46, 63, 98, 101, 268, 276, 284
   ....287, 292, 293, 294, 300-302, 309, 386, 396
fluid houses..241-251
Forest Home Cemetery...304
Forestus, Peter 109-110, 116, 118
fossarii 68
Francis, C.R. 178
Frank Leslie's Illustrated Newspaper 253
Franklin, Benjamin 221
Frantz, Frederick S..305
Frasers' Magazine for Town and Country.......................252
Frederick and Trump Corpse Cooler 222-224
Frederick, Robert 182, 222
Friedlander, Ludwig..................................52, 75, 115
"Friendly Societies"....................................... 124, 134
Frothingham, O.B. 321, 349
Frothingham, Paul R...321
Funeral or Grief a la Mode 51, 128
funeral at home.. 290, 292
funeral beliefs and practices:
   Egyptian 26-38
   Greek... 38-44
   Roman 44-50
   Hebrew 53-56
   early Christian 57-69
   German and Scandinavian 69-73
   medieval 78-110
   Protestant.. 110, 112-113
   Colonial 141-157
   19th-century American.................................279-312
   20th-century American.................................383-392
funeral badges 297, 299
funeral broadsides 145, 147, 149, 151
"funeral car" 263
Funeral Costs 74
funeral costs.......... 95-96, 146, 148, 150, 152, 154, 155-156
Funeral Customs, Their Origin and Development 50
Funeral Customs the World Over 312, 380
Funeral Customs Through the Ages 278
funeral directing:
   Egyptian 34-36
   Roman 48-50
   early Christian 66-69
   tasks described..161
   19th-century American.................................279-312
   20th-century American.................................385-387
"Funeral Director in Grandpa's Time".............................312
"Funeral Directors Since 1799" 178
funeral feasts 42, 62, 66, 88, 150, 152
funeral, feudal..123-124
funeral gifts, Colonial 146, 148

funeral home 292, 293, 310, 366, 381
.... 386-389, 392-396, 397, 398, 400
funeral invitation 125, 287, 290
funeral, medieval funeral of state 89
funeral notice, late-19th century 288
funeral offerings, Greek 42, 44
funeral oration, Roman 49
funeral ostentation 95-96
funeral pattern in modern America 383-392
funeral procession:
    Egyptian 35-36
    Greek 40, 42, 43
    Roman 47, 48-49
    Hebrew 54
    early Christian 62-63
    medieval 79, 81, 86, 89
    Protestant 112
    Colonial 148, 152
    and the hearse 255-256, 258
    19th-century American 265, 268, 294-295
    20th-century American 272, 275
funeral sermons:
    Roman 48
    early Christian 63
    Protestant 112
    Colonial 145
    19th-century American 290, 295
Funeral Service Bureau of America 369-370
Funeral Service Foundation 371
funerals:
    of an abbess 87
    of the Archduke of Brussels 81
    of Henry V 89
    of Queen Elizabeth I 97
    of St. Edward the Confessor 81
funeral undertaker 122-123
furnishing-undertaker 164, 166, 168, 174-175, 178

G

Gabriel, Ralph H. 158, 251
Galen of Pergamon 109, 110
Gallo-Roman Mourning Scene 71
Gamer, Helena, M. 78, 86, 113, 114
Gannal, J.N. 105, 115, 120, 228, 251
Gardner, Andrew 163
Garrison, Fielding H. 116
gasoline powered hearse 266, 268-278
Gasquet, Francis 74
Gaskell's *Compendium of Forms* 290
Gaussardia, J. Anthony 236, 237, 238
Gawler, J.A. 239
Gebhart, John C. 62, 74
general public-health movement 317-319
Genesis 73, 114
Gentleman's Magazine 107, 116
German funeral sacrifice 71

Germans 69-73
Gherkin, Henry 303
Gilbert, Paul 312
Gilligan, Harry J. 218
Gilmore, George W. 73
Giraldi, Lilio 82
Gish, Jacob 240, 242
glass casket 200-201, 211
glass coffin 200-201
Gleason 118
Gliddon, Thomas 324, 325, 326
"Glimpses Into Funeral History" 278
Globe Casket Manufacturing Company 242
Goede Vrouw of Manan-ha-ta 159
Good, John 222
Goodyear Rubber Company 251
Granja, Edward 238
Grant, U.S. 197, 199, 253
Graphic News 252
"Grave, The" 132, 138
grave linings:
    cement 208, 210, 212, 227
    clay 212
    concrete 208, 210, 212, 214, 216
    metal 208, 209
    slate 210
grave robbery 184
grave symbols 44
Graves, Frank P. 40, 52, 59, 74
graves, Hebrew 55-56
Gray, James A. 185
"Great Migration" 280
Greek funeral lot 43
Greek funeral procession 40, 42, 43
Greek mourning scene 41
Greeks, ancient:
    burial practices 39-44
    coffins and tombs 42, 44
    death beliefs 38-39
Greek Popular Religion 51
Greenhill, Thomas 26-27, 35, 50, 51
.... 116, 128, 130, 131, 137
Greenwood Cemetery:
    Chicago 303
    New York 303
    Milwaukee 305
Griffith, Howard V. 224
Guide to the Egyptian Collections
    in the British Museum 51
Guilds of the City of London, The 115
Gupton-Jones School of Embalming 355

H

Habenstein, Robert 58, 74, 134, 138, 152
.... 158, 159, 280, 312, 320, 332, 349, 350
Hahn Rodenburg Advertising Agency 372

INDEX

Harlan, Richard 115, 226, 228, 251
Harold the Saxon 72
Harpers Weekly 253
Harris, W.W. 336
Harvard Theological Review 52
Harvey, William 118, 119
Hawley, Sylvanus 324
Hawthorne, Nathaniel 152
Hayes, Rutherford B. 318
Heal, Ambrose 126, 137, 182, 184, 218
hearse 255-278
    chassis 274
    Colonial 258-260
    and funeral cars 263
    gasoline powered 266, 268-274
    horse drawn 260-266
    limousine 272, 274, 275
    sizes and colors 274, 276
    stationary 256, 257
    and tasks of funeral directors 276-278
heart burial 104-106
Heart Burial 115
Hebrew:
    burial customs 54-55
    death beliefs 53-54
    interment 56
    mourning customs 55
    place of burial 55-56
Hellenists 57
Henry V 89
Herodotus 28, 30, 35, 44, 51, 92, 109, 114
Herrick, George S. 312
Hess and Eisenhardt Co. 278
Hess, Emil W. 270, 274, 278
Hill Chemical Co. 242
Hill, Edward 242, 246
History of Ancient Egyptians, A 50
History of the Art and Science of Embalming, A 51
History of Chicago 312
History of Embalming 115, 228, 251
History of Epidemics in Britain 50
History of Greek Religion 51
History of Medicine 113
History of Milwaukee 312
History of Mourning 113
History of the Persian Wars 114
History of Surgery 116, 120
Hobbies 312
Hogarth, William 93
Hohenschuh, W.P. 325, 336, 353
Hohenschuh-Carpenter College of Embalming 356
Holmes, Thomas 226, 229-233, 234, 236, 238, 239
                240, 241, 242, 251, 252, 253, 254, 283
Homans, George C. 137
home services, late-19th century 290, 292
Homeric times 38

Homrighous, John 202
Howe, Julia Ward 252
Huizinga, J. 101, 106, 107, 115, 116
Hulberg, Fred 268, 269
Hulfish, Major 248, 250
human sacrifice among Greeks 40
Humphrey, Zephine 144, 158
Hunter, John 119
Hunter, William 119
Hurlburt, Cornelius 201
Hutton, F.A. 235, 238, 239, 240, 241, 253

I

Iddings, Warren 238
illatio mortui 83
Illinois School of Embalming 354
"immortelles" 300
Indiana School of Embalming 355
Infanson and Sons 266
injection embalming 226, 228, 238
injection, venous 118
injection pump 238, 240
Innocent VIII, tomb of 67
"Inominata" 236
Institutes, NFDA 360-361
International Cemetery, Cremation & Funeral Assoc. 371
International Conference of
    Funeral Service Examining Boards 372
International Order of the Golden Rule 372-373
intramural burial 66, 80-82
Introduction to the History of Medicine, An 116
"Inviter to funerals" 174, 287
Iowa School of Embalming 354
Irion, Paul 391, 401
Irish canons 86
Isaiah 52, 54, 73
Islam, funeral practices 390

J

Jackson, Percival 142, 143, 158
Jackson, Samuel M. 73, 75, 116
Jefferson, Thomas 318
Jeffreys, L.A. 340
Jenkins, Michael 162, 163, 175
Jenkins, William 163
Jeremiah 56, 72
John of Lancaster 118
Johnson, Andrew 318
Johnson, Edward 51, 136, 226, 251
Johnson, Edward C. & Gail R. 252, 253
Johnson, G.W.C.F. 158
Johnston, Harold W. 45, 48, 52
"Joint Conference Committee" 362
Joint Conference of Embalmers Examining
    Boards and State Boards of Health 357, 372
Jones, John Paul 184

Jones, Lewis	240
Jordan, Collins H.	240
Joshua	55, 73
Journal of the Plague Year	91
Judeo-Christian beliefs and practices	25, 53, 183, 390
Justinian	80

K

Keystone State Echo, The	349
Kher-heb	34, 35
Kilpatrick, H.M.	357
Kimball, Charles	224
Kimball Corpse Cooler	224
Kings	73
Kirk, B. Frank	163
Kirk and Nice	178
"kiss of peace"	60, 63
Knorr, Jacob	163
Knorr Undertaking Establishment	165
Krichbaum, John	204
Krieger, Wilber, M.	371

L

laborantes	68
lamps	63
Landauer, Bella C.	174, 178, 290, 312
Landauer, Bella C. collection	178
Laurel Hill Cemetery	303
law and burial	142-143
Law, John	172
Law of Cadavers	158, 382
laws, mortuary	364-367
Leagues of Prayer	85-86
Leclercq	64, 75
lectarii	68
Lekythoi	43
Lekythos	41
LeMoyne, Julius	320
Leonard, Moses	198
Leonardo, Richard	109, 116, 136
LeRoy	118
letter, black edged	290, 291
levatio corporis	66
Leviticus	73
Levy and Wilson	(see Wilson and Levy)
Lewis, Dr.	233, 234
Lewis, R.A.	134, 138
libitinarius	46, 48, 68
Library of Congress	159
licensing laws	364-366, 380-381, 399
Lechford	145
Liaison Bulletin	253
Life and Labor of the People of London	135, 138
Life and Times of Sir Edwin Chadwick	138
life signal casket	203, 205, 206, 207
life signals	202-207
limousine hearse	272, 274, 275
Lincoln, Abraham	230, 233, 240
Lincoln Park Cemetery	303
linings, grave	208-210
Lippincott, S.R.	325
livery, late-19th century	293
Lockhart and Seelye	260
loculus	92
London Gazette	258
London Tradesmen's Cards of the XVIII Century	137, 218
Lord, Francis A.	231, 232, 252
Los Angeles College of Embalming	355
Lowrie, James and Sons	263
Luke	55, 73, 75
Lukens, C.M.	246, 248
Luther, Martin	110, 113
Lyford, Benjamin A.	235, 253
"lychweake"	123

M

Maecenas	45
Magasin de Deuil	99
Makeland, Michael	121
Malphigi	118
Manual d'Archeologie Chretienne	75
Manual of Social and Business Forms	290
Marshall, Dr.	119
Martin, Nancy	221
Martin, R.G.	115
masks, Roman funeral	48-49
Massachusetts College of Embalming	250
Massachusetts Historical Society Proceedings	142, 158
Massachusetts State Board of Health	318
Massachusetts Sentinel	155
Matthew	56, 62, 73, 75
McCully, J.H.	357-358, 381
McFate, Robert	364
McGraw and Taylor Co.	190
McNeil, John T.	78, 86, 113, 114
medieval burial clubs	96
Medieval Handbooks of Penance	113
medical embalmers	117-120
Memoranda	114
memorial service	390, 397
memorial societies	398
Mencken, Henry L.	124, 137
Mendelsohn, Simon	50, 116, 136, 254
Mercerie de lutto	99
Merchant Class of Medieval London, The	114
metal vault	209, 210, 211, 212
Methodus Balsamundi Corpora Humani	119
"Metropolitan Health Bill"	319
Metropolitan Museum of Art	74
Merritt, Stephen	172
Merts and Riddle Coach and Hearse Co.	260
metallic burial cases	187-193

INDEX

Meyers, Eliab 250
middle ages 77-116
   Christian influence upon funeral behavior 78-80
   church and cemetery burial 80, 82-84
   disposal and contagion 84-85
   purgatorial doctrine 85-86
   wake 86, 88
   funeral feasts 88-89
   funerals of state 89
   sepulchral monuments 89-90
   plagues 90-92
   coffined burial 92, 94-95
   funeral ostentation 95-96
   burial clubs 96
   shroud 96, 98
   mourning colors 99-100
   widow 100
   local customs 100-101
   preoccupation with physical side of death 101-102
   sexton 102-104
   heart burial 104-106
   bone burial 106
   embalming 106-110
   Reformation 110, 112-113
midwife-undertaker 168, 170
Millard, A.J. 336
Miller, Joseph 174
Mills and Lacey 242
Minnesota, University of, 1909 embalming course 355
Minoan-Mycenaen Religion 51
Mitchell, Edwin 50, 59, 62, 73, 74
Modern Cremalist 321
Modern Funeral Home, Operating 392-396
mold for concrete vaults 210
monastic medicine 110
Mondino de'Luzzi 110
monkey spoon 152, 153
Montreal, city directory 162
monuments 46, 89-90, 305
Monument Builders of North America 373-374
Morgan, John 119, 238
"Mortuary Craft of Ancient Egypt, The" 50
mortuary education 353-364
mortuary law 364-367
Mott, Valentine 228
Mt. Auburn Cemetery 303
mourners, hired Hebrew 55
mourning:
   cards 287, 289, 290, 307-308
   colors 40, 99-100, 123, 296-297
   Egyptian 34
   Greek 40
   Roman 49
   Hebrew 55
   early Christian 61-62
   medieval 86, 88, 98-101

   Colonial 145-154
   symbols 295-302
multi-unit enterprises 379
mummy 26, 30, 35, 36, 37
*(The) Mummy: A Handbook of Egyptian
   Funerary Archaeology* 50
Murphy, George W. 240, 242
Murray, Margaret A. 50, 51
Murray, Thomas 172
Mycenae, Golden Age of 38
mystery cults 45

N

National Association of Embalming
   Schools and Colleges 362
National Association of
   General Baggage Agents 327, 344
National Board of Health 319, 328, 344-346
National Burial Case Association 327, 332, 340, 342
National Casket Co. 196
National Catholic Cemetery Conference 368
National Concrete Burial Vault Association 218, 374
National Conference Board Committee
   of Embalming Examiners 359
National Conference of State Boards of Health 344
National Council on Mortuary Education 359
National Fair of Funeral Goods 326, 327
National Foundation of Funeral Service 371
National Funeral Directors Association ....
   .... 156, 218, 248, 278, 301, 312, 313, 324, 327, 333
   .... 336, 345, 348, 349, 350, 357, 358, 359, 360, 361
   ..... 362, 369, 370, 371, 372, 374-375, 379, 381, 382, 401
National Funeral Directors & Morticians Association 376
National Government and Public Health, The 349
National Selected Morticians 360, 362, 377
National Undertaker, The 336
Nelson, Horatio 221
Nevell, Thomas 182
New Baker Patent Burglar-Proof Grave Vault 214
New England Institute of Anatomy,
   Sanitary Science and Embalming 250
New English Dictionary 124
New Kingdom 28
*New Schaff-Herzog Encyclopedia of
   Religious Knowledge* 73, 75
New York City, directory 159, 229
New York Cremation Society 320
New York Herald 194
New York Historical Society Quarterly 178
New York Journal of General Advertisers, The 162
New York Sun 194
New York Tribune 186, 252
Nice, Samuel 163
Nice, William J. 163
Nilsson, Martin P. 51, 52
Nind, J. Newton 357

Nirdlinger, Albert H. ...324
Nock, Arthur D. ...49, 52, 72-73, 74, 75
Norman burial ...79
Norman, John ...182
Northcote, J. Spence ...75
Numbers ...74
nurse-undertaker ...168, 170, 172

O

Oakes, Andrew ...164, 168, 175
Oakwood Cemetery ...303
Occupational Licensing in the States ...349
octagon metallic burial case ...188-190
Odoacer ...44, 77
"ogee" design casket ...190, 191
Old Southwark and Its People ...115
"On the Art of How to Embalm
 the Dead Human Body" ...116
operating the modern funeral home ...392-396
oration, funeral Roman ...49
"Order Concerning Embalmers" ...236
O'Reilly, John A. ...63, 66, 75
Osiris ...26, 31, 34, 36, 58
Our Lusty Forefathers ...158
Outlines of Greek and Roman Medicine ...52
outside box ...208, 212, 216
Oxford Dictionary ...122

P

pagan roots of modern funeral practice ...23-52
 Egyptian ...25-38
 Greek ...38-44
 Roman ...44-50
 German and Scandinavian ...69-72
papier-mâché caskets ...185, 201
parabolani ...68
Pare, Ambrose ...84, 120
Parish of St. Giles, Cripplegate ...115
Parish Registers of England ...114
Park, Roswell ...110, 116
patera ...92
Paton, Lewis B. ...50, 57, 73
Patrick, M.R. ...253
Pence, Paul ...212, 214
Penitentials of Theodore of Tarsus, The ...78
Pennsylvania Pocket ...182
Pepys' Diary ...144
Perkinson, C.F. ...312
Persian Wars, The ...30, 51
Petrie, W.M.F. ...50
Pettigrew, Dr. ...119
pharmacists ...241, 242, 327
Philadelphia, city directory ...170
Pierce, Bessie L. ...312
Pierce, Franklin ...318
Pilgrim Fathers ...142

Pilling, James S. ...308
Pitman, Aaron ...201
Pitman, Ben ...320
Pitman, Isaac ...320
place of burial:
 Egyptian ...27-28
 Roman ...45-46
 Hebrew ...55-56
 early Christian ...63-66
 19th-century American ...302-305
plagues ...28, 59, 61, 84, 90-92, 101, 226, 319
Pliny ...46
Plutarch ...40
pollinctores ...46, 48, 68, 104
Polson, C.J. ...114, 115, 116
Pooley, Ernest ...115
Pope Alexander V ...109, 116
Pope Boniface III ...106
Pope Gregory the Great ...79
Pope John III ...66
Porter, David ...150, 180, 183
Potter, Henry C. ...321
Powell, Rebecca ...170
Practice of Interments in Towns, The ...133
praeco ...48, 52, 62
prayers over the dead ...142, 145
Prente-Orton, C.W. ...72, 75
primitive burial customs ...59
priors of Durham ...98
Private Life of the Romans, The ...52
*Proceedings of the Massachusetts
 Historical Society* ...150, 158
procession, funeral:
 Egyptian ...35, 36
 Greek ...40, 42, 43
 Roman ...47, 48-49
 Hebrew ...54
 early Christian ...62-63
 medieval ...79, 81, 86, 89
 of Queen Elizabeth I ...97
 Protestant ...112
 Colonial ...148, 152
 influence of ...255-256
 late-19th century ...255-256, 258
 mid-20th century ...272, 275
processional dress, medieval ...85-86
"professional" card, mid-19th century ...168
professionalism, 20th-century traces of ...347-349
professional mourners, Roman ...49
professions ...317
"professors" of embalming ...242, 246
"Professor Rhodes' Electrical Balm" ...242, 350
Progression ...336
The Protestant Ethic and the Spirit of Capitalism ...158
Protestantism and industriousness ...143-144
Protestants, funeral practices ...390

INDEX

Prunk, Daniel, H. 235, 253
Psyche, The Cult of Souls and
   Belief in Immortality Among the Greeks 51
Puckle, Bertram S. 49, 50, 52, 61, 74, 75
   .... 86, 91, 100, 101, 114, 115, 116
Pulte Medical College 246
purgatorial doctrine 62, 63, 85-86, 112
Purves, William B. 162
pyramids 25, 27, 29

Q

Quacks of Old London, The 136
Quarantine Act 319
Quarter Century of Cremation in North America, A 349
Queen Elizabeth I 94, 97
Queen Mary Tudor 112
Quincy 325
Quinn, Seabury 252, 254

R

Raether, Howard C. 218, 278, 371, 375, 381, 386, 401
Ralph of Coggeshall 84, 113
Ramazzini 82
Rawlinson, George 30-31, 51
Reade, John 240
Reader in General Anthropology, A 75
Reader's Digest 218
Rech, Edward H. 256, 258, 278
rectangular casket 192-193
Reformation 51, 69, 86, 89, 110, 112
refrigeration of corpses 222-224, 225
Regino 86
regulation:
   federal 398-399
   state 399-400
Religion and Conscience in Ancient Egypt 50
religious functionaries 172, 174
Reminiscences 252
Reminiscences of Early Embalming 253
Renouard, Auguste 248, 249, 250, 326, 335, 353, 354
Renouard, Charles A. 353
Report on Intra-Mural Interments 133
"Report of the Massachusetts Sanitary Commission" 318
Representative English Plays 115
Requiem Mass 62, 63, 66, 78, 79, 85, 89, 112
responses to death in modern America 383-385
"restoration" 387
resurrection belief 38-39, 53-54, 57-58, 89
"resurrectionists" 204
Reynolds Williamsburg City Directory, The 229
Rhazes 118
Rhodes' Electric Balm 242, 350
Rhodes, George M. 242, 246, 350
Richardson, Benjamin Ward 252
Riders of the Plague 349
Riesman, David 110, 116

Road to Hel 75
Roberts, T.H. 325
Rochester School of Embalming 248
Rogers, Samuel 341, 342
Rohde, A. 38, 51
Roman:
   view of death 44-45
   burial customs 45-48
   funeral directing 48-50
   influence of burial practices 50
Roman Catholic Church 68-69, 78, 110, 112, 390
Roman Craftsmen and Tradesmen of the Early Empire ... 52
Roman Life and Manners of the Early Empire 52
Roma Sotterranes 75
Romulus Augustus 44, 77
rosemary 93, 101
rough box 216
"rousing the ghost" 88
Rulon, J.C. 240
rural funeral, late-19th century 287, 295
Rush, Alfred C. 39, 50, 51, 52, 58, 59, 60, 62, 66, 74, 75
Ruysch, Frederick R. 118, 119

S

sacred boats, Egyptian 36
sacred sledge, Egyptian 36
St. Anthony 106
St. Clair, Colin C. 238
St. John Chrysostom 61, 63, 74
St. Paul 45, 57, 64
St. Peter 64
St. Rose of Viterbo 107
Salm-Salm, Princess Agnes 253
Sammons 325
Samson, Harry G. 361
Samson, Hudson 238, 242, 243
   .... 263, 266, 283, 331, 333, 346, 361
Samuel 55, 73
Sandorf, Ivan 252
Sanitary commission 319, 349
Sanitary Conditions of the Labouring
   Population of Great Britain, Report on the 133, 138
sanitary reform 133-134
sarcophagus 31, 36, 50, 67, 92, 104, 185, 192, 194
Saturday Evening Post 313
Savage, Arthur 182
"sawdust and tar" embalming 128, 132, 220
Scandinavians 69-73
schools of mortuary science 354-356
Schroeder, Theodore 204
Scollay, G.W. 200, 238
secularization 142, 144
Seely, C.A. 238
Segato, Girolamo 119
Selected Independent Funeral Homes 377
sepulchral monuments, medieval 89-90

Sepulture: Its History, Methods and Sanitary Requisites 113
Service Corporation International 379
Sewall, Samuel 144, 145, 146, 148, 150, 154, 158, 168, 170, 178, 180, 217, 258, 278
Sewell's Diary 158
sexton 91, 102, 104, 112, 150, 155, 157, 164, 172, 173, 174, 176, 259, 285, 295, 310, 322, 335
Shadyside 336
Sharer, John H. 325
sheet-metal caskets 193
sheol 54, 55, 56
Shepherd, J.J. 164
Sherman, Charles C. 73
ship burials 70, 75
Sholl, David 198
Shorter Cambridge Medieval History, The 75
Short History of Medicine, A 116
Shroud 336, 341
Shuler, Isaac 200
Sickel, James C. 238
Signboards of Old London Shops, The 127, 137, 218
Simmons School of Embalming 355
"sin-eater" 101
Skene, Gilbert 84
Smith, William 52
Smith, William M. and Co. 190
Smithson, George 127
"Social Life in the Colonies" 159
Social Life of Virginia in the Seventeenth Century 159
"Sociological Study of the Cremation Movement in America, A" 74, 138
Solon 40
"Some American Funeral Ephemera" 178
"Song of the Coffin Drummer, The" 334
Sophocles 39
"Southern Undertakers' Union" 324
Spectator Papers 128
Spiritism and the Cult of the Dead in Antiquity 50, 73
Springfield Metallic Casket Co. 214
sprinkling with earth 49, 100, 113, 295
state anatomical gift acts 397
state boards of health 318
Statuta Antiqua 78
Steele, Richard 51, 128
Stein Manufacturing Co. 194, 196-197, 216, 286
Stein Patent Burial Casket Works 263, 286
Stein, Samuel 194, 196-197, 201
Stein, "State Casket" 197, 199, 287
Stephanus 118
Stephen Merritt Burial Co. Memorial 172, 174, 178
Stewart Enterprises 379
Stone, Elizabeth 73, 75
Stories on Stone 158, 251, 313
Story of Medicine in the Middle Ages, The 116
straight-sided casket 190

"Study of the Cremation Movement in the U.S." 349
Sullivan, Felix A. 248, 354
Sunnyside 252, 253, 254, 278, 335, 341, 343
surgeon and embalming 108-110
"Surgeons of the Short Robe" 120
suttee 44, 69
swaddled 96
Swammerdon 118
Sylvius, Jacob 118
Synodical Cases and Ecclesiastical Discipline, Of 86

T

Tatlock, J.S. 115
Taylor, Henry E. 335
Taylor, James 242
Ten Years of My Life 253
terra cotta coffin 198
"Their Last Words Had a Punch" 313
Theodolinda, Empress 79
third-party sellers 380
Theodosius, Emperor 80
Thomas, George L. 324
Thompson, C.J.S. 136
Thorpe, Alexander 166
Thrupp, Sylvia 95, 96, 114
"Timber Awl" 272, 334
"Time Stays — We Go" 312
Tobey, James A. 349
Totendanz 102
tomb:
    Egyptian 36
    Greek 42, 44
    Roman 46, 47, 50
    Hebrew 55-56
    early Christian 64
tomb vases, bottomless 51
Tompkins, E.A. 325
torchbearers 48, 49
Townsend, Job 181
trade card of furnishing undertaker 164
trade embalmers 395
tradesman undertaker 117, 125, 127-132, 161-168
Tranchini, Dr. 119
transportation 255-278
transportation of the dead 328, 342, 344-345
Traynor, A. 345
Treatise on the Art of Embalming 128, 131
Trinity Cemetery 304
trocar 241, 250, 284, 285
trolley funeral car 267, 268
Trumbull, H. Clay 253
Trump, G.A. 222
Tschniernoff, Dr. 119
Turner, Levi C. 253
Tut-ankh-Amon 32, 33, 34
Tyler, John 318

INDEX

U

uncoffined burial 54, 83, 94
Undertaker, The 335
undertaker:
    cabinet-maker as 163-164
    clergyman as 132-133
    Colonial 157, 259
    early 124-127
    Egyptian 34-35
    and the feudal funeral 127-128
    furnishing 164-168, 182, 308, 309
    late-19th century 282-294, 308-312
    midwife as 170
    nurse as 168, 170
    religious functionaries as 172, 174
    Roman 44, 46, 48, 50
    sexton as 172, 174
    town health officer as 174-175
    tradesman 127-128, 130, 132, 161, 168
    upholsterer as 162
    woman as 162, 168, 170
"undertaker" etymology 122
Undertaker's Manual 353
Undertakers' Mutual Protective Association 322, 323
"undertakers" tradesmen's cards 125, 129
unit-method of quoting prices 388-389
Unitarianism in America 349
United States Cremation Co. 320
U.S. Public Health Service 319
University of Athens 38
"upholder" 124
urn 47

V

Vandals 77
Valerian, Emperor 64
Valhalla 70
Van Bibber, Andrew 208
Van Butchell, Martin 119
Van Buren, Martin 318
Van Rensselaer, Mrs. J.K. 159, 181, 217
Vester, Franz 204
Vesalius 109
viewing the corpse 40, 46, 60, 61-62, 88
Virginia colonists 141-142

W

wake 61-62, 86, 88
Wallace, Ellerslie 228
Wallis, Charles L. 144, 158, 251, 306, 313
Waning of the Middle Ages 115
War Memories of an Army Chaplain 253
washing the corpse 40, 46, 54, 59, 61, 89
     .... 109, 120, 148, 168, 202, 283, 284
Washington (D.C.), city directory 239, 253, 254
Washington Star 253

Waterman, J.S. 164
wax chandler 122, 130
Weaver, John 200
Weber, Max 158
Webster, Noah 159
Weeden, William B. 154-155, 158, 159
weepers 86
Weidenmann, Jacob 208
Weisbord, Harry A. 312
Weller, Maynard C. 312
Western College of Embalming 356
Western Undertaker 216, 247, 270, 276, 336, 343
Wheatley, Benjamin 230, 231, 233, 239
When I Was A Boy 312
When Our Mother Was a Little Girl 312
White, Blanch 162
White, John 185
White, Trentwell M. 252
White Water Valley Coffin Company 246
Whitsett, Charles T. 340
"Who Was the Father of Modern Embalming?" 252
"Whole-man — total-funeral concept" 394-395, 401
Wickes, Stephen 82, 113
widow 87, 100, 296
William the Conqueror 72, 107
Williams, E.A. 240
Williams Institute of Mortuary Science 356
Wilson and Levy 52, 75, 86, 102
     .... 113, 114, 115, 124, 137, 302, 312
Wilson, P.W. 349
Winslow, Samuel 172
Wisconsin Institute of Mortuary Science 356
Wittig, J. 216
wooden coffins 92, 180-182
wooden outside box 208, 212, 216
"Woods Medical and Surgical Monographs" 252
woodworking and coffin manufacturing 182
Worsham College of Embalming 355
Wright, G. 138
Wright, S.P. 372
Wuest, Hermann 204

Y

Young, Sidney 120, 136, 137

Z

zinc chloride-based embalming compound 228, 229
zinc shoulder casket 192